Woodbourne Library
Washington-Centerville Public Library
Centerville, Ohio

"At a time when inner and outer peace are so essential, Barrie shows us how to create sacred space to heal ourselves and the world. Readers will be blessed with Barrie's wisdom and insights."

— Allen M. Schoen, D.V.M., M.S., author of *Kindred Spirits*

"*The Medicine Wheel Garden* combines both the deep wisdom of creating sacred space in our lives and the practical aspect of health and healing discovered by the Native peoples of North America. Hundreds of years later, I use these plants all the time in my practice as a physician. A treasure of knowledge."

— Dr. Michael Friedman, physician, Northwest Holistic Health Center, and founder of Earthmedicines

"E. Barrie Kavasch's benevolent spirit grows from these very pages. Come walk the garden paths and partake of her deep knowledge of healing plants."

— Michael J. Caduto, author of *Earth Tales from Around the World* and co-author of *Native American Gardening*

PRAISE FOR *AMERICAN INDIAN HEALING ARTS:*

"Written in a highly reverent tone, this book goes beyond most popular herbals by helping the reader experience the richness of the rituals connecting the people, the herbs, and their uses into one complex, interwoven fabric."

— Mark Blumenthal, founder and Executive Director, American Botanical Council

"A book of charm and substance: a literal teach-yourself volume on American Indian healing arts."

— Thomas E. Lovejoy, Counselor to the Secretary for Biodiversity and Environmental Affairs, Smithsonian Institution

"With her Native American ancestry, and her Western training, Barrie Kavasch is superbly qualified to teach all of us about American Indian healing arts. This book is a joy to read."

— Mark J. Plotkin, Ph.D., Executive Director, The Ethnobiology and Conservation Team

Woodbourne Library
Washington-Centerville Public Library
Centerville, Ohio

*By E. Barrie Kavasch
and Karen Barr*

AMERICAN INDIAN HEALING ARTS

Additional Books by E. Barrie Kavasch

ENDURING HARVESTS: NATIVE AMERICAN FOODS & FESTIVALS
HANDS OF TIME: SELECT POETRY & HAIKU IN FIVE SEASONS
EARTHWISE: AMERICAN INDIAN USES OF NATIVE TREES
NATIVE HARVESTS: AMERICAN INDIAN WILD FOODS
EARTHSENSE: AMERICAN INDIAN ETHNOBOTANY
GUIDE TO NORTHEASTERN WILD EDIBLES
GUIDE TO EASTERN WILDFLOWERS
GUIDE TO EASTERN MUSHROOMS
AMERICAN INDIAN COOKING
BOTANICAL TAPESTRY
HERBAL TRADITIONS: MEDICINAL PLANTS IN AMERICAN INDIAN LIFE

Books for Young Adults
THE MOUNDBUILDERS OF ANCIENT NORTH AMERICA
A STUDENT'S GUIDE TO NATIVE AMERICAN GENEALOGY
EARTHMAKER'S LODGE: NATIVE AMERICAN FOLKLORE
THE SEMINOLES: INDIAN NATIONS

Books for Children
DREAMCATCHER
APACHE CHILDREN & ELDERS TALK TOGETHER
BLACKFOOT CHILDREN & ELDERS TALK TOGETHER
CROW CHILDREN & ELDERS TALK TOGETHER
LAKOTA CHILDREN & ELDERS TALK TOGETHER
SEMINOLE CHILDREN & ELDERS TALK TOGETHER
ZUNI CHILDREN & ELDERS TALK TOGETHER

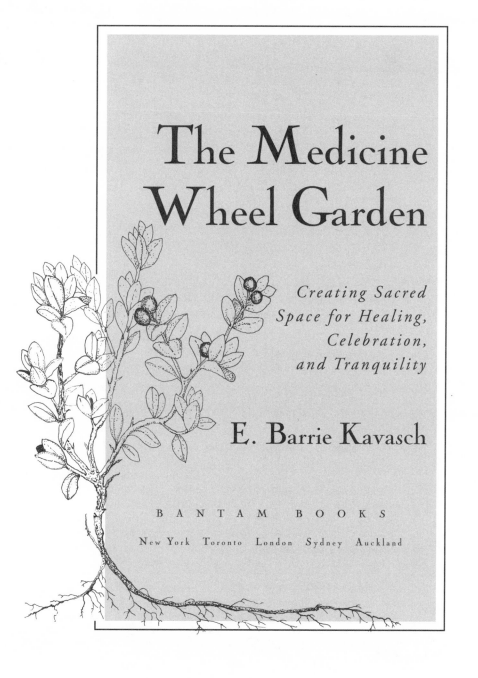

The Medicine Wheel Garden

*Creating Sacred
Space for Healing,
Celebration,
and Tranquility*

E. Barrie Kavasch

BANTAM BOOKS

New York Toronto London Sydney Auckland

THE MEDICINE WHEEL GARDEN

A Bantam Book / July 2002

All rights reserved.
Copyright © 2002 by E. Barrie Kavasch
Book design by Glen M. Edelstein
Cover photo by William Seitz Photography

Portions of the royalties from this book will go to support the Medicine Wheel Coalition, Sacred Sights, and the Association on American Indian Affairs along with the Native American Rights Fund.

No part of this book may be reproduced or transmitted in any form or by any means, electronic or mechanical, including photocopying, recording, or by any information storage and retrieval system, without permission in writing from the publisher. For information address: Bantam Books.

Library of Congress Cataloging-in-Publication Data

Kavasch, E. Barrie.
    The medicine wheel garden : creating sacred space for healing, celebration, and tranquility / E. Barrie Kavasch.
        p.   cm.
    Includes bibliographical references and index.
    ISBN 0-553-38089-3
    1. Herbs—Therapeutic use.   2. Indians of North America—Medicine.   3. Sacred space.   4. Herb gardening.   5. Traditional medicine—North America.   6. Healing.   I. Title.
    RM666.H33 K393 2002
    615'.321—dc21   2002018500

Published simultaneously in the United States and Canada

Bantam Books are published by Bantam Books, a division of Random House, Inc. Its trademark, consisting of the words "Bantam Books" and the portrayal of a rooster, is Registered in U.S. Patent and Trademark Office and in other countries. Marca Registrada, Bantam Books, 1540 Broadway, New York, New York 10036.

PRINTED IN THE UNITED STATES OF AMERICA

RRH   10 9 8 7 6 5 4

To everyone who creates sacred space
and holds a sense of the sacred in everyday life,
especially to Kim and Chris, Mom, and
our sacred circle of family and herbal compatriots

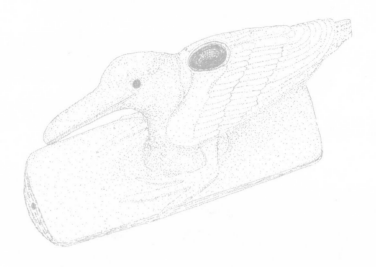

This book is a reference work on the history and current uses of Native American healing practices. The information found in this book should not be used as a substitute for the advice and care of a health care professional in dealing with medical ailments or conditions. In particular, pregnant and nursing women and individuals who are taking medication or have existing medical conditions should consult a physician before trying any of the treatments discussed in this book.

Herbs are complex chemical factories and can interact with prescription medicines, sometimes causing harm rather than healing. If you are taking a prescription drug, it is important to talk with your doctor or nurse-practitioner about the use of herbs in order to avoid any drug-herb interaction.

The author and the publisher are not responsible for any adverse effects resulting from the use or application of the information contained in this book.

CONTENTS

INTRODUCTION:
WELCOME TO THE MEDICINE
WHEEL GARDEN

THE MEDICINE WHEEL GARDEN is a guide to creating your personal sacred space and filling it with plants and objects that will offer pleasure and renewal. With American Indian medicine wheels as foundation and inspiration, this book aims to open a new door to garden design that is ancient and modern, healing and spiritual, simple and sophisticated.

A medicine wheel is a central circle, spiral, or cairn of stones from which lines of other stones radiate, often as "spokes" to an outer circle of stones. Since ancient times, American Indians have created many such arrangements of stones and held them sacred. Planted with healing herbs, the sacred space of a medicine wheel can also become a special kind of garden: a private ecosystem and a small sanctuary for the birds, butterflies, and animals whose natural wild spaces are at risk. Or the medicine wheel garden can take a larger form as a unique community area or even an outdoor classroom.

The creation of sacred space—how we set apart and arrange a certain spot and imbue it with reverent feelings—is at the core of this book. Whatever our religious beliefs, creating a medicine wheel garden outdoors or a smaller space in the form of an altar

In many ways this circle, the Medicine Wheel, can best be understood if you think of it as a mirror in which everything is reflected. "The Universe is the mirror of the People," the old teachers tell us (the teachers being Cheyenne ancestors), "and each person is a mirror to every other person." Any ideal, person, or object, can be a Medicine Wheel, a mirror for Man. The tiniest flower can be such a mirror, as can a wolf, a story, a touch, a religion, or a mountaintop.

—Hyemeyohsts Storm, *Seven Arrows*, 1972

inside the home will enhance them. Both draw us closer to nature and native peoples and affirm our personal ties with the earth. However we approach it, the medicine wheel garden can move each of us into new healing and spiritual realms.

My own lifelong interest in nature and Native American lifeways has made the medicine wheel garden a powerful magnet for me. Decades ago I visited my first medicine wheel site high in the mountains of southern Colorado and felt an amazing shift in my personal energy. This beneficial, clarifying experience was a "felt sense" not easily explained, yet exciting and unforgettable.

A few years later, the continuing force of this feeling led me to construct my own private medicine wheel beside a wildflower meadow, where I regularly spent time observing nature. This peaceful site beneath an old apple tree, set in a wild hedgerow near a quiet pool, was not planted with anything, although in time I did move in small patches of various mosses to cover bare ground in shady spots. I would go there daily to pray and meditate, and I would often come away with surprising new clarity about projects I was working on.

Amazing things began to happen in my little sanctuary. Deer and rabbits would sometimes come right up to me while I was meditating there, and curious songbirds always surrounded me. Large flocks of wild turkeys trooped through the meadow daily and headed straight to my medicine wheel.

I continue my daily visits to my medicine wheel to pray and express my gratitude to the Creator. I especially feel the need to "walk my medicine wheel" when I am troubled about something or having difficulty working out certain situations. As I walk slowly around the low central altar of stones, I ask for guidance, or healing for someone, or better understanding of issues I am not seeing clearly. In this special space I have received remarkable insights. I also walk around the outer boundaries of my medicine wheel in meditation or sit on the earth inside the surrounding ring of stones to contemplate a difficult challenge.

It was while meditating within this medicine wheel that the inspiration came to design and create a medicine wheel garden, planted with healing herbs. I later realized that I had admired just such a place many years before in Ithaca, New York, at the home of an elder herbalist. I suspect that the idea of a sacred space uniting healing herbs and stones had grown deep inside me long before it came to the surface of my mind. I have spent a lifetime working with native plants, both in the wild and in gardens, and for years I have taught courses in landscape design with native plants and healing herbs. I raised my two children on natural home remedies, garden foods, wild edibles, and herbal products. We often laugh about our many successful adventures shared with numerous friends and school classes. These are the resources that have shaped us into the healthy people we are today.

I like to think that my connection with healing herbs and native plants is in my blood. I come from many generations of farming folks in Tennessee and Alabama. My Scotch-Irish, English, and German ancestors settled in the early seventeenth and eighteenth centuries in the Southeast. Some of them intermarried with Cherokee, Creek, and early Powhatan Indians, blending our bloodlines and strengthening our ties to the land and healing herbs. Grandpa Ferguson farmed the rich southern Tennessee earth and wildcrafted medicinal plants for early pharmaceutical companies in the Tennessee hills. He collected striped pipsissewa, mayapple, ginseng, and trillium, always taking care to leave enough behind to continue growing a colony for the next season. Grandpa McLemore and Grandpa Morris, on my father's side, hunted and planted in the northwest hills of Alabama with a fierce love of the land that holds their relatives there today.

Generations later, of course, wildcrafting is no longer the same business it once was, because wildflower and medicinal plant populations have been sadly depleted. As conservationists, we must now protect endangered species and cultivate them in our own gardens, and a medicine wheel garden offers them safety and appreciation—the perfect design for keeping these precious plants close at hand.

American Indian herbalists have long followed this route, bringing wild herbs into favorable situations where they could flourish and produce larger, dependable crops. Pipsissewa, bloodroot, lobelia, yellow dock, and other vital herbs for treating heart,

When you dig for roots, you don't dig them all. You leave a few so the next time you come, you know where to find them.

—Sabinita Herrera, Hispanic *curandera*, 1982

Forms of the Medicine Wheel exist all around the globe from the great stone circles of Europe to the mandalas of India. All of these are reminders of our past when the world was guided by the law of right relationship, and humans respected themselves and all their relations: mineral, plant, animal, and spirit—on Earth Mother. Learning about the medicine wheel can help you remember your connection with all these aspects of the universe. Each stone in the Medicine Wheel is a tool to help you understand your ties with the ancient past that molds both personal and planetary present and future.

—Sun Bear (1929–1992), of Chippewa descent, founder of the Bear Tribe

liver, and respiratory disease seem to have been planted near settlements, as were trillium, cohosh, and violet for assisting with pregnancy, childbirth, and infant care.

Medicine wheel gardens are also places for celebrating and teaching. Some American Indians go alone to the medicine wheel for vision quests, prayer, and personal renewal. Others see it as a place to gather people together for drumming, fire ceremonies, and singing.

With my great affinity for these American Indian practices, I felt a growing impulse to help bring more medicine wheel gardens into being, to extend their use for teaching knowledge of healing plants, enhancing spiritual awareness, and cultivating a deeper appreciation for sacred space. I could see this idea developing into a movement destined to enrich our practical and spiritual needs. My energies in this direction have led to creating a medicine wheel garden on the grounds of the Institute of American Indian Studies in Washington, Connecticut, and another beside the Herb Shop in the center of Sherman, Connecticut, as well as others at botanical gardens and on private property. The one established at the American Indian Museum has multiplied itself in true garden fashion, as many people have taken the idea and my plans and created their own medicine wheel gardens at group homes, civic centers, and other community facilities across the United States and Canada.

As we cultivate and multiply sacred space, we also honor our ancient native traditions. In the spirit of this understanding, many of my American Indian friends have shared with me their tribal wisdom and ceremonial ways, confident that the knowledge they impart would be deeply respected. Each of us can adapt special aspects of these spiritual practices without pretending to be Lakota, Cree, Cheyenne, or Cherokee. The sense of reverence imbued in a medicine wheel garden transcends specific tribal practices.

Benefiting to the full from these gardens does not require drawing on them to provide your own natural medicines. Rather, let the presence of select healing herbs enhance your understanding of their value, and feel comfortable depending on a health food store or other reliable source for medicinal quantities of these herbs as needed. Those in the medicine wheel garden can best remain there to contribute to the conservation and propagation of endangered species whose habitats are shrinking. Some selective harvesting from this garden may well provide for foods and health care recipes, as you will see in Part III of this book. However, the most important thing is to feel a close association with the healing plants.

The chapters that follow describe in detail the steps, practical and ceremonial, and the resources needed to design and plant a medicine wheel garden or indoor altar that best meets your personal goals for creating and using a sacred space. They also provide profiles of a wide variety of native plants you can choose from, identifying the healing properties, other uses such as recipes, and the soil/sun/water requirements of each. The cultivation and propagation requirements of each plant are also detailed, along with different varieties of medicine wheel gardens that could inspire gardeners in various regions of the country.

In this book I will lead you to some of the most revered American Indian medicine wheel sites and other sacred sites. My accompanying pen-and-ink illustrations are intended to make the wonderful native plants more vivid than words alone can hope to do and to emphasize and enhance the spirit of the book.

My goals in this book are simple: to touch some vital chords in each reader and inspire the motivation and energy to create your own sacred space, outdoors or indoors, alone or with others, for spiritual and educational fulfillment. I hope you will receive as much joy and satisfaction from your medicine wheel garden as I do from mine.

"Even if two otherwise warring tribes came together on Medicine Mountain, they always went there in peace. This relates to how Medicine Mountain gets its name. Tribes coming out of the Southwest, the North, the Southeast, they always brought the medicine that grows in their area, and left that when they got to Medicine Mountain. Then the local tribes from this area brought medicines from here for the district tribes to take with them . . ."
—Francis Brown, Northern Arapaho Elder, regarding the Big Horn Medicine Wheel

ACKNOWLEDGMENTS

MY SACRED CIRCLES OF appreciation embrace the creators of the ancient medicine wheels and their descendants. My gratitude to the ancestors who first created sacred space and imbued it with a power that continues to inform and inspire.

I am grateful to my circle of family and relatives who support this work. My admiration to Kim and Mike, Chris and Fran, and my four grandchildren, Derek, Sarah, Jeffrey, and Brooke, who share our passion for the earth. Special love to my mother, who helps create these visions.

Heartfelt gratitude to my many students over these past thirty-five years. You have also taught me a good deal. I am particularly grateful to the many institutions where I have offered courses, talks, and seminars. The Institute for American Indian Studies, the Institute of Ecosystem Studies, the American Museum of Natural History, various botanical gardens, Teva Learning Center, Mohonk Mountain House, Mercy Center at Madison, the Norwich Inn and Spa, and many different colleges, universities, schools, and American Indian reservations deserve special praise.

My great thanks to the initial collaborators and guardians of this book: Betsy Amster, Toni Burbank, and Peggy Cooper for trusting, cultivating, and believing in this whole process, and sculpting and guiding it through to completion. Everyone at Bantam has earned my enduring gratitude and praise, especially Toni Burbank's superb team. Special appreciation to Peter Dubos for spiritual guidance and moral support all along the way. Georgia Middlebrook, Beth McCormick, and everyone at the Institute for American Indian Studies in Washington, Connecticut, have long shared the visions and compassion to make the creative processes even richer and more educational. My immense gratitude to the various libraries and helpful librarians who have worked tirelessly with me to gather fine details.

The Medicine Wheel Garden would not have been possible without the help of many supportive friends who have enriched my work throughout this long, creative process. Foremost, my praise to Dr. Rolf Martin and Barrie Sachs of Happy Rainbows Tea and Apothecary Shoppe, Dr. Mary Miller, Sandra and Maya Cointreau of Earthlodge Horse Herbals, Audrey O'Connell, Kim Kavasch of Body Wisdom, Ellen Carr, Georgia Middlebrook, and the Herb Society of America. Mother Catherine, Mother Placid, Mother Margaret Georgina, and everyone at the Abbey of Regina Laudis in Bethlehem, Connecticut, along with Sister Eugenie Guterch and everyone at Mercy Center Madison, all deserve great praise for their support, time given, and helpful energies. My gratitude also to each member of our IAIS Drumming Circle, Native American Spirituality Circle, Medicine Wheel Study Circle, and Shamanic Drumming Circle, as well as our special Healing Circle. You continue to enrich my pathways in more ways than you could know.

My gratitude to Peg Streep, Laurie Stein, and John Glover for your wonderful treatment of the IAIS Medicine Wheel Garden and my work in your book *Spiritual Gardening: Creating Sacred Space* (Time-Life, 1999). I also want to thank the thousands of visitors who come to the medicine wheel gardens we have created and feel the magic.

Think not of yourselves, O chiefs, or of your own generation, but think of future generations, your children, your grandchildren and those yet unborn whose faces are still beneath the earth.

—The Peacemaker, founder of the Iroquois Confederacy

PART ONE

Creating Sacred Space: A Medicine Wheel Garden

Every part of the earth is sacred to my people . . . every shining pine needle, every sandy shore, every light mist in the dark forest, every clearing . . . and every winged creature is sacred to my people. We are part of the earth and it is part of us. The fragrant flowers are our sisters; the deer and mighty eagle are our brothers; the rocky peak, the fertile meadows, all things are connected like the blood that unites a family.

—Chief Seattle, Duwamish, 1854

CHAPTER ONE

The Circle Is Sacred

The Ancient History
of Medicine Wheels

CIRCLES IN NATURE DRAW our attention. I see the concentric circles within the faces of flowers and their ovaries, fruits, and seeds. I study the geometric spiral in the face of a sunflower, like the patterns in pinecones and acorns. The growth rings radiating from the heartwood of a tree, which we count to learn its age, are classic circles of life. I am drawn to the circular rosettes of lichen colonies on tree bark and old stone walls. Patterning in nature seems to be a mosaic of circles.

The circle symbolizes many ideas for different people and provides healing, too. We are awed by the prehistoric circle of great standing stones at Stonehenge, in England, which relate to the perceived annual movements of the sun, and by the detailed circularity within pre-Christian labyrinths and Roman mosaics on temple floors. In our lives, the sacred protective link represented by a wedding band is a universal symbol. Hindus represent the great Wheel of Existence within a circle, and the Chinese, too, fashion the symbols of active and passive forces within the yin and yang of the universal circle. Tibetan lamas create a sacred universe within the circle of an intricate sand painting, as do Navajo sand

The life of man is a circle from childhood to childhood, and so it is in everything where power moves. Our tipis were round like the nests of birds, and these were always set in a circle, the nation's hoop, a nest of many nests, where the Great Spirit meant for us to hatch our children.
—Black Elk, Oglala Sioux holy man and medicine man

Labyrinths

Labyrinths are circular pathways within the great outer circle reflecting the spiritual journey of life. This ancient sacred geometry embraces a meandering but purposeful path to the center from the outer circle. Walking a circuitous labyrinth path in meditation is a powerful tool for transformation, as it quiets the mind and opens the soul, evoking a feeling of wholeness and mindfulness. The path can be three, seven, or eleven circuits around the center within the great outer circle. Unlike in a maze, there is no wrong way to walk a labyrinth. This mystical ritual, thousands of years old, is a metaphor for one's journey to the center of understanding and to God. Labyrinths can inspire change, a sense of peace, and a deeper connection with the divine. The labyrinth is a sacred place, like the medicine wheel, and a universal symbol of peace. Some labyrinths are planted with special herbs between the paths.

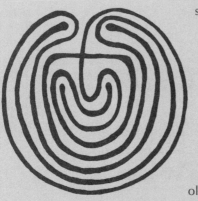

Ancient Hopi medicine wheel—labyrinth petroglyph representing Mother Earth

The Papagos' Elder Brother, I'itoi, who gave the desert Southwest homelands to the people, the O'odham, is pictured within another ancient form of Native American labyrinth woven in their classic spiral basket tray. This traditional design is repeated on many objects in order to remind the people of the importance of their walk through life.

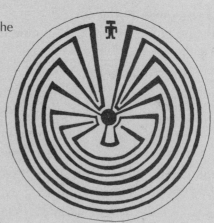

Traditional Papago spiderweblike design woven into sacred baskets

painters pouring healing energies into their lengthy Chant Way ceremonies blessed with cornmeal.

The sacred circle has long been a basic form in American Indian artwork, dwellings, clothing, and dances as well as in healing practices and rituals. Sacred drums, rattles, dream catchers, and bull roarers embody the circle and mirror the shape of the sun, moon, and earth. The year's passage of time comes full circle and continues. Wherever we look, circles embrace us and teach us about the interconnections of all life.

ANCIENT STONE CIRCLES

Great stone circles are considered feats of ritual architecture. These are terrestrial and celestial markers on the landscape that have forever changed the land. Some authorities believe certain of these sites were solar calendars that regulated work and hunting among the people of these regions under the protection of the ancestors and gods. These ancient ruins have a certain spell about them that affects everyone who journeys to see them.

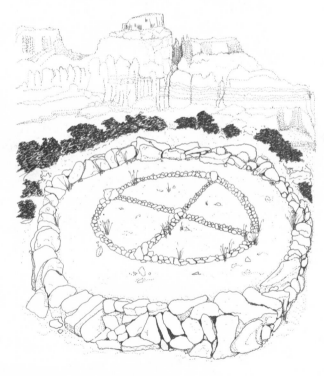

Ancient medicine wheel overlooking the Long Canyon in the red rock country of Sedona, Arizona

Striking parallels may be found between the prehistoric stonework of Europe, Africa, South America, and North America. Amazing similarities exist between the Celtic menhirs (tall standing stones), Mayan stelae, and the great standing stones of Easter Island in the Pacific, all marking sacred ritual sites. Also, stone cairns—stones carefully placed in a pile as a marker—are one of the earliest human constructions found around the world.

Many ancient stone medicine wheels still dot our landscape from Canada to Mexico and from Florida to the Rocky Mountains. Across North America, they can be found from the Cree homelands on the plains of Alberta and Saskatchewan in southern Canada to the Ute territories in southern Colorado, Pueblo Indian sites in New Mexico, and east into the ancient Mound Builder sites along the Mississippi floodplains. They are usually located on prominent features of land, such as the summits of hills, plateaus, and ridges—places often hard to reach but well worth the effort of doing so. Earlier people must have journeyed great distances to reach these sites. Perhaps those journeys, much like pilgrimages, served to heighten the importance of such sacred places.

Scientists studying these enigmatic configurations in the late nineteenth century called them medicine wheels because of their similarities to the Plains Indian symbols commonly used in ceremonial artworks. For centuries, these Indians have made beautifully quilled circles with a simple cross in the middle. Plains Indian warriors often wore such a power symbol fastened to a war shield, their horses' manes or bridles, or their own hair. Early settlers thought these resembled great wagon wheels.

Plains Indian medicine wheel ornament

Whatever the location of the medicine wheel, at its heart is the circle, spiral, or cairn of stones. From this radiate lines of stones, and the ends of these lines become points on an outer stone circle. Sometimes the outer circle is closed, but it usually has one or more openings. The size, the form of the center, and the number of spokes vary in different medicine wheels, but the sacred circle is a constant theme.

It is this place that holds our memories and the bones of our people. . . . This is the place that made us.

—A Pueblo elder

Created over the course of the past 5,500 years, medicine wheels guard the mysteries of their ancient origins and uses, while tantalizing us to want to know them better as a vital part of this continent's heritage. These stone circles continue to draw people to them for sacred, ceremonial, and healing necessities. Many seem to exude sheer power and energy, as I sensed so clearly during my visit to the medicine wheel site in Colorado.

The Sun Dance

The Sun Dance was born of visions and evolved out of ancient American Indian ceremonies. It flourished in the 1800s during the golden age of Plains Indian life. For some of the more than twenty Plains Indian tribes the Sun Dance was (and still is) the most important period of ritual and the only time of year when their people all gather at the same place. Elaborate ceremonies vary from tribe to tribe across the West, yet they all center on sacrifice and self-denial among the adult men and women. The Sun Dance may last four days and more, yet requires many days of preparation before it begins. Medicine Lodge and Spirit Lodge are also names given to the Sun Dance and certain of its aspects by some of the tribes.

Quite a few also have been found to have astronomical significance. The famous Big Horn Medicine Wheel in Wyoming, for example, is believed to act as a calendar device, much like Stonehenge in England.

Creating sacred space in which to pray, fast, seek visions, focus on group needs, or predict the seasonal behavior of game animals or the weather was natural for people living close to nature in much earlier times. They must have employed a variety of techniques to honor the land from which they drew sustenance. The prehistoric medicine wheel sites, mounds, and earthworks in North America suggest the heightened spiritual quality of particular places, "power spots" that seem to have served as primal cathedrals—shrines on the land. We need to reconnect with this.

There is clear evidence that Plains Indians camped at some of the medicine wheel sites over time. Remains of stone tipi rings and blackened earth from campfires exist at some sites. Elder tribespeople recall various stories and events celebrated around the medicine wheel. In some family traditions, people camped at the medicine wheel long before the introduction of the horse, when Plains Indians still used dogs to pull their travois. Some tribal historians claim that the medicine wheel symbolized the layout and design of the Great Medicine Lodge for the Sun Dance rituals. The Plains Indian scholar George Bird Grinnell wrote extensively about this connection, relating that the medicine wheel

At the center of the Earth stand looking around you, recognizing the tribe, stand looking around you.
—Song fragment from the
Lakota Sun Dance

is the place "where the instruction is given to the Medicine Lodge makers and from which the Cheyenne Medicine Lodge women carry the buffalo skull down to the Medicine Lodge."

THE MOST FAMOUS MEDICINE WHEEL

Noted for its distinctive design and remoteness, the Big Horn Medicine Wheel is set high in the Big Horn Mountains near Sheridan, Wyoming. As you make your way up to this austere location, you can hear the constant call of the wind. Rugged junipers and prairie grasses hug the upper slopes, their foliage whispering in the strong wind. This famous site was sacred to the early Crow, Sioux, Arapahoe, Shoshone, and Cheyenne Indians who lived as nomads across the region. Some of their earliest ancestors probably constructed it. Distinctive features include the twenty-eight stone spokes radiating from the center and three cairns placed beyond the outer stone circle, all thought to have astronomical significance.

Big Horn Medicine Wheel in Wyoming

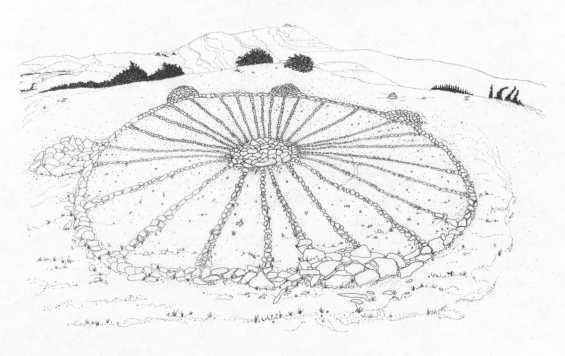

Studying medicine wheels for many years, especially the Big Horn site, astronomer John Eddy has concluded that they could have been used as horizon markers to identify the rising or setting of selected celestial bodies. He notes that the spoked pattern resembles a common sun symbol and comments that a Crow name for the Big Horn Medicine Wheel was "Sun's Tipi." Supporting this idea, Eddy also notes, one Crow legend reports that the sun built Big Horn "to show us how to build a tipi."

The Big Horn Medicine Wheel is made of limestone slabs and boulders and is about ninety-eight feet across. The central cairn is about twelve feet in diameter and over two feet high. It was constructed on this high mountain plateau at an elevation of 10,500 feet in the early 1400s. This huge earth altar was used for many things, especially as a solar and stellar marking point.

The three outlying cairns at Big Horn align with three stars prominent in the summer sky: Aldebaran in the constellation Taurus, Rigel in Orion, and Sirius, the Dog Star, in Canis Major. These three stars appear as the biggest and brightest in the sky at the latitude of the Big Horn Mountains. Eddy explains that this site must have been an important mountain observatory in the twelfth to fourteenth centuries. The three stars rise almost twenty-eight days, or one moon, apart from one another, suggesting a connection with Big Horn's twenty-eight long spokes. And in line with the idea that the medicine wheel inspired the design for the Great Medicine Lodge for the Sun Dance, there is persuasive evidence that Big Horn is a good marker for the summer solstice along the alignment of the central stone cairn with the distinctive outlying one. That is the time when many tribes came together to hold their Sun Dance ceremony with its days of ritual, fasting, feasting, and prayer.

Set in a windswept, rugged location some 425 miles from the Big Horn Medicine Wheel is the Moose Mountain Medicine Wheel, in southern Alberta, Canada. It bears such a striking resemblance to Big Horn that, according to scholars who study these sacred sites, it might have been built from the same set of plans. Constructed 1,700 years ago, it aligns with the same three

They believed in gods, chief of which was the Sun, and consecrated their lives to them; and their eternal happiness would be complete in the great Happy Region where all is bright and warm. The great wheel or shrine of this people is eighty feet across the face, and has twenty-eight spokes, representing the twenty-eight tribes of their race. At the center or hub there is a house of stone, where Red Eagle held the position of chief or leader of the god of plenty, and on the southeast faced the house of the goddess of beauty; and due west was the beautifully built granite cave dedicated to the sun god, and from this position the services were supposed to be directed by him. Standing along the twenty-eight spokes were the worshipers, chanting their songs of praise to the heavens, while their sundial on earth was a true copy of the sun.

—From a sign-language account describing the Big Horn Medicine Wheel, by an elderly Sheepeater Shoshone Indian woman in 1913

stars' risings and the sun's position as the Wyoming structure, to mark the summer solstice.

The stones are Earth's bones. They are not dead at all, and anything that has life still retains the life when you use it. I gather pieces of soapstone from a quarry that Indians used for pots 8,000 years ago. I take the pieces they left behind, and I can feel the hands of the ancient people upon these pieces still.
—Tsonakwa, Abenaki artist and storyteller, 1980

VISIONS, REMEMBRANCES, AND CEREMONIES

Crow Indian traditions tell that vision quests were held at or in the immediate vicinity of medicine wheels. Certainly these would be places of immense power for visioning. You have only to sit quietly at one of these sites and meditate for a time to feel the site's strength and energy.

Research has revealed that some Plains Indians (especially the Northern Blackfeet; Dakota, Nakota, and Lakota Sioux; Mandan; Hidatsa; and Crow) also created monuments to memorable events by piling stones in cairns and by using simple outline effigy figures. These constructions are sometimes found within, but usually outside, the medicine wheels as ancillary features. A few tribal elders recalled that certain medicine wheels were constructed as death markers to honor a great chief. According to Blackfeet traditions, medicine wheels were created to mark the residence or grave of a warrior chief during historical memory. Their word for the medicine wheel is *atsot-akeeh': tuksin,* which generally means "from all sides, a small marker of stones for remembrance."

I heard that when they buried a real chief, one that the people loved, they would pile rocks around the edge of his lodge and then place rows of rocks out from his burial tipi. The rock lines show that everybody went there to get something to eat. He is inviting someone every day.
—Adam White Man, Southern Peigan

Canadian Inuit people constructed ancient rock markers they called *inukshuk.* Similar to cairns, these rocks were piled up to look like a person from a distance. They used these as guideposts and trail markers.

Some of the stone cairns that have been examined contained offerings of both ceremonial and utilitarian objects. These suggest that the cairns were vital in the buffalo-hunting sequences in these regions. For example, two striking sites in Alberta, Canada, the Majorville Cairn and the Moose Mountain Medicine Wheel, both on windy hilltops, contained numerous prehistoric tools, many of which were used for scraping bison hides. Along with a number of pipes, scientists also found *iniskim,* fossils used as bison-calling fetishes by the Blackfeet, as well as beads. Evidently, earlier people made valuable offerings in the cairns at the various medicine wheel sites. Such offerings might well have been part of a ceremonial event.

We don't know whether ancient medicine wheels included plantings of healing herbs—in exposed, windswept places such as the Big Horn site, many would not do too well—but some tribal traditions point to a strong link between medicine wheels and healing. The ancient medicine wheel in the Red Rock country of Sedona, Arizona, rests on a high overlook above Long Canyon. These are the homelands of the Hohokam and Sinagua people of ten thousand years ago, distant ancestors of the Yavapai. They called this remote site Wipuk, meaning "at the foot of the rocks." Their cosmology tells of how these people originated here at Wipuk, where the Creator taught them singing and dancing, which are forms of prayer. The creation story describes how the first human, Sakarakaamche, descended to earth on lightning flashes and sang a healing song as he knelt on the ground, causing medicine plants to grow wherever he touched the earth. The Yavapai say that as long as the songs are sung and the stories are told, the land will continue to live and flourish.

Certainly medicine plants merit a central place in a modern medicine wheel ceremony, adding their power to the other features of the design and the occasion. I have participated in such ceremonies, outdoors as part of a large group and indoors with a smaller number of friends and colleagues, especially when the weather is forbidding. We always begin with quiet smudging in the smoke of fragrant herbs such as cedar, sweetgrass, bearberry, and sage for cleansing. Usually everyone is asked to bring a grapefruit-size stone to place in the medicine wheel's outer rim and smaller stones to add to the prayer cairns. Each of the larger stones can be designated to represent a celestial body: the sun, the moon, or a star or planet. A large stone each for Mother Earth and Father Sky hold the center. As people walk within and outside the medicine wheel circle, they contemplate their own life path and sense of destiny and commitments to their own

To you, Sun, I offer tobacco. You blessed me after I had fasted for five days and you told me that you would come to my aid whenever I had something difficult to do. . . . To you, Grandmother Moon, I also offer tobacco. You blessed me and said that whenever I needed your power you would aid me. To you, Grandmother Earth, I too offer tobacco. You blessed me and promised to help me whenever I needed you. You said that I could use all the best herbs that grow upon you, and that I would always be able to effect cures with them.
—Warukana, Winnebago Shaman, ca. 1923

To you, who are in charge of the Snake Lodge, you who are perfectly white, Rattlesnake, I pray. You blessed me with your rattles to wrap around my gourd and you told me after I had fasted for four days that you could help me. You said that I would never fail in anything that I attempted.
—Warukana, Winnebago Shaman, ca. 1923

goals, asking for clarity and vision. Time for sharing afterward often brings additional clarity.

OTHER CEREMONIAL SITES

The medicine wheel has particular appeal for us today, because it is a powerful spiritual structure that we can create for ourselves and fill with plants that give it additional potency. Yet many other kinds of sacred places abound throughout the Indian Americas.

Two millennia ago, along the rivers of what is now southern Ohio, a complex Native American culture arose, known today as Hopewell. The Hopewell culture flourished for over five hundred years, leaving behind mounds, earthworks, and dazzling artifacts as evidence of its existence. The Mound City Group in southern Ohio preserves the site of a major Hopewell ceremonial, and possibly social, center.

Another spectacle of the Hopewell site is the Great Serpent Mound. This impressive earthen structure represents a giant uncoiling snake; the oval embankment at the end may represent the snake's open mouth as it strikes. This is the largest and best serpent effigy in the world: its sensuous shape curves and slithers across a quarter mile of lowland meadow on a ridge above Brush Creek. The Great Snake appears to be swallowing a large circle, perhaps an egg. Many North American mound sites are associated with burials and celebrations of the afterlife, but the Serpent Mound holds no human remains. The symbolism and ceremonial purpose of this inspiring structure remain a mystery.

We do know that the serpent, like the circle, has important meanings around the world. For Native American people, the serpent symbolized great power and energy, and among some tribes it signified one of the "keepers of the land." The Hindus took the serpent as a symbol of enlightenment; for Christians it meant forbidden knowledge; the Greeks took it as a symbol of the life force

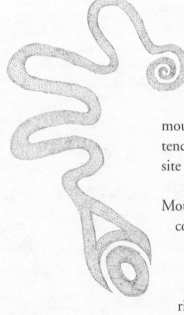

The Great Serpent Mound in south-central Ohio

on the physician's staff. For the Chinese and Japanese, the serpent force circulates energy, both in the body (where it is known through the ancient science of *qi*) and throughout the earth (where the practice of feng shui helps us draw upon it). The Toltec and Mayan peoples embellished their temples with serpents symbolizing wisdom and life force.

Today we instantly recognize the caduceus, two serpents intertwined around a staff, which has become the symbol of modern medicine. This comes from the ancient winged staff with two serpents that was carried by Hermes, Greek god of commerce. So much of our modern symbolism is based upon ancient inspirations.

Numerous other sacred sites are also worth exploring. Hundreds of effigy mounds (man-made earthen structures) in the shapes of birds, bears, men, cylinders, and flat-topped pyramids rise on the North American landscape. Effigy Mounds National Monument, in Iowa, preserves almost two hundred earthen structures ranging from simple mounds and cylinders to the forms of a bird, a bear, and various human shapes.

Other effigy mounds can be found from Georgia and Florida to Wisconsin. Ancient petroglyphs and pictographs, such as the Great Spiral petroglyph in Saguaro National Park, Arizona, evoke a mysterious presence, a complex sense of the divine, expressed by ancestors who once peopled this continent.

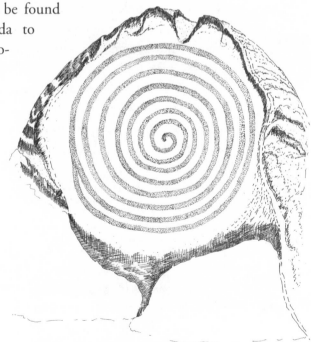

Ancient spiral petroglyph in
Saguaro National Park, Arizona

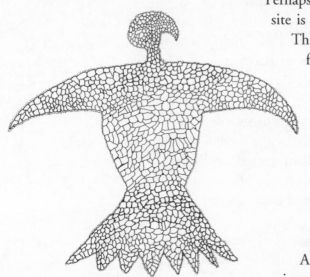

5,000-year-old Rock Eagle stone mound effigy, Eatonton, Georgia

Perhaps the most unusual stone effigy mound site is Rock Eagle, near Eatonton, Georgia. This enormous bird effigy, with a 120-foot wingspan, is composed entirely of white quartz boulders. Created more than five thousand years ago by distant ancestors of the Cherokee and Creek Indians, Rock Eagle is older than the Great Pyramid of Egypt. Ancestral builders who created this site carried white quartz boulders and cobbles here from great distances. And like so many Native American sacred sites, this one is most impressive when viewed from the air. Many medicinal herbs surround this site, creating the impression that such places might have served as important healing centers.

The spectacular Chaco Canyon National Historic Park, in New Mexico, holds many tantalizing ruins of a sophisticated ancient culture whose sense of ritual continues to impress us. Numerous multiroom dwellings and carefully built kivas—large circular ceremonial chambers, partially underground—occupy the site. At many pueblos, great kivas like these still serve as healing centers wherein herbalists and ceremonialists come together for periodic festivals of renewal. This early desert city reflects the sedentary lifestyle of successful gardeners. Their advanced society included "sky watchers," who observed celestial changes. The Anasazi, the Ancient Ones, the people of a Pueblo culture, pictured three particular symbols: a large star close to the crescent moon and a human hand nearby. Scientists conjecture that this painting represents their observation of a supernova widely observed around July 4, 1054.

Thousands of years before our European ancestors proclaimed their "discovery" of a new world, our Native American ancestors knew this ancient world was filled with countless spirits. They followed ritual practices to placate them. Clearly, the ancient sites were sacred space wherein the earth and the people were honored. We can only guess about ancient ceremonies and honoring rituals. And these sites still exude a source of power that many visitors feel upon visiting them.

From Chaco Canyon to the Great Serpent Mound and the Big Horn Medicine Wheel, many of the sites constructed by American Indian ancestors and sacred to their descendants are now managed and protected by the National Park Service; with great respect for Native American uses and sensitivities, they are open to the public. Others are on private property and not available to visitors. American Indians return to the medicine wheel sites for many reasons, often to seek a vision and endure a traditional vision quest. Each site remains a unique geographical feature of cultural, spiritual, and scientific significance.

> *For who but the people indigenous to the soil could produce its song, story, and folktale . . . who but the people who loved the dust beneath their feet could shape it and put it into undying ceramic form . . . who but those who loved the reeds that grew beside still waters and the damp roots of shrub and tree could save it from seasonal death and weave it into timeless art.*
>
> —Chief Luther Standing Bear, Lakota

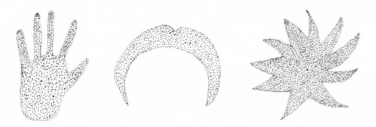

Anasazi supernova pictograph,
Chaco Canyon

CHAPTER TWO

Centering Earth Energies

Designing Your Medicine Wheel

Then I was standing on the highest mountain of them all, and round about me was the whole hoop of the world. And while I stood there I saw more than I can tell and I understood more than I saw; for I was seeing in a sacred manner the shapes of all things in the spirit, and the shape of all shapes as they must live together like one being. And I saw that the sacred hoop of my people was one of many hoops that made one circle.

—Black Elk, Oglala Sioux
holy man

THE STRIKING LOCATIONS OF ancient medicine wheels show us that choosing the right site is an important part of creating a sacred space. Living across large territories, American Indian ancestors could seek, or perhaps come upon, unusual natural sites that proclaimed their appeal. Whatever the size of our much smaller living spaces today, we can follow the same principle, finding just the right spot for our medicine wheel gardens.

In my own case, before I could even begin thinking about choosing the perfect site for my first medicine wheel garden, the site actually chose me. I was clearing away unwanted growth around a small pool shaded by an apple tree, intent on improving this little area of my property. This spot beside a sunny wildflower meadow was choked with old rosebushes and bittersweet vines. Working to clear the tangle, I realized the unique beauty of the location—an appeal not lost on the wildlife continually visiting the site.

Each day the site drew me back. As I continued clearing away tangled undergrowth, I watched the various activities of ground animals and birds. I also noticed a lot of white quartz rock chips in the soil surrounding a large rock I sat on to rest. This little area became more and more compelling to me, and I could feel its particular energy and peace. It was during a brief rest break and meditation, sitting on my rock, that I got the idea to construct a small medicine wheel here using the white quartz and other native stones.

I worked a few hours on my project each day, morning or evening, and soon I had constructed a small stone circle, five feet in diameter, with a tiny stone altar in the center. I brought a few clumps of fresh moss to press into spots of bare soil. The moss has spread and carpeted this protected circle. Creeping wild strawberry and speedwell plants have "volunteered" here, and sweetgrass and jewelweed grow around the medicine wheel circle. In the same way that I encouraged the natural quality of the site to reveal itself as I cleared it, I encouraged the natural growth of local native plants to create a garden in and around my medicine wheel. This old medicine wheel garden has become my favorite place to meditate and work out new ideas.

We now plant a Tree whose tops will reach the sun, and its branches spread far abroad, so that it shall be seen afar off; and we shall shelter ourselves under it, and live in Peace, without molestation.
—Mohawk chief to Lord Effingham, 1684

CHOOSING YOUR SITE

While some sites, like mine, seem almost magically to declare themselves special, it is more likely, in particular if you have limited outdoor space, that you will need to do the choosing.

Whether your yard is large or small, flat or sloped will help determine the best size and location for your medicine wheel garden; rely on the ancient medicine wheels for inspiration. Walk your property carefully, thoughtfully, in a meditative mood. Visualize a large circle on the land, perhaps twenty or thirty feet in diameter, with paths making a cross through it. Imagine that each quadrant is planted with five or more of your favorite healing herbs. Envision a peace pole standing in the center of the crosswalk with long colored ribbons fluttering from it in the breeze.

If you are an apartment dweller without land, you can choose a balcony, a windowsill, or a tabletop on which to create a miniature medicine wheel garden. Condense this vision into a miniature form that will be easy for you to make and enjoy.

Whether your garden will be small or large, indoors or outdoors, you may want to fashion a prototype altar before you create the real thing on the landscape. This way you can move things around. For example, you could create a miniature garden or altar out of clay on a large tray using tiny stones and dried plant materials and mosses to simulate the real thing.

Besides considerations of size and of slope (which affects soil drainage), it is important to orient the garden to the path of the sun. The movements of the sun across the sky can influence the growth and blossoming of the plants, especially if your plot has partial shade. An area that is shady in one season may be bright and sunny in another. Make a solar and lunar study of your plot of land.

Cultivating sacred space in tune with the seasons is another way of honoring nature's ongoing cycles, rhythms, and needs. It is also a way of gardening for your soul. As the Haudenosaunee (the Iroquois or Six Nations) say in their traditional Thanksgiving address: "We are all thankful to our Mother, the Earth, for she gives us all that we need for life. She supports our feet as we walk about upon her. It gives us joy that she continues to care for us as she has from the beginning of time."

Your choice of site will also naturally involve the ceremonial, aesthetic, or other purposes you envision for your medicine wheel garden. Do you want to see it from one or more windows of your house, or do you feel that a secluded setting would be more in harmony with its spirit? Would you like to approach it as you walk past a different group of garden plantings, or do you think of it as a space separated from all others? Study what is already growing in the space you are thinking of selecting. If you have herbs there, they can form a basic part of your medicine wheel garden, as they are already at home. Would that please you, or would you prefer to transfer them elsewhere and start afresh? Perhaps you want to make your medicine wheel garden an artistic, therapeutic "classroom," where you will teach others about healing herbs and medicine wheel rites. The answers to all these questions help to shape your plans.

Your medicine wheel garden can be a "show garden" in the front yard, serving as an intriguing welcoming space. I have several friends who planted their medicine wheel gardens outside their front doors; these designs work beautifully, as the medicine wheel embraces the front walk, radiating out around it on either side. Now everyone who comes to the door walks through the medicine wheel and is blessed by it. I know others who have created the medicine wheel as a sort of outdoor "room," a healing space filled with their good energies and favorite plants. Some people might even want to center their house within the medicine wheel and have the garden extend all around it. (This plan works best for small cottages.) The visual and spiritual effects are quite wonderful, depending upon how you design and plant the garden.

On the other hand, you might decide to create a medicine wheel sanctuary without adding healing plants, as I first did, waiting to see what herbs come into this new space naturally. Or maybe a Zen garden concept, with stones alone, appeals to your sensitivities. These dry landscape gardens create a meditative microcosm of the universe, and they too venerate the nature spirits and the ancestors—rocks play an extremely important role in the creation of sacred space.

Think through these many possibilities, practical and spiritual, and take your time about reaching a decision, weighing how

Asian Concepts of Energy and Space

The ancient Asian art of feng shui and the science of *qi*, life force or energy, have much in common with the Native American medicine wheel. *Feng* means "wind," and *shui means* "water"; the practice maps the forces responsible for determining health, prosperity, relationships, and good luck. This mystical art of placement is thousands of years old and has attracted many modern students. It recognizes five elements: earth, fire, water, metal, and wood, which compose *qi*. This life force or energy animates all things. We consider this energy well in planning the medicine wheel garden. Most people have their own innate sense of good feng shui.

well the features of different sites fit your personal concept. Once you have made your choice, sit down beside the site or within it. Listen to it. Feel it. Reach out in your mind to the trees and other plants there and discover the influence of their presence. What are the plants here telling you about the soil and sun? Do a simple meditation in this space and pay close attention to which animals form part of the environment, from grubs and worms to chipmunks and songbirds. Spend an hour or more doing this.

Go back often to your chosen location to get a clear sense of the patterns of sun and shade, the comings and goings of wildlife, and other subtle details. Look again at the rocks, large and small, protruding tree roots, and any other special features of the space. All these aspects are important to help you choose the most suitable plants to place within your medicine wheel and to enhance its design. You may want to keep a journal about your thoughts and experiences.

BLESSING THE SPACE

It is important to ask the nature spirits to give permission for use of the plot of land you have chosen and to bless it. As you build your communication with and within this space, your creativity will take on a special quality. With sacred intent at work in your space, all your energies will reap greater rewards. Before you begin the work of preparing the ground for your garden and setting the medicine wheel stones in place, you must also bless the space yourself.

My words are tied in one with the great mountains, with the great rocks, with the great trees, in one with my body and my heart.

—Yokuts Indian prayer

Select an offering substance such as cornmeal, tobacco, sweetgrass, bearberry, cedar, or sage. A pinch of one or more of these sacred plants "feeds" the earth and shows the Creator that we remember to give thanks for everything. We must nourish the place we plan to create within, and this form of consideration is just as necessary as putting compost on a garden and fertilizing the plants. Offer a silent or spoken prayer or song.

While giving your blessing to this site, also give a prayer to the

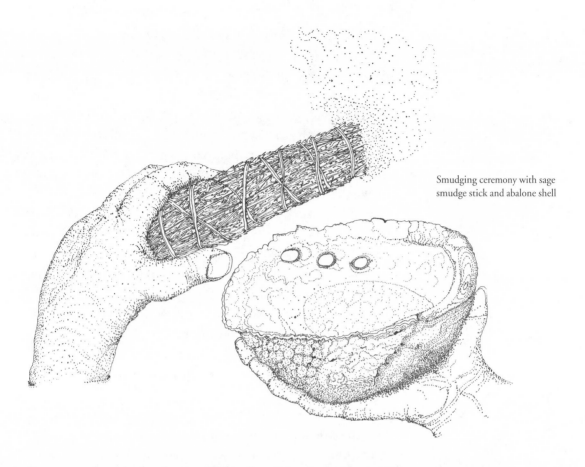

Smudging ceremony with sage smudge stick and abalone shell

Creator and to the land you will be disturbing in order to create your medicine wheel garden. Afterward, remain silent and sense the spirits of the land and the existing plants that already grow all around you here. Ask for their approval to move forward with your project.

Do a ritual smudging for this area. Ignite some sage, cedar, rosemary, or lavender in a small fireproof clay dish or shell. Extinguish the flame so that the botanicals just smudge or smoke. Bathe yourself in this fragrant smoke, wiping away all anxieties and ill feelings. Now walk slowly around the whole area, smudging it while offering thoughts of gratitude. Finally, sit down on the ground with the remaining smudge. Allow it to burn out completely. Then carefully empty the ashes onto the ground. Plan to repeat this whole process when your medicine wheel garden is completed.

Knowing the quality of the soil in your chosen site will help you create a successful medicine wheel garden. Healthy soil that encourages plant growth contains fairly equal proportions of clay, sand, and silt. Pick up a handful of soil and compress it into a ball. If it keeps its shape, that suggests good clay content to hold in moisture. If it crumbles apart, the soil may be too dry or sandy.

A simple home test will show you how the soil in your site sorts out. Dig down six to eight inches below the surface to the root zone in the middle of the site and take a generous trowelful of soil. Sift this sample through a medium-mesh screen to remove any stones and clumps of organic matter, and place the soil in a straight-sided jar, like an old peanut butter or mason jar. Add one tablespoon of dishwashing detergent, which will coat the particles and keep them separate. Finally, add enough water to fill the jar, screw the lid on tight, and shake the jar vigorously for about three minutes.

She went down to the river and got some mud, just like the mud dauber did, and she made a little bowl. And she put it out in the sun and let it dry until it got real hard.
—Kathi Smith Littlejohn, Eastern Band Cherokee storyteller, North Carolina

Set the jar on a flat shelf for a few days to allow all the soil particles to settle into layers. Sand particles, the heaviest, will settle to the bottom quite rapidly. The next layer will be the silt, which is darker than the sand. Clay, much finer in texture and lighter in color, has the lightest particles in the mix and will slowly settle on top.

Kitchen and Garden Recycling

Powdered lime and crushed eggshells and seashells dug into the top three inches of the soil will counteract soil acidity, while decayed leaves, coffee grounds, and used tea leaves scratched into the surface will help soil that is too alkaline. Banana peels decompose in the soil to release additional potassium for plant roots and leaves. Cuttings of nettles and comfrey act like "green manure," feeding the soil beneath them, so place these clippings around select plants in the medicine wheel garden. Grass clippings placed around beneath the plants also act as green manure and help keep the underneath of the plants clean during watering and rainfall. Yarrow clippings spread on the soil surface help to sweeten it.

Study your sample to discover your soil type. Are the three materials present in fairly equal proportions, or have you too much of one compared to the others? If your soil tends to be a silt-clay mix, for example, you may want to add some sand. You will want to add some organic materials to increase its fertility and the drainage around roots.

With the same kind of soil sample, you can also learn the pH factor of your soil, indicating whether it tends to be acid or alkaline. Soil test kits for this purpose are available from many garden centers and from state cooperative extension service offices, some of which also test soil samples and provide reports on the result. Check your telephone book for the office closest to you. For this test, you will need about a cup of sample soil. Well-balanced soil will come out somewhere near the middle of the pH scale.

Unless your soil conditions tend to be seriously out of balance, most kinds of plants will manage to grow. With or without tests, the best help you can give your soil and your plants is to follow organic gardening methods. Organic gardening techniques involve building up the soil's life and vigor while avoiding chemical pesticides. The permanence of reliable nutrients in your soil that this approach provides are an especially vital necessity for food and medicine plants. Loosening the soil is important, too. When you get ready to plant your medicine wheel garden, spade your soil deeply.

For a successful medicine wheel garden, the key word is *compost*. A compost pile can contain discarded kitchen scraps, grass

Take a handful of earth, hold it, squeeze it, smell it. . . .

I come from the Bear Clan, known as a medicine clan to most tribes. In the Mashpee Tribe it has been one of mystery and spiritual pursuits. When the elders speak about members of my clan, they tell strange stories of direct communication with living spirits of plants, animals, elements, water beings, winged ones, and, of course, human spirits. Information gathered from these spirits revealed correct uses of herbs, mineral substances, elemental combinations, and a wealth of medicine ways for the people to maintain health.
—Ramona Peters (Nosapocket),
Mashpee Wampanoag artist
and traditional leader, 1996

Once I was digging roots . . . and I got very tired. I made a pile of earth with my digging stick, put my head on it, and lay down. In front of me was a hole in the earth made by the rains, and there hung a gray spider going up and down, up and down on its long thread.

—Maria Chona, Papago medicine woman, 1930

This really happened through the aid of the medicine man, and some of the leaders of the tribe would get together, and they would learn these things. And if anyone wanted to employ the Little People—in Cherokee, nunnehi—*they're not born, they don't die,* nunnehi. *They're like spirits, and they could implore them to come, and there are some who have seen them.*

—Robert Bushyhead, Eastern Band Cherokee elder and storyteller, North Carolina

clippings, dead leaves, garden debris, even paper. Keep adding to it, turn it over from time to time, and within six months to a year it will yield a rich humus. Compost adds nutrients and organic matter to the soil while supporting a healthy soil life of beneficial nematodes and other soil organisms.

ORGANIC PEST CONTROL

Beneficial insects and valuable soil organisms are critical to successful gardening. As I have said, it is valuable to spend time getting to know your birds and insects around the medicine wheel garden. Some of the more delicate and less seen insects can be highly beneficial. The green lacewing and the praying mantis are the gardener's best friends because they eat most harmful insect pests that might harm your new plants. We are not always lucky enough to have these insect populations living in our home ecosystems. An investment of less than twenty dollars can buy sufficient egg cases of these two beneficial insects to stock most small gardens.

Fortunately there are a growing number of earth-friendly enterprises devoted to helping us in this respect. Many home gardeners, like many responsible commercial greenhouses, are using integrated pest management (IPM) systems—wherein beneficial insects and soil amendments attack their harmful counterparts while working to build healthier environments. Two of the best resources for home gardeners are Gardens Alive and Arbico; both have toll-free phone numbers and Web sites, plus informative catalogs to reassure you that good garden health is achievable. Check their various biological controls and beneficial soil amendments, as well as colorful predator controls. (See Appendix 1 for fuller details.)

CHAPTER THREE

Making the Medicine Wheel

Ground Plans and Garden Styles

THE POINTS OF FOCUS in a medicine wheel garden are the center and the four cardinal directions—north, east, south, and west. Many Native Americans also add three more directions: zenith (above), nadir (below), and here. Welcoming ceremonies and sacred rites always honor the four or seven primary directions, as you will do in your own medicine wheel garden. These directions are the places of the spirits of the winds, the forces that govern life. A peace pole placed at the garden's center marks zenith, nadir, and here. Similar cardinal poles can be anchored along the medicine wheel garden's outer circle to mark the north, east, south, and west points.

Many cultures have imbued the four directions with larger meanings. East, the start of each day's light and activities, is the place of sunrise, new beginnings, and birth. South is the place of warmth, nurturing, creativity, understanding, and youth. West is the place of sunset, arched rainbows, freedom, spaciousness, and maturity—natural connections for the direction where daylight

The Four Directions are within me, for when I look within and when I look without, I perceive the resplendent beauty of the great living Medicine Wheel.

—Mary Summer Rain, author of Dreamwalker: The Path of Sacred Power

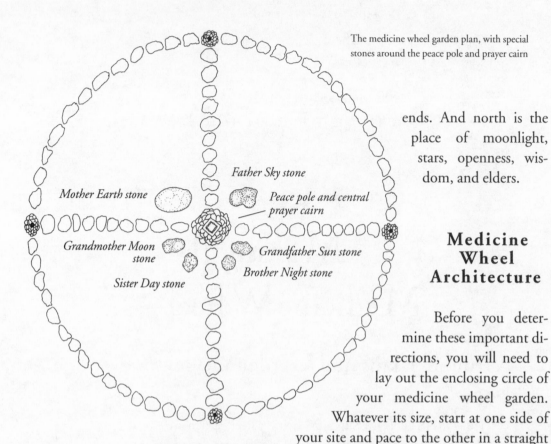

Father Sky stone

Mother Earth stone

Peace pole and central prayer cairn

Grandmother Moon stone

Grandfather Sun stone

Sister Day stone

Brother Night stone

ends. And north is the place of moonlight, stars, openness, wisdom, and elders.

Medicine Wheel Architecture

Before you determine these important directions, you will need to lay out the enclosing circle of your medicine wheel garden. Whatever its size, start at one side of your site and pace to the other in a straight line, counting your footsteps. Turn around and follow your footsteps back, stopping when your count reaches the midpoint. If you have taken fifty steps, for example, stop at twenty-five. That is the center of your medicine wheel. Mark this spot by sinking a short temporary pole in the ground.

The stone center, outer circle, and directional cross of a medicine wheel garden give this sacred space its basic form. Some of the herbs you plant will be colorful and grow quite tall, but they should always be arranged so that the stone architecture remains clearly seen.

Tie one end of a long, strong cord around the pole. Holding the cord, pace from the center to the edge of your site (twenty-five steps in our example). Stretch the cord taut and tie a knot in it to establish your distance from the center. Now hold the cord at the knot, keeping it stretched taut, and begin walking in a circle around the center pole. As you walk, place a fist-sized stone or anchor a stake every few feet in your path. When you have completed your circle, take time to look over the site more than once and make sure that the size is just right for you. At this point, it's easy enough to change your mind and make the circle larger or smaller, following the same procedure.

Depending on the size of your circle, you will need quite a few stones to mark the entire rim, a central circle, and the interior lines connecting the east-west and north-south points on the outer circle. When you begin planning for your medicine wheel garden, it's a good idea to start a rock pile at the same time. According to where you live, your area might be rich in glacial stones, river cobbles, or other types of native rock. If too few stones turn up on your land, look for local sources that supply builders, or you can substitute brick or even wooden logs, if necessary. You may even find "cultured stone" available locally. (See Appendix 2 for resources.) Keep the temporary center pole in place until your medicine wheel architecture is complete.

Once your outer stone circle is in place, you can mark the cardinal directions. You already know in general the east-west direction from observing the daily path of the sun across your site. For a more accurate reading, dust off your magnetic compass. Stand at the center of your medicine wheel and find north on the compass. Holding the compass steady, so that the needle moves as little as possible, walk a straight northward line to your stone circle. Set a temporary pole at this point on the circle. Repeat the same procedure to find south on the circle, placing another temporary pole. Now tie the cord you used before to one of these two poles and carry it across the circle to the other one. When you stretch the cord taut, you know you've done things right if it passes across the center of the medicine wheel. Place marking stones along the path of the cord as a guide for making the giant interior cross, which will divide your medicine wheel garden into quadrants. Take the same steps for finding east and west on the outer circle.

Your medicine wheel pattern is now set. You can place more spokes in the wheel if you wish, by again following the procedure that you used to establish and connect the cardinal points.

We emerged from our land. . . . This is our medicine chest—full of our sacred plants, our remnants of wild prairie, our wild rice, the best of our maple syrup trees. This land is filled with deer, moose, and fish, once even sturgeon, the chief of all fish.

—Winona LaDuke, Ojibwe, founding director, White Earth Land Recovery Project, northern Minnesota

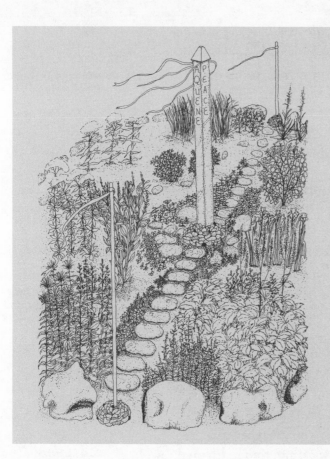

Peace Pole

The heart of the medicine wheel garden is the tall peace pole planted at the very center. Here you offer pinches of sacred cornmeal, tobacco, and your prayers. Your prayers might be for peace, healing, wellness, compassion, understanding, humility, and gratitude, or whatever seems most pertinent to you. Every person who comes into this garden and to the peace pole is invited to bring a small stone to place at its base with the thoughts: "I lay here my prayers for peace and understanding." Soon this central area becomes a prayer cairn around the peace pole.

GARDEN DESIGNS

The simplicity of the circle with its interior spokes opens a world of possibilities for each gardener. While this book focuses on native American plants, you may easily substitute Eurasian, African, or Chinese plants to suit your own unique needs. Perhaps you want to create an Ayurvedic medicine wheel garden or a traditional Chinese medicine (TCM) wheel. I offer here several kinds of garden styles for you to choose from. Or you might want to use one or more of these styles as a springboard for designing a unique garden plan of your own.

Whichever garden style you choose or invent, you'll want to be careful not to overcrowd plants. Allow them room to grow. Also consider the maximum height of each plant you want to include: take care not to start tall plants where they will overshadow smaller ones, unless the smaller ones are shade-loving varieties. Consider the whole ecosystem of the garden, too. Perhaps you prefer to plant a large clump of one kind of plant to give a grounded, mature feeling to the garden space. It would certainly be interesting to see ten moccasin flowers blooming en masse, or ten jack-in-the-pulpits in a lively colony.

Native traditions connect particular colors to each cardinal direction. Most often, gold or yellow relates to east, blue or purple to south, red or magenta to west, and white or silver to north. But this can vary from one tribe to another. You may have your own vision or color sense for the cardinal (directional) poles.

The Classic Medicine Wheel Garden

The crossed lines connecting the cardinal points on the medicine wheel circle form directional quadrants, which define the spaces between north and east, east and south, and so on. You can fill each quadrant with clusters of healing plants whose color at some stage of development—blossoms, fruit, or foliage—coordinates with the colors symbolic of the related cardinal direction. According to your preference, appropriately colored plants can be

CLASSIC MEDICINE WHEEL

East (yellow or gold)	South (blue or purple)	West (red or magenta)	North (white or silver)
Arnica	Blue flag	Bergamot	Sweetgrass
Evening primrose	Heal-all	Cardinal flower	Sage
Prickly pear	Blue lobelia	Ginger	Clematis
Goldthread	Blueberry	Strawberry	Boneset
St. John's wort	Elderberry	Poke	Fairywand
Rudbeckia	Blue cohosh	Echinacea	Pipsissewa
Yellow lady's slipper	Skullcap	Bloodroot	Wintergreen
Jewelweed	Pennyroyal	Joe-pye weed	Bayberry
Yellow dock	Sage	Indian turnip	Cleome
Witch hazel	Hepatica	Chili peppers	Purslane
	Wild bergamot	Bearberry	Elderberry
	Joe-pye weed		Bristly cucumber
	Black cohosh		

grouped around the dividing line representing the direction, such as east, or plant groups can be combined—for example, by placing those with colors appropriate to north and east in the northeast quadrant. You decide what will give you greatest pleasure.

One approach would be to choose five kinds of plants for each of the four quadrants, with low, ever-blooming strawberry plants placed around the central peace pole. Start with conservative selections chosen to suit the soil and climate of your site. Each season

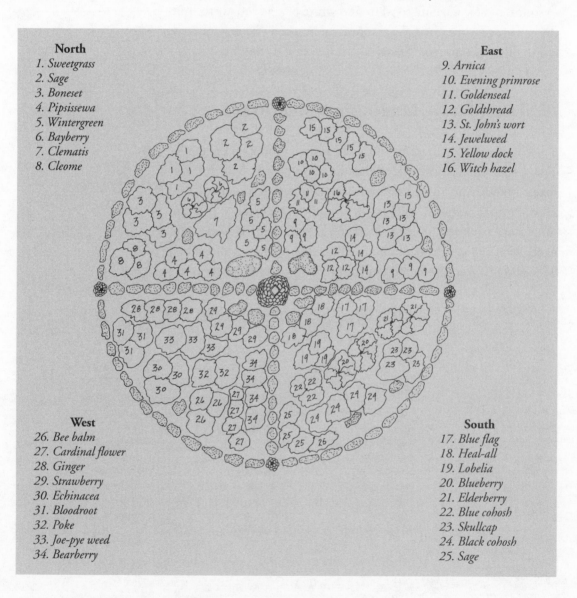

North
1. Sweetgrass
2. Sage
3. Boneset
4. Pipsissewa
5. Wintergreen
6. Bayberry
7. Clematis
8. Cleome

East
9. Arnica
10. Evening primrose
11. Goldenseal
12. Goldthread
13. St. John's wort
14. Jewelweed
15. Yellow dock
16. Witch hazel

West
26. Bee balm
27. Cardinal flower
28. Ginger
29. Strawberry
30. Echinacea
31. Bloodroot
32. Poke
33. Joe-pye weed
34. Bearberry

South
17. Blue flag
18. Heal-all
19. Lobelia
20. Blueberry
21. Elderberry
22. Blue cohosh
23. Skullcap
24. Black cohosh
25. Sage

you may add a few; the medicine wheel garden has much to teach and share as we cultivate it and grow with this project.

The Coastal Medicine Wheel Garden

This garden features rugged coastal plants that can withstand sea winds, salty air, and sandy soil. The East and West Coasts both have appealing plant species. You might wish to cultivate low, creeping herbs in this garden, including rugged ground covers such as ajuga, alumroot, antennaria, bearberry, blue-eyed grass, bird's-foot violet, false heather, windflower, woolly thyme, vinca, heal-all, rabbitfoot clover, moneywort, hens and chicks, and sedum—all add their own spirit to the garden design. Both native and introduced plants can intertwine here for textural diversity.

Spread broken clam, oyster, and mussel shells saved from seafood dinners and beachcombing expeditions among your plants. The shells will serve to sweeten your soil as lime slowly leaches out of them.

Perhaps you are lucky enough to have an oak tree or some bayberry and blueberry shrubs nearby. Look around for the wild onions, wild leeks, lamb's quarters, nettles, dandelion, and chicory plants that may fill the hedgerows. These "garden escapes" from centuries earlier are now considered weeds, yet their healing benefits are considerable, and they fit in well with other selections for this medicine wheel garden. Many of these will simply jump borders and turn up in freshly disturbed soil.

COASTAL MEDICINE WHEEL

East (yellow or gold)	South (blue or purple)	West (red or magenta)	North (white or silver)
St. John's wort	Heal-all	Ginger	Sweetgrass
Cinquefoil	Blueberry	Bearberry	Bayberry
Moneywort	Skullcap	Bloodroot	Sweet fern
Hens and chicks	Pennyroyal	Strawberry	Pipsissewa
Purslane	Seaside lavender	Dwarf seaside roses	Sage
	Ajuga		Dwarf seaside beach plums
			Rabbitfoot clover

XERISCAPE MEDICINE WHEEL

East (yellow or gold)	South (blue or purple)	West (red or magenta)	North (white or silver)
Cinquefoil	Hollyhock	Prickly pear	Night-blooming cereus
Prickly pear	Desert lavender	Ocotillo	Milk thistle
Hollyhock	Passionflower	Cenizo	Anemone
Jojoba	Wild gloxinia	Desert willow	Sangre de drago
Chaparral	Vervain	Ratany	Yerba mansa
Desert senna	Apache plume rose	Sumac	Puncture vine
Anil del muerto	Agave	Red root	Sage
Prickly poppy	Mesquite	Pineapple weed	Shepherd's purse
Cliff rose		Mallow	Epazote
Stillingia		Indian root	Yucca
Turkey mullein			

The Xeriscape Medicine Wheel Garden

A xeriscape garden is a beautiful choice for people living where rainfall is scarce. The word *xeriscape* comes from the ancient Greek word meaning "dry." Xeriscape gardening has its roots in our arid west and in Israel, where expanding populations depleted the already limited water supply, forcing farmers and scientists to explore alternatives. It also draws on ancient gardening wisdom of the Hohokam and their descendants, the Tohono O'odham or Pima and Papago Indians. Making the most of drought-resistant plants, the xeriscape can become a showplace and teaching center. We all need to learn to use less water and natural resources while creating lovely gardens.

You can actually create a microclimate using the careful placement of rocks to help hold the soil in place, act as windbreaks, shade more delicate plants, and keep the underlying soil cool. Careful site inventory will help you determine your soil structure, terrain, and sun exposure and how to work to best advantage with these conditions. Choose the rugged native plants that thrive in your area, and group plants together within the medicine wheel to achieve low maintenance and water use.

Mulching in this garden is essential to retain moisture, maintain a reasonable soil temperature, control wind erosion, and inhibit the growth of weeds. Organic mulches break down over time and contribute to soil quality and water-holding capacity. Select the mulch carefully to contribute to the appearance of the surrounding landscape and site design. You might wish to double-mulch, using select stone groupings over an organic mulch. See Chapter 6 for details.

The Desert Southwest Medicine Wheel Garden

Like the xeriscape garden, the desert Southwest garden grows on a dry landscape and uses the same system of frugal water and soil applications, relying heavily on rugged native plants. The enduring charm of this garden is that it embraces so many native plants that thrive in the desert Southwest.

Do your site evaluations carefully, with an eye to the rocks and other natural features you can use in this design. Any large boulders can become major focal points within or beside your medicine wheel garden. Perhaps you may want to bring in rocks from other places to create special effects.

As with the xeriscape garden, mulching is an important factor in nourishing these plants. Select mulches that harmonize with your environment and add interest as well as protect the fragile root systems of newly planted herbs. There are a number of distinctive stone mulches, for example, that might be layered over an organic mulch. Double-mulching in this case might be valuable. More details are offered in Chapter 6.

DESERT SOUTHWEST MEDICINE WHEEL

East (yellow or gold)	South (blue or purple)	West (red or magenta)	North (white or silver)
Rabbit bush	Desert lavender	Echinacea	Oregon grape holly
Coreopsis	Prairie larkspur	Poppy mallow	Angel's trumpet
Wild sunflower	Vervain	Shooting star	Sage
Cliff rose	Hollyhock	Ocotillo	Antennaria
Prickly pear	Pasque flower	Prickly poppy	Candle anemone
Antelope milkweed	Leadplant	Dwarf sumac	Windflower
	Passionflower		Prairie false indigo
			New Jersey tea
			Yucca

WOODLAND MEDICINE WHEEL

East (yellow or gold)	South (blue or purple)	West (red or magenta)	North (white or silver)
Goldenseal	Pennyroyal	Cardinal flower	Sweetgrass
Goldthread	Blueberry	Bee balm	Sage
Coreopsis	Elderberry	Poke	Purslane
Yellow dock	Juniper	Strawberry	Pipsissewa
Tobacco	Blue cohosh	Bearberry	Wintergreen
Rudbeckia	Black cohosh	Bloodroot	Boneset
Evening primrose	Skullcap	Ginger	Bayberry shrub
Arnica	Heal-all	Spicebush	Angelica
	Blue flag		
	Passionflower		
	Blue lobelia		

The Woodland Medicine Wheel Garden

Plants that do best in the shade are a prime feature of the woodland garden. Often this type of garden is created near or surrounding a tree. Many of the unusual native medicinal plants thrive in rich, shady soil. Our first medicine wheel garden at the Institute for American Indian Studies in Washington, Connecticut, is bordered by a tall, old oak tree and partially surrounded with sumacs and witch hazel shrubs that help to cool the space through hot summer days. Do your site planning for this garden with an eye to how natural rock features can be used to hold the soil and protect it from erosion. You may also want to use tree rounds or logs as "sit-upons" in the garden and to help shade and cool some low-growing plants.

The Prairie Medicine Wheel Garden

The prairie is known for hot sun, and a prairie garden features species that thrive on this. It might feature a combination of rugged grasses, yuccas, milkweeds, echinacea, and sages. Many native prairie plants could be situated here to portray prairie lands' diversity of stunning wildflowers and grasses.

PRAIRIE MEDICINE WHEEL

East (yellow or gold)	South (blue or purple)	West (red or magenta)	North (white or silver)
Helianthus (western sunflower)	Regal blue lupine	Prairie blazing star	Sweetgrass
False heather	Horsemint	Prairie rose	Sweet vernal grass
Turk's cap lily	Prairie phlox	Prairie smoke	White prairie clover
Prickly pear	Violet prairie clover	Columbine	Culversroot
Night willow herb	Prairie turnip	Queen-of-the-prairie	Goatsrue
Dwarf buttercup	Blue-eyed grass	Ironweed	Rabbitfoot
Gayhead coneflower	Bird's-foot violet	Echinacea	Flowering spurge
Cup-plant	Big bluestem prairie grass	Indian grass	Rattlesnake master
Goldenrod	Poppy mallow		Shooting star
Prairie milkweed	Spiderwort		Prairie larkspur
Puccoon			New Jersey tea
			Yucca
			Alumroot

You want to first lay out the classic medicine wheel design on the land, as previously described. Perhaps you will create the great wagon wheel design with twenty-eight spokes, and choose eight different plants for each major quarter of the medicine wheel garden. Or just choose three or four plants for each quadrant of a smaller garden.

The Medicinal/Culinary Medicine Wheel Garden

The medicinal/culinary garden combines vegetables with favorite culinary herbs. Make sure the deeply dug earth is well fertilized and balanced with sand, as most of these old favorite herbs are Mediterranean in origin and will thrive in sandy, neutral soil and full sun. Colorful carpets of nasturtiums might be planted to encircle the peace pole and cairn in the center.

GARDENING WITH CHILDREN

American Indian children often worked in the family fields and gardens, where they had assigned tasks. Young children were

A curandera *is more than a doctor. The* curanderas *cure with their minds, with their experience, and with herbs. With love to the people.*

—Gregorita Rodriguez, *curandera y sobradora,* Santa Fe, New Mexico

MEDICINAL/CULINARY MEDICINE WHEEL

East (yellow or gold)	South (blue or purple)	West (red or magenta)	North (white or silver)
Thyme	Lavender	Red sage	Tarragon
Marigold	Rosemary	Pineapple sage	Basil
Summer squash	Anise hyssop	Chili peppers	Mint
Epazote	Heal-all	Cherry peppers	Garlic
Fennel	Heart'sease	Cherry or plum	Parsley
Dill	Sage	tomatoes	Cilantro
Horsemint	Purple kale	Beets	Angelica
Dwarf sunflower	Chard	Scarlet runner pole beans	Egyptian walking (top)
Teucrium	Garlic	(tipi)	onions
Yellow cherry or pear	Blueberry	Red oak-leaf lettuce	Cuban basil
tomatoes			Mexican sweet herb
			Strawberry
			Bearberry

responsible for driving predatory birds and animals, such as crows, ravens, and chipmunks, out of the spring gardens where young plants were sprouting. The children would gather piles of small stones to throw at these garden thieves to oust them.

Growing children and growing gardens are natural complements. Children can closely experience the nurturing of seeds and roots into plants, and then into foods and health care aids. Gardening becomes an all-around learning experience. Training vines and pruning sucker growth from some plants is a responsible part of plant culture. As Halloween approaches, fun in the garden means watching the pumpkins and gourds grow to maturity.

Many of the healing herbs in the medicine wheel garden have glorious blossoms that attract bees, hummingbirds, and butterflies, along with a range of beneficial garden spiders. By midsummer, the garden becomes a colorful quilt of life with many insects to learn more about. Pollination, which is continually demonstrated in the summer garden, becomes a tangible theme for study. Building compost bins and carrying out the daily compostable remains from the kitchen adds another dimension to gardening and garbage disposal. Children like to watch the natural process of how, with their help, garbage recycles itself into usable garden humus.

The **Mother Goose Garden** is named after the old Mother Goose nursery rhyme popularized by Simon and Garfunkel in the hit song "Scarborough Fair." The refrain "Parsley, sage, rosemary, and thyme" gives us the stalwart herbs for inclusion here. There are many hybrid varieties of each of these four classic Mediterranean herbs, so this garden will be colorful as well as highly fragrant.

Consider how children like to touch and sniff, and use this opportunity to enlighten, educate, and just have great fun in this summer garden. Because the carefully stroked foliage of each plant has a distinctive aroma and feel, this project can also be used as a fragrance garden for people with impaired vision.

The aromatic qualities of herbs have long served to stimulate the mind, ward off illness, season our foods, provide sweet perfume, and serve as valuable insecticides. The picked foliage of these plants, especially sage, rosemary, lavender, and onions, effectively chases stinging insects away when worn in a scarf or hat or tied in a bandanna around one's neck. Children can make a pet's collar, using a bandanna to hold several sprigs of herbs, twisted and loosely tied around the pet's neck— the leaves are particularly effective there. Like all natural products, they need to be refreshed often, but what a pleasure!

Plants tell stories and stimulate new stories to be told. It is fun to investigate the origins of each plant and learn more about how it traveled the world, intersecting with the beliefs and economic and medical needs of different peoples.

With the classic medicine wheel design, you might place the parsley, sage, rosemary, and thyme each in a separate quadrant. You may want to place stepping-stones among the plants so that children can move easily within the garden without compacting the soil. Select several varieties of sage; perhaps pineapple sage, silver sage, golden sage, tricolor sage, and bronze sage plants might cluster around the most familiar one, the garden or kitchen sage, *Salvia officinalis*. Or you can plant multiples of just one species for attractive foliage and spring/summer blossoms.

Several delicious types of parsley and cilantro, and even celery and fennel, would create a fancy showing in the next quadrant of the garden. Parsley and other herbs with shiny dark green leaves

These stories are traces of native reason and memories as the birch trees are traces of the catkin, and salmon are memories of the rivers.
—Gerald Vizenor, Chippewa author of *The Heirs of Columbus*

favor slightly more acid soil, whereas the gray-leaved herbs (sage, rosemary, and thyme) favor a sweeter, more alkaline soil. You may want to do some simple composting for these herbs by adding used coffee grounds and tea leaves to the acid-lovers' soil, and crushed eggshells for the alkaline-lovers. Scratch these well into the soil and distribute them well around the plants.

For the last two quadrants of this garden, finish one with a selection of upright and weeping rosemary plants and the other with a grouping of various thyme plants. You can never have enough thyme! The thymes vary from soft gray to variegated (green and gold, or green and white) and deep green. All varieties have tiny oval leaves, and when stroked they release a heavenly fragrance.

If you choose to plant a wagon wheel garden with multiple spokes, you might add lavender, strawberry, heal-all, wintergreen, bearberry, and pennyroyal. Other childhood favorites are the tiny antennarias, the dense, cosmopolitan pussy-toes, or cat's paws. My mother remembers these small plants were called rabbit tobacco in rural Tennessee when she was a child growing up. Or you can choose your own regional favorites to plant within your design. Perhaps you will encourage the children to construct a twig tipi to stand in one quadrant of the garden to support a hops vine or passionflower vine for shade and added interest.

A good school project might be to establish a version of this garden as an outdoor classroom and adopt certain plants to study during the year, writing papers and doing research on each one as well as

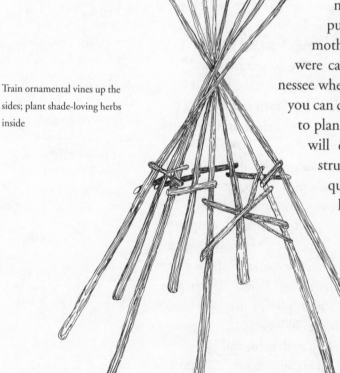

Train ornamental vines up the sides; plant shade-loving herbs inside

caring for it in the garden. This is an excellent exercise in nurturing and creating sacred space. It might also be an interesting stretch to design and plant a **Three Sisters Medicine Wheel Garden,** focusing on regional varieties of corn squash, pumpkin, and beans, along with their "fourth sister," the great varieties of chili, sweet, and hot peppers.

AROMA GARDENS

Fragrances are alluring pleasures. Many of the herbs we grow in our medicine wheel garden release their aromas in the summer heat when you brush by their foliage and blossoms. Capturing the volatile oils (the quickly escaping fragrances) in concentrated essential oils is an art that has been practiced for thousands of years. Many ancient cultures knew that fragrances can trigger emotional and healing responses in people. In fact, archaeological evidence reveals the use of essential oils in ancient burial sites.

René Maurice Gattefosse, a French chemist who investigated the chemical constituents in essential oils that aided the healing process, popularized the term *aromatherapy* in 1920. Many different essential oils provide amazing healing potential when smelled and rubbed on the skin. For this reason, and for pleasure, aromatherapy has become enormously popular.

American Indian sweat lodge rites include the fragrance of sage, pine, or juniper in the steaming mists rising off fire-heated rocks. Beyond sweat lodge rites, fragrance also played a role in diverse medicines and ceremonial rites. Many of the healing plants in the medicine wheel garden give particular aromas that perfume various healing applications. Bergamot (bee balm), American pennyroyal, bayberry, sage, sweetgrass, wintergreen, and yarrow are some of the most prominent. These herbs and their fragrances have antiseptic and antibiotic qualities.

Inhaling certain fragrances can bring back memories and stir emotions. Some fragrances, such as sage, sweetgrass, and yarrow, can be relaxing and grounding; other aromas, including the per-

One of the most noted herbalists among the Massachusetts Indians was Dr. William Perry of the Fall River Band. He traveled among the people performing miraculous cures and he was well known not only in Massachusetts but also among the Indians of Rhode Island and Connecticut. Frequently he was called upon to minister to a number of white families.

Dr. Perry was a psychic and a practitioner of the old school of Massachusetts Indian belief attributing his success to the power and guidance of the Great Spirit through the agency of Granny Squannit. His cures were secret and he never told what herbs he used.

—Gladys Tantaquidgeon, Mohegan medicine woman, writing in 1928 on traditional Algonquian healing

fume of bee balm, sweet flag, and pennyroyal, can be invigorating and cleansing. Think of the intoxicating fragrances of ripe strawberries, vanilla, and chocolate.

A **Fragrance Medicine Wheel Garden** might feature selections from over two hundred herb-scented geraniums in the genus *Pelargonium*, which originated in South Africa. These highly perfumed ornamentals exhibit diverse foliage and blossom types. Their aromas mimic everything from nutmeg, strawberry, lemon, and lime to gooseberry, old rose, pine, ginger, orange, crème de menthe, chocolate, apricot, peach, and much more. Their leaves are used in teas, tisanes, creams, and lotions, and as insecticides. The geraniums are tender perennials in most zones, where they must be replanted from new stock each year. Many of us collect them, always adding to our favorite varieties when we find a new one.

TWO MEDICINE WHEEL GARDENS

One of my medicine wheel gardens is situated in full sun on a knoll, with deep loamy soil. My original goal was to have five different species of healing plants in each quadrant, for a total of twenty classic herbs in this large space. Preliminary plantings centered around the four sacred plants: tobacco in the east quadrant (yellow blossoms), sage in the south (lavender blossoms), bearberry in the west (red berries following pink-white blooms), and sweetgrass in the north (white blooms). I placed large standing stones by each of the four special groupings, because these were my accent features and points of strength in the medicine wheel. I planted four of each species in a simple natural clump to encourage healthy growth.

I always want to start the medicine wheel garden with the four sacred plants—tobacco, sage, bearberry, and sweetgrass—and give them particular care and attention. I offer special prayers and dig them in with extra cornmeal blessings and songs.

I based my next choices on what native medicinal plants would really do best in that garden site. I selected these additional

In the prayers of my people are prayers for grass, for the renewal of the earth, and for deer. And if we do this . . . then all of this life and all of this spirit will go on forever.

—Tsonakwa, Abenaki artist and storyteller, 1986

plants in groups of two and three for each species: epazote and shrubby cinquefoil in the east quadrant; blue flag and sweet flag in the south; butterfly weed, bee balm, and pineapple sage in the west; Cuban basil and jimsonweed in the north. I planted extra bearberry in the west-central sector around the peace pole and followed with strawberry for the north, creeping cinquefoil for the east, and heal-all for the south. I even found a stunning red-blossomed strawberry that is ever-blooming and ever-bearing, which I added in the west and north quadrants.

I made a special area in the north quadrant for a good-sized colony of my best broadleaf plantain, *Plantago major*. This old Eurasian healing herb is one of my reliable favorites. I use the sturdy green leaves as "innersoles" in my sandals and shoes because they relieve leg and foot fatigue and leave my feet feeling healthier. I even take small plastic bags of these leaves when I travel. A chewed leaf, or portion, will relieve stomach cramps and queasiness. In summer I roast the fresh seeds, grind them, and add them to vegetable dishes, as plantain seeds help soothe and regulate the digestive system. I also brought dandelion into the eastern quadrant, but I prevent it from going to seed. I used chicory in the south and purslane in the west quadrant because these, too, are valuable nutriceuticals (see more about this in Chapter 11).

In the much larger medicine wheel garden at the Institute of American Indian Studies, I followed the same plan. This garden is situated on a stone-ridden, shady western slope with slightly acid soil, suggesting different choices from those in my personal medicine wheel garden. Considering these conditions and the soil enrichments I had added, we planted the east quadrant with native species of arnica, St. John's wort, and yellow dock. The south received sage, blue flag, and wild bergamot. For the west I selected bee balm, red-stemmed native angelica, and butterfly weed, and for the north quadrant mayapple, bloodroot, and sweetgrass. Again, we planted four of each species in a healthy little colony.

A big medicine wheel garden like this one, more than thirty feet across, can support a shrub in the middle of each quadrant, supplying extra shade for sun-shy native wildflowers planted be-

I was now more sure than ever that our ancient Indian wisdom and knowledge was the surest source of safety, salvation, and success in life. The priest preached against love medicine, but even devout Catholics continue to use it. They cannot be shaken in their belief that the spiritual herbs are blessings that God bestowed upon our ancestors centuries ago.

—Christine Quintasket, (Mourning Dove), Salish, Colville Confederated Tribes of eastern Washington State

neath it. Remembering our colors, we included a witch hazel shrub in the east quadrant, an elderberry shrub in the south, a bayberry shrub in the north, and a sumac in the west. These shrubs provide wonderful perches as well as seeds and berries for songbirds and game birds. To keep them looking their best, each of these shrubs needs to be lightly clipped or pinched back several times during the growing season.

Regardless of her supernatural contacts, a woman always knew the many uses of various herbs for medicines, for curing childhood ailments like tummyaches, earaches, or toothaches, and for the different personal upsets. . . . Oregon grape roots and tops strengthened the blood in the spring and made the body more hardy. Red willow bark made into a tea cures sores on the face of a child or wounds on an adult. Pine pitch served the same purpose or was diluted in warm water to cure a cold or weak lungs. Another cold cure was a brew of mentholated sagebrush.

—Christine Quintasket (Mourning Dove), Salish, Colville Confederated Tribes of eastern Washington State

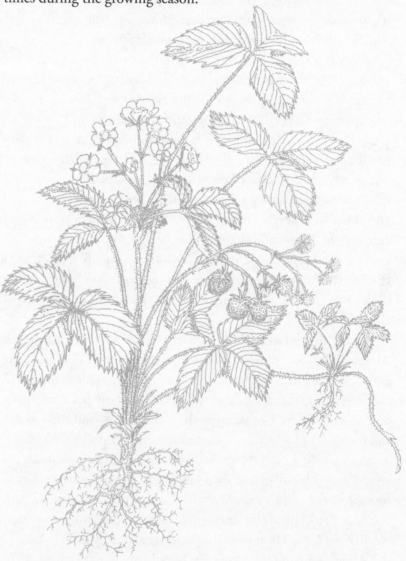

CHAPTER FOUR

Planting the Medicine Wheel Garden

Securing Sacred Space

AFTER YOU HAVE DECIDED on the garden style that best suits your regional and local environment and your personal preference, planting your medicine wheel garden should be a great pleasure. The fun begins with choosing the most harmonious group of native healing plants for each quadrant of your medicine wheel. The plant profiles in Part II of this book can serve as a basic guide, enlarged by your own knowledge and further investigations of the many possibilities.

As you make these exciting choices, the important point is to think ahead. Gardens change with both the seasons and the years. Innocent-looking seedlings can shoot up to unforeseen heights. Make careful choices among the short and tall species and plan your arrangements so that the tall plants will not deprive the smaller ones of needed sun. Consider also which plants will fill their spaces most quickly, and don't overplant. Leave open spaces.

Tending my own medicine wheel garden, I have noticed how many plants—including yarrow, angelica, and mayapple—jump

The Medicine Wheel Circle is the Universe. It is change, life, death, birth, and learning. This Great Circle is the lodge of our bodies, our minds, and our hearts. It is the cycle of all things that exist.

—Hyemeyohsts Storm, *Seven Arrows*, 1972

Both the design and use of sacred space are processes that draw on both the conscious and unconscious levels of mind and spirit. We learn as we create and we change as we garden. Let the process inform your spirit.

—Peg Streep, author of *Spiritual Gardening: Creating Sacred Space Outdoors*, 1999

boundaries and expand their growth areas, while others such as sweetgrass, sweet flag, and blue flag emerge early in spring and barely expand their colonies. Yarrow strengthens the other plants that grow nearby, so I tend to leave it alone and appreciate its gifts, but I may weed out and give away the oversupply of some other expanding populations. I always hope that the angelica has self-sowed, although I usually have to chase after these seedlings and transplant them back into the quadrant reserved for them. Plants are continually teaching me many things about their spirits and personalities.

ADDING WILDFLOWERS

For delicate beauty and strong healing qualities in your medicine wheel garden, wildflowers have an appeal often unmatched by their hybrid cousins. Most wildflowers have special therapeutic benefits. An increasing number are now being "farmed" to produce quantities for the burgeoning health food industry. One grower, Hsu Ginseng in Wisconsin, has more than a thousand acres planted in ginseng! Our native Jerusalem artichoke and lupine are grown in increasing amounts to provide their beneficial flour—ground from the processed roots and seeds, the flour goes into healthier, more digestible pastas and breads for those with dietary sensitivities. Many other wildflower species are being considered by growers for their unique beauty as well as therapeutic attributes. Some possess healing constituents not yet isolated in the laboratory.

Leading examples of wildflowers with important healing attributes include species of echinacea, arnica, evening primrose, ginseng, lobelia, goldenseal, goldthread, moccasin flower, mayapple, hellebore, and yarrow.

When I walk through my meadows of yarrow, blue flag, wood betony, black-eyed Susan, lobelia, daisies, and Queen Anne's lace, I realize how fortunate I am to live in Connecticut's northwest hills and take part in the growing wildflower conserva-

When making your color selections, keep seasons in mind, again—not only the blossoms but buds, leaves, and fruits may develop striking colors as the year progresses. As color of one group of plants passes, another will take over, keeping the garden beautiful with its bright quadrants of sacred colors.

Living Color

Throughout the blossoming season, the medicine wheel garden can also attract many colorful pollinators tantalized by flowers especially appealing to them. Flowers particularly favored by hummingbirds, butterflies, and moths include species of bee balm, cardinal flower and other lobelias, jewelweed, opuntia, sage, skullcap, tobacco, and yucca. These welcome visitors will also dip into many other flowers to sip nectar, especially boneset, fairywand, joe-pye weed, mint, and evening primrose.

tion movement. Farmland restoration work in my region is looking to new ways of saving old New England dairy farms by using valuable acreage to propagate medicinal plants. This fledgling movement may coax to abundance more native species while preserving and using the land in new ways rather than leaving us to watch old farms disappear into building lots and housing developments.

Each state has its symbolic official wildflower, and there are many wildflower conservation organizations, botanical societies, branches of the Herb Society of America, and garden clubs. One of my early enthusiasms, thirty-five years ago, was working for wildflower preservation in our local garden club. Little did I know then that this interest would become a lifelong devotion, leading me into all my other areas of writing, gardening, teaching, and museum work.

I have enjoyed speaking at various wildflower conferences in places from Massachusetts to Oklahoma, where thousands of people support their state wildflower societies and devote countless hours to propagating wildflowers, photographing them, and writing about them, especially the medicinal plants still in use—educating us all about their many benefits. And we are all beneficiaries of the movement, led by Lady Bird Johnson, to maintain the vitality of native wildflowers by planting them along roadsides, in national parks, and in other welcoming open spaces where they brighten every season.

The medicine wheel garden is a perfect place to develop new colonies of wildflowers as their numbers diminish in the wild habitats. High on the list of possibilities are native orchids, such

How long we will have the maple is up to the people. How long we will have the strawberry is up to the people. How long we will have water to survive is up to the people. Every individual can make a difference!

—Audrey Shenandoah, clan mother of the Onondaga nation and respected elder, 1992

as moccasin flower and trillium, blue cohosh, sweetgrass, goldenseal, goldthread, and maidenhair fern. As some of these herbs become established in your garden and multiply, you can help them by moving new young plants into other gardens and giving some to friends.

But with conservation in mind, a strong word of caution is necessary. Unless you are doing salvage botany and retrieving plants from an active building site (with permission), do not remove plants from wild areas, where their survival is continually threatened. The resource list in this book suggests a number of reliable suppliers for ordering living plants or seeds. Be aware, however, that the seeds of some wildflowers take three to four years to become well-established plants under the best circumstances. It is wisest to rely on plants or good healthy roots. You can order hard-to-find species from Richter's, in Canada, as I do, until you can propagate your own colony. See Appendix 1 for plant suppliers.

You can also choose hybridized, cultivated forms and varieties of many wildflowers for planting in your medicine wheel garden. They may not have the same level of healing constituents in all cases, but hybrid forms of species such as yarrow and lobelia add cheerful color and charm to the garden and may beg for inclusion.

BREAKING GROUND

You've made your wonderful choices and obtained your batches of plants. Now it's time to get out your spading fork, rake, and trowel. Keep a wheelbarrow handy and wear good gardening gloves to protect your hands. Also prepare a small bag of fine cornmeal and one of tobacco to use as offering substances to the land and to each plant. This step is important to honor and activate the best energies surrounding your work.

Before you begin creating your garden, light a small dish or wand of sage or cedar or lavender stems and smudge the whole area and yourself. Walk around the whole outer circle area of your medicine wheel with this fragrant smudge, while thinking how your project will beautify the area. Establish a new balance here with love and gratitude for the land and the little creatures it supports.

Spade deep into the earth and turn it over, breaking up large clods of soil. Look at the soil you have exposed. Study the little organisms and worms that make it so alive. Use the spading fork to dig deeper and turn more soil. If you can, rototill your garden by hand, turning over a section of the circle at a time. Allow the earth to open to the sunlight and breathe. Pick up a handful of earth; hold it, squeeze it, smell it. As you work, contemplate the beauty of your project and concentrate on making a successful, healthy medicine wheel garden.

Every spoonful of healthy soil contains millions of beneficial microscopic organisms: good species of fungi, nematodes, and bacteria. Far from causing disease or becoming pests to the plants growing there, they unlock many nutrients in the soil that stimulate root growth and development. Healthy soil with a good diversity of microbial nutrients also will inhibit root rot and the types of fungi that can damage roots and cause plants to wilt and fail. Nutrient retention occurs when bacteria and fungi multiply and increase their populations. These organisms are extremely rich in protein that is made from nitrogen. When they work in balance within your garden, your plants will be healthier, with less need for fertilizer and pest control.

When you have prepared the garden soil, place stepping-stones within your work area. If you can move from stone to stone, staying out of the freshly dug soil, you minimize the likelihood of compacting it. Always try to stay out of the garden during (or immediately following) rain or when it has just been watered. Plant roots need room to "breathe" underground, and working in the garden at these times can hasten soil compaction.

Later, you will encourage the health of your medicine wheel garden plants by working each year to enhance the soil's tilth—the crumbly, light, rich nature that allows for the best root system development and water retention. The easiest way to achieve and maintain this quality is to make a compost pile and add this

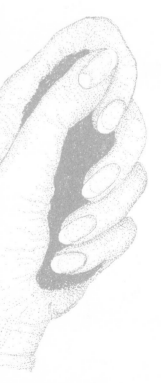

And this time of year our Mother Earth has worked all winter long in making her dress, beautiful dress, but it's green. 'Bout the early spring she adds some wildflowers to it. And whenever she gets ready she drops her skirt down the mountain side, you can see it across the mountain downhill, her skirt is full with all the flowers—all kinds of flowers. That's our Mother's skirt that she had worked on all winter long.

—Edna Chekelelee, Cherokee storyteller from the Snowbird community, Qualla Boundary, North Carolina

humus to your garden each spring and summer. After the garden becomes established, you will also want to top-dress the soil each spring with well-decayed compost and leaf mulch, scratching it in with a trowel or hoe.

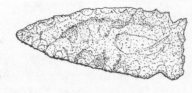

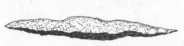

Special spirit stone (*sicun wotawe wotai*); prehistoric spear point found in Bridgewater, Connecticut

The Manitou comes from the place of its abode in the stone. It becomes roused by the heat of the fire, and proceeds out of the stone when water is sprinkled on it. It moves up and down and all over inside the body, driving out everything that inflicts pain. Before the Manitou returns to the stone it imparts some of its nature to the body. That is why one feels so well after having been in the sweat lodge.

—William Jones, Mesquakie (Fox), 1905

PERSONAL SPIRIT STONES

As you break ground for your medicine wheel garden, look for a special stone. Lakota author Ed MaGaa Eagle Man teaches about the importance of finding your own *wotai,* your special stone, which will serve as *wotawe,* a personal charm guiding your work. This special stone will draw your attention and can take any form that appeals to you. You may already have such stones. Perhaps you have a special crystal or geode that you keep on your altar or a small stone that you wear in your medicine bag. You may even see a special animal or plant shape or symbol within this stone that helps you to identify with it.

Your stone has *sicun,* its own soul or spirit. *Sicun wotawe wotai* is Lakota for "a special stone whose spirit is obvious and comes to the bearer in a special way." It can be a touchstone and protector for you during this time.

Several years ago, while I was digging in an old peony patch in my front garden, my shovel struck a small stone. This was not at all unusual in our stony New England soil—in some places every shovelful of earth is filled with stones. Yet something about the sound of this stone, lodged well underground, made me stop and reach down for it and pick it up. As I rubbed it between my fingers to release the caked dirt around it, I could see that it was a projectile point. My heart was pounding with excitement as I realized that this was an ancient flint spear point, too large to be an arrowhead. And the flint was not native to my region.

Specialists at the nearby Institute for American Indian Studies dated my spear point at about four thousand to five thousand years old. It is a fine example of a Late Archaic side-notched spear point, possibly a Brewerton, named for a type of prehistoric American Indian site in Brewerton, New York. The stone, which has a distinctive smoky green composition, is a Dutchess County flint, commonly used by prehistoric Indian toolmakers in the Northeast. Another season, while working to repair our old stone wall, I found a large, old hammer stone of primitively worked native granite. Many such ancient Indian objects do turn up in old stone walls, where they were simply thrown in with the other rocks. As a "rock hound," I continually learn more about what stones and rocks have to teach me.

I should add that I live in a small farming community where Indian artifacts like these continually appear in the soil. Indians gardened corn, beans, squash, peppers, and tobacco in this area more than a thousand years ago. Long before then, they hunted across this region. The town workmen tell me that they each have a shoebox filled with arrowheads they have found while digging to put in fence posts and highway signs. Many of the old cornfields that are plowed each spring still yield occasional crops of arrowheads. Country folks walk the furrows in the fields each spring and pick up white quartz spear points, drills, and arrowheads. In this respect, our New England region doesn't differ much from other regions of the country. Native Americans hunted and fished all over this continent for many centuries before our European ancestors came to live here. Maybe your spirit stone, like mine, comes from prehistoric hands.

Penobscot legends tell of earliest times when the Creator first made native people out of rock. When this did not work, he broke the rocks, which then became *manogemassak,* little spirits.

The mother of my mother was noted for her knowledge of herbs and her skill at making love charms. The Colville and Okanogan paid her large sums for love charms. Many asked her to "make medicine" for them, trying to get her secret formulas, but none ever succeeded.

—Christine Quintasket (Mourning Dove), Salish, Colville Confederated Tribes of eastern Washington State

PLANTING AND BLESSING

The usual rule of thumb for planting is to do this work after the sun leaves the site for the day or on an overcast day. Hot sun beating down on newly installed plants can cause even healthy specimens to wilt and go into shock. Herbs whose aboveground parts are most vital for healing should be planted between the new moon and the full moon, while the moon is on the increase. Plants whose food or healing value is concentrated in the roots should be planted during the waning moon, between the full moon and the new moon. You will achieve your greatest gardening success if you abide by the wisdom of the moon signs.

Healthy plants dug into the medicine wheel garden will provide your showiest results, though seeds, root divisions, and stem cuttings are also valuable additions. Before removing the plants from pots or flats, place them in the prepared garden at the spots where you plan to dig them in. See how they look. Now is a good time to rearrange groupings. As you move about in the garden, remember to walk on your stepping-stones or along the criss-crossing paths.

When you have placed the new plants to your satisfaction, you can begin to dig them in one by one. Prepare the holes, digging each hole carefully and loosening the soil all around and beneath where the root system will rest. Sprinkle a pinch of cornmeal or tobacco in the hole with a prayer or song. Carefully

Plants That Spread Easily

Once you have developed a healthy colony of angelica or blue flag iris, for instance, you hope these plants will continue to self-sow and thrive in this same space you have so carefully given to them. Don't be surprised, however, to find that many sow their seeds beyond the quadrant you designated as home. Plants, like people, love to wander and jump across borders and defy boundaries. You may enjoy resetting young seedlings in the medicine wheel garden, placing them in other garden beds of yours, or giving them to friends.

Many of us keep "friendship gardens" where we cultivate plants given to us by various friends. As we gain new plants, we also enjoy giving some away.

nest each plant into its new location and pat more soil around its base. Water it well enough to soak it. Do not smother it, but make sure its roots are properly covered. Try to purchase and plant three or four of each kind of plant. Work to establish little colonies of your favorite herbs. If you begin with seeds or tender seedlings, careful planting work is especially vital. Most seeds should be started in flats and transplanted to the garden when the new seedlings have grown strong and healthy.

As you plant each herb, think about how it will fit into the

An Offering to Granny Squannit

On Cape Cod, Nantucket, and the nearby smaller islands, as well as in southern mainland New England, Granny Squannit was the leader of the Little People, who predominate as unseen forces throughout the Northeast. Many Algonquian women believed that these Little People, the *makiawisug* of the Mohegan, aided the growth of corn and healthy medicine plants. Today, storytellers and medicine people continue to honor these magical little beings and leave tiny offerings of cornbread in their gardens for Granny, as no one wants to incur their displeasure. Says Gladys Tantaquidgeon, Mohegan medicine woman and historian, "Granny Squannit gave to the Indians the knowledge of medicinal properties found in certain plants and also knowledge of how to prepare roots for use in curing certain diseases."

ecosystem of your medicine wheel garden. What are its strengths and needs? Think about it enhancing your own sacred space.

Planning a medicine wheel garden can be a perfect opportunity to invite friends to share the pleasures. Working together harmoniously for a few hours or a day is a memorable experience. Native people have always found the greatest benefits in sharing labor. They learned long ago that many hands and hearts make work go quickly. And people working together create a garden with very special energies. Everyone's energy becomes part of this creation.

Invite each friend to bring a special stone to begin building the prayer cairn and a special rock to place in one of the quadrants. Friends may also wish to bring a prayer tie—a long ribbon or narrow strip of cloth on which prayers for success and renewal are painted or written. You might also suggest that they bring a potluck dish for sharing a communal meal to celebrate after the work is accomplished.

Whether you are working alone or with friends, give a special little blessing to each plant, silently or aloud, as you place it in the ground and offer the ground itself a pinch of tobacco with gratitude. This small blessing engenders the plant's energies to grow successfully.

As we listen in the wind, we can hear the sounds and songs of our ancestors, and as we walk on the ground, we are walking on the faces of those yet unborn. Let us make a beautiful dream, full of hope, clean water, good land, and a good way of life for them.

—Winona LaDuke, Ojibwe, founding director, White Earth Land Recovery Project, northern Minnesota

CHAPTER FIVE

Finishing Touches

Peace Poles, Wind Horses, and Prayer Cairns

They talked medicine. There are stories of the plants that were here before my grandmother was born. The spirits tell stories. They are the ones that molded me. . . . I am best known as the Flower That Speaks in a Pollen Way. I am the explainer of the ceremonies. My specialty is teaching.

—Annie Kahn, Navajo medicine woman

N OW COME THE EXCITING steps of accentuating all your hard work. Stand back and admire the medicine wheel garden. You may feel that it is already "talking to you" and giving you ideas about what to do next.

When I have finished planting a new medicine wheel garden, I'm certainly tired—I just want to go wash and relax. I can see that the work is done and well accomplished, yet I cannot quit. The garden seems to tease and beckon me to pay attention to this path or that corner, or move in more stones, or stand them up here and there, sheltering some of the more fragile plants against strong sun and wind.

I've learned that others experience the same amazing reaction. Once, after creating a public medicine wheel garden in Sherman, Connecticut, I stood with the small circle of friends who remained to admire our accomplishments. We were tired, hungry, and ready to call a halt. Yet even after the garden looked finished and right, it still held us. As we worked for several hours longer, we were surprised at the renewed energy we felt as we created little paths, moved stones, and beautified the whole area. We kept going to the prayer cairns we had built up as a group to place more small stones with special prayers. A certain magnetism develops around these sacred spaces. It makes everyone feel good just to be there.

SETTING THE PEACE POLE AND DIRECTIONAL POLES

With plants, paths, and stones in place, the important finishing touches to make your medicine wheel garden complete will be best added on another day. These are the central peace pole and the directional poles with their adornments. These final steps, both simple and profound, signal the garden's unique structure, serving as keys to its purpose and focusing the color themes of the plants you have set in the ground.

You will want to obtain or create and prepare your poles to fit your garden plan and your personal desires before the day for planting arrives. Getting them ready requires creative thought, good energies, and a peaceful spirit.

The peace pole that rises in the very center of your garden should declare itself prominently. A fine four-by-four post (four inches square and eight feet long) of cedar or spruce will fit well into many garden sizes. A carved cedar newel post is also a nice peace pole. You can obtain a suitable post from a local lumberyard or buy a peace pole beautifully decorated by the World Peace Prayer Society. This worthy organization offers you a choice of words from many languages, all meaning "May peace prevail on earth," printed on the sides of the pole. (See Appendix 2 for address.) If you prefer to do your own decorating, you can embellish your peace pole with four American Indian tribal words for "peace," one word for each side of the pole. Make your selections from the following list and carefully write your chosen words on the post, using a pencil to write the letters of each word vertically, in descending order. This step is important to work out the spacing and clarity of the letters.

When you are satisfied, the words can be permanently carved or burned or painted into the wood. I have found it easiest to use a

After you've set your last batch of plants in its quadrant and you stand back to admire the result of all your hard work, it's more than likely that your medicine wheel garden will keep you there a bit longer, and you'll feel a new surge of the energy you need to adjust what it's telling you to do.

Words of Peace

Achwangundowagan	Delaware (Lenape) for "lasting peace"
Aquenne	Southern Algonquian for "peace"
Aquenne-ut	Wampanoag for "place of peace"
Awige	Northern Algonquian for "peace"
Her'kv	Muscogee Creek for "peace"
Hozhqqji	Navajo for "blessing way"
Ikachi techqua	Hopi for "blending with the land and celebrating life"
Langundowagan	Delaware (Lenape) for "peace and amity"
Laule'a	Hawaiian for "peaceful, happy time"
Malu	Hawaiian for "peace"
Mitakuye oyasin	Sioux for "with all things we are related"
Onen	Iroquois for "peace be with you"
Waunakee	Great Lakes Algonquian for "we have peace"
Wetaskiwin	Alberta Cree for "hills of peace"
Wowalj'wa	Lakota for "peace"
Wulangundowagan	Delaware (Lenape) for "peace"

simple wood-burning tool with a beveled stylus, available at craft shops, which readily helps me to form clear, beautiful letters. Using this tool on a cedar post also releases the aroma of the wood.

Select a cap for the top of your peace pole. Many hardware stores provide a choice of plastic, wood, or metal caps, easily attached to the top of the pole for a nice, neat look. To anchor the post firmly, you may wish to get a metal post base to sink into the ground.

For the cardinal direction poles, choose five- to six-foot cedar or pine posts. Or, if you are feeling ambitious, you might harvest and trim young hickory, ash, or alder saplings to serve as your poles. If you like lots of color, you can paint each pole with its directional hue and add plant symbols and animal totems, painted or burned in or both. For this style of decoration, I like to use acrylic all-weather paints, and I choose bright colors.

You might also wrap each pole in satin ribbons of its cardinal direction color, with matching ribbon streamers or banners flying at the top. Tied into place, the ribbons will naturally flutter in the breeze and fly in strong winds. The Tibetan use of colorful prayer

Symbolic Animals in the Garden

Many of us feel strong animal association with each cardinal direction. I visualize bear and coyote in the north and the wolf and wild turkey opposite in the south, with the deer and red-tailed hawk guarding the eastern door juxtaposed with the eagle and mountain lion guarding the west. Many other animal and bird symbols are also embraced within the medicine wheel garden as protective influences and guardian spirits. I draw my personal medicine wheel mandala and adorn my spirit shield with some of these traditional spirit animals. See Chapter 14 for fuller details.

flags strung along cords, which they call "wind horses," inspires this thought. What could be more perfect than committing your prayers to the wind so that they can be swept around the world?

Your wind horses may be adorned and painted with special prayers before you tie them to the cardinal poles. Setting the poles in the ground and making sure that they stand properly vertical is easier and more fun when done in company. Invite a few close friends to share in this rewarding activity, and encourage each person helping you to write or paint a personal prayer on a ribbon or banner. Later, on major occasions, additional banners may be painted with prayers and tied to a shrub or tree near the medicine wheel garden. This observance is especially meaningful on the solstices and equinoxes. Perhaps, too, you will want to designate a shrub, such as an elderberry or bayberry, in your medicine wheel garden to receive prayer ties.

When the poles are fully decorated and ready to be installed, begin with the peace pole. Walk to the center of your garden, taking care to use one of your stone paths and your stepping-stones rather than treading on the soil. Remove the temporary pole you placed there while creating your medicine wheel garden. Then, if necessary, enlarge the hole to accommodate the peace pole. The hole will probably have to be made deeper, in any case, for an eight-foot pole to stand in it securely. The peace pole can be carried by two people or possibly pushed on a wheelbarrow along the cross paths to the edge of the prepared hole. If you are using a post base, attach it to the peace pole and carefully lower the pole into its hole so that its four sides face the four cardinal directions.

Partially fill the hole so that the pole stands upright but can be adjusted. Use a level, holding one end of the level against a side of the pole to make sure that the pole is standing vertically, not at a slant. Now pack the dirt firmly around the pole, filling the hole completely. Use the same method to install your cardinal direction poles. Offer a ceremonial blessing to the pole and earth.

When you stand back with your friends to admire your finished medicine wheel garden, you'll have a lot to celebrate! It's a fine time for a circle of prayer and a potluck lunch or supper.

ADDING STONE CAIRNS

Around the world, stone cairns are among the most ancient landmarks we know. They signify different things to different people: In some places, they may have served as trail markers, and in others as markers of sacred places. In the arctic region, where survival long depended on the food and materials that the caribou supplied, cairns indicated the migratory paths of these animals, which tend to follow the same route year after year. In some places, cairns marked human burial sites, and they also topped some Native American mounds, accentuating the importance of these unusual structures on the landscape.

Algonquian people commonly placed stones in piles to commemorate places where remarkable events happened. We still visit these places and add yet more stones, reinforcing our sense of identity and shared history. Schaghticoke and Mahican Indians living near Stockbridge, Massachusetts, in the eighteenth century added stones to a cairn ten cartloads high, because it was the custom of their fathers. Wampanoag Indians also observed this tradition because their fathers and grandfathers and great-grandfathers did so, and charged all their children to do so. These customs express a deep belief in the power of special places on the land and in the spirit present in stone.

Cairns certainly deserve a significant presence in the medicine wheel garden. In earlier chapters, I have suggested honoring the

Stone People

One, two, or three stones stacked and balanced upon one another become Stone People, solid guardians of my medicine wheel garden and my yard. They stand like wise sentinels, surveying everything and making no comments. They are good garden friends.

garden by asking each person who comes there to add a small stone to existing prayer cairns. These cairns can be created around the garden's central peace pole and the base of each cardinal pole. After each pole is secured in the ground and the earth tamped down around it, begin placing stones around its base. Each stone placed on the cairn represents a person's prayer, and everyone who comes into the garden and adds a stone contributes a prayer and energy to the growing cairn. It won't take long before all the poles have attractive piles of varied stones around them.

If you have decided to leave some sizable rocks standing in your garden, make the most of them. In creating my own medicine wheel garden, I designated one big, smooth stone near the center as the Mother Earth stone and another as the Father Sky stone. Smaller stones like these joined them to encircle the center as Grandmother Moon and Grandfather Sun along with Sister Day and Brother Night.

They remind me of various Native American legends about the First People, the Stone People, who the Great Manitou created before making the five-fingered beings who were our ancestors. Earthmaker first made a race of giants, who were the ones that helped shape the land. Then she made the Stone People, destined to guard things on the surface realm. The magical Little People, whom she created after this, are just as strong and inhabit a mystical realm in the underworld. They can come and go freely between the realms, yet none but the most astute gardeners can ever see them, unless the Little People are in a happy mood. Then they might change themselves into fireflies and butterflies and dance all around. They have the greatest freedom of all.

The Stone People stand guard over special plants and bring creative earth energy into the medicine wheel garden. Stone Peo-

The rocks are manitou asseinah, *literally "spirit rocks" where God abides.*

—Eastern Algonquian saying

ple catch the sunlight, moonlight, and starlight. They look fabulous in deep snow when the garden is slumbering, yet the medicine wheel is filled with energy and delight. Stone People have become little "personalities" in and around my medicine wheel gardens and around the property, and they are always a source of conversation when folks visit. They have inspired countless copies, as folks go away thinking, "Well, I can do that!"

You can see a number of my Stone People on the cover of this book. The old tree logs are wooden "sit-upons" where visitors and I pause to rest. It is important to create a spot or two within the medicine wheel where you can sit and reflect or meditate and simply be with the plants, prayers, and healing therein.

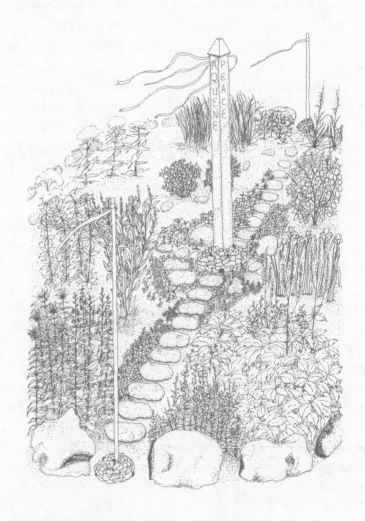

CHAPTER SIX

Mulches

The Garden's Conservationists

NOT SURPRISINGLY, THE MEDICINE wheel garden's showy top layers of colorful flowers, berries, and bright foliage consume most of our attention; when we say "garden," we think of the plant parts that we can see. To sustain the vitality of these visible layers of growth, however, the more mysterious underground plant layers require careful nurturing. The root zone is a labyrinth of essential nutrients and movement that enable the whole plant to thrive and look its best. Mulching can favor all layers, from bottom to top.

Covering the earth, even lightly, prevents the soil around sensitive roots from drying out too rapidly. By conserving moisture, mulching eliminates the need for frequent watering, which is impractical in many regions—and wherever you live, saving water is desirable and important. If your garden rests on a slope, mulching will help to check erosion by water runoff and wind. Some mulches also provide valuable soil nutrients.

Top-dressing the garden soil around the plants is a perennial activity for many gardeners. Mulches protect and preserve your plants and also enhance the attractiveness of the plants and garden layout. Yet another part of their duty is to keep the undersides

The whole process of gathering had a ceremony, no matter what you were using. There are proper ways to be observed in the preparation of the materials. I'm extremely grateful that my grandmother showed me these things.

—Tu Moonwalker, Apache medicine woman and basketmaker

of the plants clean during rain and watering. When selecting mulch, consider your garden's special needs: the type of soil, the lay of the land, and the plants you have chosen. The design and style of your garden may dictate use of certain mulches.

Mulches can be divided into organic and inorganic types. Organic mulches, such as aged compost and leaf mold, serve as temporary soil covering and enrich the plants and earth as they decompose through the seasons. Inorganic mulches are more permanent, especially if properly installed. For example, a cover of river cobbles over a layer of landscape fabric can last for decades and requires little maintenance beyond removing dead leaves and plant clippings as needed.

ORGANIC MULCHES

Rapidly decomposing mulches, such as compost, leaf mold, straw, and hay, are very valuable for all soil types. If your soil is light and sandy, mulches such as these, especially compost, will enrich it and add moisture retention qualities. If your soil is heavy with clay, organic mulch can help to lighten and loosen its texture over time. Even if your soil is just perfect—loose and dark with humus—mulch will add nourishment and protect it from rapid drying.

Compost is a universal, increasingly valuable soil enricher. The health and vigor of many gardens can be improved by top-dressing with good compost each spring. Compost begins with garden waste and food scraps that can range from discarded vegetable and fruit parts to eggshells, coffee grounds, and tea leaves layered with grass clippings, leaves, and straw or hay. Over time, these materials break down and become humus. This can be created quite rapidly in compost bins, where the mixture should be turned over often. You can also create large compost piles or bins that are not turned and slowly decompose. You can dig the rich humus from underneath, at the side of the pile.

Many gardeners in our eastern states, including those managing public gardens and large estates, chop and recycle autumn leaves and choose *leaf mold mulch* as their free, sustainable preference for building good soil. Like compost, leaf mulch breaks down quickly and needs to be replaced each year. Some mixtures of leaves tend to be acidic. If a test shows a change in the soil pH, a dusting of lime or broken eggshells and chopped yarrow scratched into the leaf mold and soil will help.

Two other good seasonal mulches, straw and hay, both decompose rapidly and can be turned into the soil and replenished. *Straw mulch,* which consists of the stem bottoms from the wheat harvest, is best kept loose and spread several inches thick around the garden. It is an excellent soil enricher but should be used with caution around food and medicinal plants, because wheat fields are treated with herbicides. With *hay mulch,* if possible choose young green hay or salt hay, as mature hay is full of seeds and can introduce vigorous weeds into the garden.

A number of organic mulches derive from tree bark or wood. Some of these have an appealing decorative quality as well as protecting the soil. Red cedar, *Juniperus communis,* is a common "weed" tree in many states and can be easily culled from the ecosystem without harm to other organisms. *Cedar bark mulch* and *red cedar shavings* come mainly from residue of cedar furniture and fencing manufacture. The fragrant mulch of red bark will last throughout the season if the shavings are applied several inches thick over the ground. Cedar mulches are insect-resistant, so they can be laid close to the house or other buildings where insect pests might be a problem.

Mulches made from red cedar add a showy look when used with other mulches for textural diversity and strong color. Their fragrance is wonderful!

Pine bark mulch and *pine nuggets* come from plantations and natural stands of pine that have been clear-cut and debarked for paper or lumber. Both these mulches are good soil modifiers and will last several years if not used in pedestrian areas and if put down over landscape fabric, not directly over soil. Laid around permanent plantings, the pine nuggets are the more decorative of the two.

Attractively straw-colored and without obvious odor, *cypress mulch* is also long-lasting. After young cypress trees are ground and planed in furniture manufacture, the leftovers are shredded to make this mulch. (Old-growth cypress is not used.) Different textures of cypress mulch are available; the finer particles hold a slope better in washout areas, while the larger particle size lasts longer.

Nugget-sized bark renderings from trees such as oak and sycamore provide *hardwood mulch*. Unlike insect-repellent cedar mulches, this one could become a home for insects like carpenter ants or termites and should not be placed too near the house. It is great beneath shrubs, trees, and tall herbs, especially in woodland gardens. In some settings, this mulch may last a couple of years before needing replacement. Usually a coarsely shredded, random mix of shrub and tree materials, *wood chip mulch* from landscape and clearing projects is often widely available. While useful for footpaths and many garden areas if applied several inches thick, it can leach vital nitrogen from the soil for the first year or two until it decomposes and returns the theft by enriching the area.

When environmental conditions are right, wood chip mulch may produce a range of fungi after rain—an extra benefit. Fungi are the ultimate decomposers.

Cocoa bean hull mulch is a renewable resource that when fresh has a wonderful fragrance and rich brown color. The small size and uniformity of the hulls make it visually appealing. A good conditioner for clayey and sandy soils, it lasts only about one season, as it biodegrades into the soil, and it should be replaced each spring.

Cottonseed hull mulch comes from the cottonseed residue after cotton and oil are removed. *Composted cotton burrs* are the prickly husks from the outer cotton boll. Both these mulches are short-lived but excellent soil conditioners. They work best when applied two to three inches deep and kept fairly moist. Caution: Because cotton is an intensively treated crop, composting may not remove enough of the residual chemicals for safe use of the burrs with food and medicinal plants.

INORGANIC MULCHES

These extremely elegant mulches are often used for Japanese and xeriscape gardens, especially in the desert Southwest, southern California, and Florida. Along with stones of various kinds, this group includes mulches made from dead coral, seashells, and beach glass. These permanent mulches are more expensive than others.

Stones smoothed by long contact with water have a particularly "finished" appearance for use as mulches. Water-smoothed stones selected for *river rock mulch* rank as one of the best permanent mulches, especially when applied over a layer of landscape fabric. This mulch is most suitable for applications around shrubs or trees, in meditation gardens, and for footpaths. *Beach stone mulch* is beautiful, but large-scale removal of choice beach stones has damaged many picturesque beaches. Removing stones from some beaches is now forbidden. Other stony waterfronts willingly give their cargo for landscape use, but the stones must be washed repeatedly to remove the salt. For use on garden paths, the salt residue is no problem, as it suppresses weed growth.

In contrast to stones shaped by water, *lava rock mulch* is porous and rough-textured. Produced by volcanic activity, lava rock is perceived by some American Indians as coming from the heart of the Earth and the passion of creation. Mined from surface pits in western states, it is used primarily for road building and garden adornment in the Southwest. This mulch is tough on hands and plant stems and it traps falling leaves and plant debris, but if you clean the surface carefully, it will maintain a carpet of permanent, interesting textures.

Despite its name, *white marble rock mulch* is not actually marble or even stone, but gypsum (calcium sulfate), a chalky mineral mined from surface pits. This mulch is excellent to delineate footpaths and walkways in the garden and to spread between large flagstones and fieldstones. It is most attractive in deeply shaded areas and on bright moonlit nights year-round. Ideally, white rock mulch should be put down over a sheet of landscape fabric, yet it

Japanese gardeners have a highly developed vocabulary for the rocks and types of stones used in various gardens. Similarly, American Indian traditionalists perceive rocks and stones as each having a spirit that can tell us certain things.

eventually may look dingy as it acquires mineral salts from its surroundings. It also traps falling leaves and other plant materials and should be cleaned by hand each season or, in some locations, top-dressed with additional thin layers of white rock once a year.

While collecting beach stones is widely discouraged, *sea coral* and *seashells* for mulch, salty gifts from the sea along storm coasts, can be collected freely in most areas. These mulches look beautiful in coastal gardens, especially on bright moonlit nights when they catch the moon's glow and reflect it back. They also provide a somewhat musical crunching noise beneath the feet. Chipped shells from shellfish farms or your last great oyster and clam bash can be artfully used in narrow beds around the house and on footpaths, providing wonderful walkways through the garden. These arrangements recall historical uses in Nantucket, Martha's Vineyard, Cape Cod, and coastal Maine. Wash and rinse these mulches thoroughly before putting them down. Gardeners want the lime they contain but not their salty qualities, unless used for pathways.

Beach glass mulch is a colorful, renewable resource for small paths and decorative garden areas. This mulch is best applied over a cover of landscape fabric for cleaner, long-lasting permanence. The small, smooth pieces of glass also look beautiful spread around potted plants. In states where glass bottles are not recycled, you can toss bottles into a small cement mixer with several shovelfuls of sand and small stones and tumble them for a few hours to make your own multicolored "beach glass"—the ultimate in recycling.

When making your choice of mulches, there is no need to restrict yourself to only one type. Our big, public medicine wheel garden at the Institute of American Indian Studies sits on a steep woodland slope. During the fall and winter, we top-dress the garden with leaf mulch and compost, digging it in around the big perennial plants. Each spring we apply fresh red cedar mulch to the four main quarters of the garden. This colorful mulch is easily put down and spread around colonies of perennial herbs. We spread it about one inch thick so that new plants can emerge without being smothered.

The four main pathways into the center of the garden are top-dressed with white rock mulch, which is also renewed each spring. This combination of mulches produces a vivid white cross surrounded by deep red and rimmed with large white quartz and marble boulders.

Oriented to the four cardinal directions, the early spring garden looks like a sacred jewel on the landscape. Later on, the profusion of blossoms and leaves almost masks the garden's artistic layout, and by late summer, the medicine wheel garden looks like an herbal classroom filled with healthy plants and winged pollinators. The garden remains a cathedral for hummingbirds, butterflies, and butterfly moths until the first frost, when, as we cut back the mature growth and dress the garden for the winter, the medicine wheel pattern emerges again.

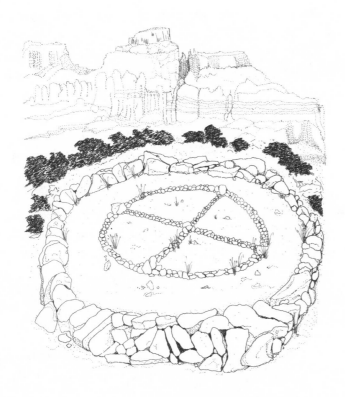

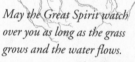

CHAPTER SEVEN

Personal Altars

Creating a Medicine Wheel Indoors

May the Great Spirit watch over you as long as the grass grows and the water flows.

—Cherokee song

WITH ITS HEALING PLANTS, sacred directions, and prayer cairns, the medicine wheel garden is truly an altar, laid out on the earth. Everything you add to it for its beauty and renewal enhances its efficacy. Similarly, the creation of a miniature medicine wheel indoors can provide a special focus for remembrance, renewal, and prayer. When you create this little personal altar, you will be in tune with long-standing American Indian spiritual practices. Native people create altars, large or small, prominent or discreet, temporary or permanent, for countless needs, and they have done so for many centuries. Traditional American Indian altars are usually created on the earth and open to nature.

But indoor medicine wheels can be especially rewarding for use in winter, during stormy weather, or as a gift for friends and family members, especially people who are elderly or shut in.

SELECTING SPECIAL STONES

As with the outdoor medicine wheel garden, the circle of special stones carefully placed on a favorite plate or round tray sets

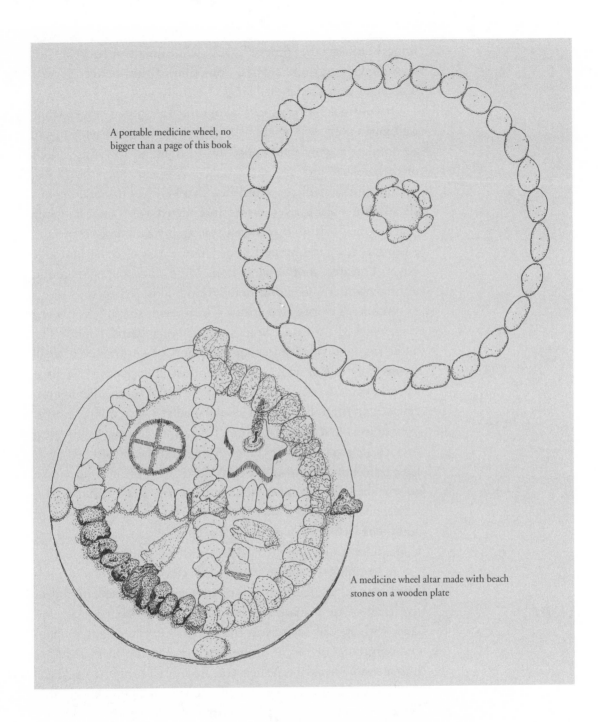

A portable medicine wheel, no bigger than a page of this book

A medicine wheel altar made with beach stones on a wooden plate

the basic form for your miniature medicine wheel altar. Hiking along backcountry roads or beachcombing, I pick up stones along the way that look special to me. Some days I'll light on dark, smooth stones; other times I'll select white quartz or feldspar with jagged edges and odd shapes. Sometimes I find perfect garnets with eight smooth, beveled sides.

If you make a habit of looking out for special stones while walking in your own neighborhood and when you travel, you will accumulate a wonderful collection to draw on for your indoor medicine wheel altars.

One small medicine wheel altar that I created has an outer circle of shiny black river stones intermixed with smooth white beach stones. Within this circle I placed tiny Zuni fetishes around a central "sun face" stone resting upon a bed of cedar and sage leaves. I created another altar from white coral fragments found during a winter walk along a Hollywood, Florida, beach.

Another favorite altar is one I made with small, select beach stones picked up from shores around Long Island Sound. The outer ring is divided into four quadrants of ten or eleven small stones each: one of white quartz, another of black or gray quartz, a third of gold feldspar nuggets, and the last of speckled conglomerates. For the inner cross I chose smaller white quartz stones. Very unusual red and pink stones I encountered on a visit to New Mexico are stacked in the center. A small candle, my quilled medicine wheel ornament, my special spirit stone spear point, and a cowrie shell fill the inner quadrants of this altar. I change this arrangement often and vary it according to what my meditations and focus seem to dictate. I made a small leather bag to hold my altar stones, and I take them with me when I travel.

A stunning medicine wheel altar can be created with polished gemstones. Perhaps your outer circle will accommodate five each of rose quartz, clear quartz, leopard-skin jaspar, and jade, with special crystals in the center. Or you might want to choose groups of special stone beads and string them together into a simple necklace. When you are not wearing the necklace, you can lay it out as the rim of a small medicine wheel altar. Whatever your choices, it is important to change this small altar often. Wash all of the stones and clean the other elements that you add to your altar. Each time you do this you add more of your own personal energy to this creation.

COMPLETING THE ALTAR

Inside the altar's stone circle, an arrangement of fresh or dried herbal blossoms, leaves, seeds, or roots can embody some of the vital healing plants that grow in the outdoor medicine wheel garden. Pinches of sage, tobacco, sweetgrass, and bearberry or cornmeal, representing the sacred plants, can be set in tiny bowls in the four quadrants. Or you may evoke the four elements: Four more tiny bowls, one in each quadrant, can hold water, a candle symbolizing fire, a pinch of earth, and a small feather to symbolize the wind.

Placing sacred foods on the medicine wheel altar can help you or someone close to you when experiencing digestive problems. Separate tiny bowls can hold bits of the "three sisters": cornmeal, dried beans, and dried or fresh squash or pumpkin. Or you might choose tiny bits of your own choice foods. You will want to offer a daily prayer to invoke the spirit of the foods with the spirit of healing.

Small *milagros* can further bless your altar arrangement. *Milagros,* "little miracles," are tiny symbolic offerings that express gratitude for an important need in your life fulfilled or hope for fulfillment of such a need. A *milagro* may be made of silver, gold, tin, brass, or other alloy and can take the form of anything from a roadrunner or a car to an arm, leg, breasts, or a kneeling angel. If you have visited churches in the Southwest, you have probably seen entire walls covered with these offerings of faith and thanksgiving.

A candle in the center of your medicine wheel altar or several candles within the arrangement of other offerings will help focus prayers and healing energies. Small candles in suitable colors can mark the cardinal directions: yellow or gold for east, blue or purple for south, red or magenta for west, and white or silver for north. Fragrant candles are an especially nice touch, especially for meditation. I always set a clear glass or bowl of water nearby to catch the reflections of the candle flames. If you live in a place where white birches grow, you may want to add small strips of fallen birchbark collected in the woods to hold the names and

One dear friend of mine was given a tiny *milagro* of a pair of human breasts inside a small medicine bag filled with prayers and sacred herbs before she faced breast cancer surgery. She credited this charming amulet, along with the many prayers she was given, with smoothing her passage through a scary period of her life.

prayers of loved ones. You can also use slips of paper wrapped in sweetgrass for this purpose. But make absolutely certain not to place these materials close to burning candles—they are highly flammable.

A MINIATURE MEDICINE WHEEL GARDEN

In an eagle there is all the wisdom of the world.
—John Fire Lame Deer, Minnicoujou Sioux medicine man

You can create a miniature medicine wheel garden with living plants indoors, perhaps in a round basket or clay dish or shallow bowl. I do this seasonally for the pleasure of having the small, fresh plants nearby—I especially enjoy the fragrance of plants, earth, and stones when I mist the garden. This kind of miniature garden also makes a lovely gift.

Recently I assembled a miniature Mother Goose garden in a shallow, round bamboo basket lined with a clear plastic tray. I selected young parsley, sage, and thyme plants, set in small plastic pots, for the outer rim of the tray and placed a nice young rosemary plant in the center. I used clumps of Spanish moss to cover all the little pots. Quartz cobbles and crystals, carefully placed, added a particularly festive feeling. I tied a quilled Plains Indian medicine wheel ornament to the basket's handle, fastening it in place with a tiny bundle of sage and sweetgrass. A shiny red ribbon set off everything proudly.

This tiny garden is the center of my spring altar for the May full moon to honor the regeneration of my full-scale medicine wheel garden outside. To pay my respects to the four cardinal directions, I placed a small, hand-carved Zuni fetish of deer (for the east), wolf (for the south), eagle (for the west), and bear (for the north) on the quartz cobbles. These are the "power animals," along with crow, that guard my work, especially my gardens.

Just as our country chose the eagle over the turkey as its national symbol, and each state has an animal and bird symbol, many people are drawn to one or more animals that for them symbolize strength and confidence.

Before first frost in autumn, I create a similar indoor altar centerpiece using selected cuttings of a few choice plants that I have rooted from my outdoor medicine wheel garden. I plant the cuttings in fine soil in a large, shallow clay dish more than a foot in diameter and about three inches deep. (The kind of plastic tray with low sides that is set under a large garden pot will also serve this purpose.) I like to have young cuttings of sage, sweetgrass, bearberry, and strawberry, and a few little tobacco seedlings. Like my large medicine wheel, this miniature garden features its tiny peace pole in the center surrounded by pretty little pebbles piled in a cairn. The four cardinal directions are marked with trimmed stems of goldenrod or yarrow and adorned with thin ribbons of appropriate colors. Small beach stones mark the crisscross pathway and larger beach stones surround the rim of the clay dish. I treat these plants in bonsai fashion, clipping them judiciously to keep them small and misting to prevent them from getting leggy.

Black crow or raven platform pipe, Hopewell culture, Mound City, Ohio

THE POWER OF FETISHES

My living garden altars often feature my tiny Zuni fetishes, each on a small piece of white quartz. A fetish is a small object whose form resembles a living being. It may be made of bone, ivory, stone, or shell. Many are carved of semi-precious stones. Sometimes they are adorned with tiny arrowheads, or pearl or stone amulets. When honored and treated with respect, the fetish becomes a helpful amulet for the person who possesses it.

Native American clans and bands have always felt a close kinship with the birds and animals around them and have long had sacred animal totems and affiliations. Fetishes are one way of representing these affiliations. In some tribes, members of the Badger Clan were the fiercest fighters, while the Deer Clan had the swift runners and good providers. The Panther Clan wore the mark of supernatural powers, swift hunting abilities, and special medicine powers. The Kit Fox Society of Plains Indian warriors were noted

Since you were good to me, I have taught you, the women of the Wolf Clan, all the cures of the forest. And from this day forward, you, the women of the Wolf Clan, will be the doctors of the communities and the reservations.

—Freeman Owle, Eastern Band Cherokee storyteller, recounting part of an old Cherokee medicine story

hunters and skilled diplomats. In many tribes, members of the Bear Society were the medicine people. Of course, this varies from tribe to tribe.

Shamans in particular had, and have, power animals that serve as their special guardians and spirit helpers in the otherworld. Animal and bird symbols are often painted on their drums, rattles, whistles, and ceremonial clothing. Native people felt an equally close kinship with the cosmos—the sun, moon, stars, comets, and plants—and it was the strength of the power animals that allowed one to journey to the outer cosmos.

Some sacred Native American sites honored the vital animals so respected in their beliefs. Effigy mounds especially have immortalized the eagle, bear, snake, and lizard for all time. We look at these sites today as ancient reminders of an earlier reverence for the myriad powers in nature. They are truly amazing earth altars imbued with ritual ceremonial energies.

Eagle medicine, like bear medicine, is especially powerful, and the eagle or the bear is often a central figure in medicine ceremonies. Skilled healers who know the sacred formulas have handed them down, over many generations, among different tribes. Wearing or carrying the fetish or claws of either of these two animals was a sign of great power. Traditionally, the right to wear eagle feathers or bear claws was earned by acts of valor and sacrifice. It was understood that one could not lie or commit misdeeds in the presence of a bear claw or an eagle feather.

Both the eagle and the bear are considered sacred beings. Eagle feathers represent courage and honesty, bear claws strength and courage. And both are symbols of good fortune. Many tribes believe that the bear and the eagle also bring healing and wisdom, and each can mean a great deal more to those for whom they are totems and guides.

Perhaps you have a special animal, domestic or wild, prehistoric or contemporary, that comes to you in your dreams and visions. You may even carry a fetish of your totem animal(s), or wear it in your medicine bag for clarity and protection. If so, you may wish to find a way to incorporate a representation of this animal on your medicine wheel altar.

The power of a fetish is the spirit it contains, not the fetish itself. The earliest fetishes were pieces of stone, coral, or bone with natural shapes suggesting animal forms. Such objects continue to be a favored type of fetish as well as a valuable omen. If you stoop to pick up a worn stone that somewhat resembles a bird, bear, or other creature, it is considered to be a good sign that you have this energy traveling with you in your journey through life.

Prayer Sticks and Prayer Ties

I am inspired by the Zuni ceremonial practice of making prayer sticks and prayer ties for sacred events and at times of special needs. For example, the Zuni have a specific prayer for preparing prayer sticks for the winter solstice. These objects are usually placed in a special spot on the land or in the house or given to a person who needs particular help.

Let a person decide upon their favorite animal and make a study of it, learning its innocent ways. Learn to understand its sounds and motions. The animals want to communicate with us.

    —Brave Bull, Lakota medicine man

Winter Solstice

This many are the days since our Moon Mother.
This many days we have waited.
Appeared, still small:
When but a short span remained till she was fully grown,
Then our daylight father, Pekwin of the Dogwood Clan,
For his Sun Father, told off the days.
This many days we have waited.
We have come to the appointed time.
My children, all my children, will make plume wands.
My child, my Father Sun, my Mother Moon,
All my children will clothe you with prayer plumes.
When you have attended yourselves in these,
With your waters, your seeds,
You will bless all my children.
All your good fortune you will grant to them all.
To this end my Father, my Mother:
May I finish my road; may I grow old;
May you bless me with long life.

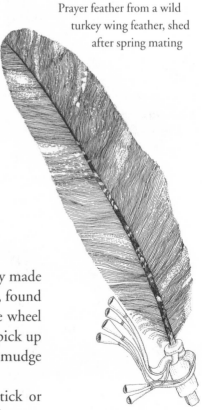

Prayer feather from a wild turkey wing feather, shed after spring mating

Miniature prayer sticks or prayer feathers can be readily made to fit the scale of your medicine wheel altar, using feathers, found materials, and small harvests from your outdoor medicine wheel garden. On my countryside and beach walks I will often pick up feathers from various birds to wash and clean, carefully smudge with sage, and save for special offerings.

To make a prayer stick or prayer feather, select a stick or feather that appeals to you. Make a tiny smudge stick of fragrant herbs from your garden: perhaps a sprig each of sage, pennyroyal, sweetgrass, and wood sage that you tie up with a red string or bit of red wool yarn. Any color will do, but red has particular value as a sacred color. Tie the little herbal smudge stick to the stick or feather. You might even add a small bead or *milagro* for extra emphasis. There are more directions in Chapter 14.

OTHER TYPES OF ALTARS

Among American Indians, each major or minor event and special gathering invites the creation of an altar. Such altars vary greatly from tribe to tribe. The Oklahoma Pawnee place a long, narrow table against the wall and dress it with a fine, bright cloth. On top they arrange their finest crafts and traditional foods. Two or three cloth dolls, adorned with colorful beadwork necklaces and bracelets, stand as sentinels. Four beautiful blue bowls are filled with sacred foods for the four cardinal directions: cornmeal, whole dried corn kernels, sage leaves, and dried beans. Branches of juniper bring the promise of evergreen life, and whole ears of corn placed on the altar reassure the people that abundance will continue along with their prayers and blessings.

Pueblo Feast Day altars honor their sacred foods, sacred plants, selected kachinas, and prayer sticks. Ornate basket trays and traditional drums and rattles flank the central offerings. This arrangement and presentation will vary from one home to another, and changes seasonally. Such altars assure the spirits that the people still remember the sacred traditions.

Sweetgrass and cornmeal altars of the eastern Algonquian and Iroquois people might also feature coastal seashells and wampum beads, or bone and wood carvings and prayer feathers. Fine curly baskets woven in the shape of an ear of corn or a bowl serve as emblems of outstanding craftsmanship, especially the tightly woven strawberry and blueberry baskets trimmed with sweetgrass for which these eastern tribes are famous.

Altars should be changed and refreshed often. Each gathering

Sometimes I sit down and make a whole bunch of prayer sticks and prayer feathers with the materials I have been assembling and delicate clippings from my medicine wheel garden. They make wonderful little gifts for a circle of spiritual friends—my drumming circle, for example.

or celebration necessitates different displays of ingredients and seasonal produce, fresh flowers, and prayer feathers.

Our regular drumming circle, which meets monthly at the Institute for American Indian Studies, always makes a central altar that everyone contributes to, and we drum around it each month when we meet. Surrounding this altar's central lighted candle and smudge shell we place various rattles, drums, Tibetan singing bowls, and bells. A sweetgrass braid, some sage, and white cedar also adorn the altar, along with a photograph of the drum group. Sometimes we create a prayer basket in which we place the names of loved ones and friends who need extra prayers for healing and help, understanding and guidance as they endure difficult times. Remarkable things can occur when good people work in concert around the altar that they have created.

My friend Irene awoke from a dream and immediately went outside and built a small sacred altar near her garden. She saw the altar precisely in her dream. Its natural earth elements are drawn from the surrounding environment. It now rests at the base of a hickory tree. A medley of carefully selected stones is placed in this special clearing. Everything in and around this sacred space seems energized!

Vision is something that is hoped for but not yet seen. The vision is what leads you on, what directs you and points the way. In the old times, each young man was encouraged to seek a vision, and native women were also free to do this. In seeking the vision, one would go out and pray. "What shall be my purpose in life, Great Spirit? How can I best serve the needs of my people? What is my part in the universe?" With the vision comes the power of direction.
—Sun Bear, medicine man of Chippewa descent, founder of the Bear Tribe

Sunpath in the Stars
Time takes me on its wing and I travel to the sun and am consumed by fire.
Time takes me on its wing and I travel to the river and am drowned in water.
Time takes me on its wing and I travel into the earth and am a mountain not yet risen.
Each place I go others have gone before me.
That is why the sun dances, the wind weeps, the river leaps and the earth sings.
Neither the sun nor the wind, the river nor the earth did these things
Before man was placed in this world to believe it.
                                        —Taos Pueblo saying

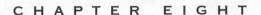

CHAPTER EIGHT

Celebrating Your Medicine Wheel Garden

Seasonal Healing Rituals

When the old rituals were restored to us and I was able to participate in the Sun Dance, it was not easy for me. I remember that the need to cry filled my heart the first time I danced in the Sun Dance circle. Those first real tears ran down my face and spilled into my soul. Out there in that great circle, I realized how truly humble I was in all the universe.

—Delphine Red Shirt, Lakota author, *Bead on an Anthill*, 1998

WORKING IN THE MEDICINE wheel garden, you will feel in balance with the rhythms of the earth and the cycles of the seasons. Handling the individual plants, their roots, the earth, and the rocks brings you closer to an earth-based wisdom and deepens your intuitive connections with nature. For some individuals, the medicine wheel garden becomes a mirror of life and soul. Within its sacred stone circle, you may discover insights into the powerful path to self-discovery. In some ways, this special garden is like a giant sun face that radiates healing—a road map for spiritual change.

My time in my own medicine wheel garden is always enlightening. I work hard cleaning and weeding my garden's quadrants; I sit and reflect on all the vigorous beauty here; I build more Stone People that stand as guardians within and around this sacred circle. Every plant and stone has a spirit of its own. I can stand here in the deep snow of frozen winter and feel a peaceful kinship to my dormant plants. At any season I often come here at dawn to do my yoga and sing the sun up. I chant this song softly:

O Spirit of the Dawn, bring us your light.
O Spirit of the Sun, give us your warmth.
O Spirit of the Day, guide us with love.
O Spirit of the Night, nurture our dreams.

Whatever the time of day, walking or working in the medicine wheel garden helps me get out of my head and into the more intuitive and caring mode of my heart. As I let go of my own needs and broaden my focus, I can see and feel the larger picture of nature and realms beyond what I see before me. I can connect with the plant and mushroom spirits and other nature spirits in my vicinity. They tell me remarkable things and can help me see into the future. You will be able to accomplish this too if you really want to.

American Indian herbalists make offerings to and pray to the plant spirits before they harvest a plant to use for healing. This way the medicine has a far greater synergistic effect when used. Indeed, some say that the failure to make this offering renders some plant medicines far less useful. A gift of song, or prayers, with a pinch of cornmeal or tobacco in exchange for the medicine plant's healing power is part of our compact, our continuing dance of reciprocity with the plants we depend on in so many ways.

When you chant properly, you take in the energy of the earth through your body, magnify it, and send it out to all of your relations on the planet. This means that you should feel the chant throughout your body, not just in your throat. It should cause a vibration that touches all your energy centers. It does not matter if you do not think you can sing. Chanting is a way of centering and sending energy, not a way of proving your vocal ability.

—Sun Bear, medicine man of Chippewa descent, founder of the Bear Tribe

WALKING THE WHEEL

Walking the wheel is a way of honoring the medicine wheel as a universal symbol of balance and reflection. As you walk around and into your medicine wheel garden, you direct your thoughts inward, to your heart and spirit, and outward, to Mother Earth and the healing plants that surround you. This flow of thought can take the form of a personal meditation. It is important, too, to become more sensitive to the space that surrounds your medicine wheel, which can serve as an immense earth altar, infusing everything in the area with new respect. While working within this garden space, or walking around it, you are walking with the Creator to your own center and to a new centered peace within yourself. Many people see the medicine walk and work as similar to walking the labyrinth's circuitous paths with God. The Sacred Circles Institute in Washington State gives special instruction in "walking the sacred wheel" as a year's journey of initiation in sacred practices, incorporating American Indian tribal wisdom and earth-based wisdom into teachings from around the world.

For me, walking the wheel is an aspect of personal growth and deepening. I receive remarkable gifts of awareness, special insights that enrich my gardening as well as my life in many ways. Approaching my medicine wheel garden, I take a stone—rubbed with good energy and my prayers of gratitude for this day—and place it on the eastern prayer cairn. Then I step into the garden at the "eastern door," the opening at the eastern cardinal direction pole. I begin with a simple smudging of dried cedar, bearberry, or sage leaves, or a combination of all three. I smudge myself from head to toe, especially my hands and arms; then I turn and offer a smudge blessing to each of the seven directions.

As I smudge, I quietly say or silently think:

Great Mystery, behold our beautiful work and make it good.
Spirits of the East, illuminate our work in every way.
Spirits of the South, warm our vigorous growth.
Spirits of the West, strengthen our garden's health.
Spirits of the North, ripen our labors with fruitfulness.
Spirits of the Sky World, wash us with vital sun and rain.
Spirits of the earth, ground our work in fulfillment.
Spirits of the sacred center, embrace us with protection.
Great Mystery, our gratitude and love for all you share.

Carrying the smoking herbs in a smudge dish, or a large abalone shell, I walk around the garden three times just inside the perimeter, using a feather fan to direct the smoke around and into the garden. The smudge secures the garden from any negativity and also serves as a fine insecticide. I pause to watch the wind horses fluttering or flapping on the peace pole and the cardinal direction poles; each tells me more about the day.

Listening intently, I heighten my sense of awareness by paying particularly close attention to sounds and sights in nature all around me. I try to be sensitive to which birds are nesting nearby and foraging here for food. I need the songbirds to eat the harmful plant pests in the medicine wheel garden, so I often maintain a small birdbath within the medicine wheel near the water-loving plants. The catbirds that nest in the hazelnut shrub nearby seek continual relief in the birdbath! I enjoy watching and listening to them.

I check for other signs. Deer and rabbit droppings alert me to the overnight and early-morning presence of these abundant animals. They like to graze on herbal foliage and eat the echinacea, and I am prepared to share with them, as they live here, too. They generally prefer tender hybrid plants and do not ravage the native wildflowers as much. Yet I must protect the moccasin flowers from these predators, so each evening I set a large basket over these plants, weighting it on top with a sizable rock. The deer also eat Indian turnip, so I set out various repellents, especially Milorganite, which is also an organic fertilizer.

I check for garden spiders and their webs in the garden, as these allies of the Little People provide healing in their bodies and spin this into their webs. When placed on the skin, spiderwebs can calm skin irritations and stop bleeding. A spiderweb rolled into a tiny "pill" and swallowed can relieve a headache or fever. But I'm aware that if annoyed, spiders can also deliver a nasty bite or sting. I invoke Grandmother Spider's powerful spiritual protection as one of the native creation figures. I ask her to be well and at home in this garden.

The Connecticut Mohegan believe, as do many tribes, that the east-to-west passage of spirits, following the movement of the sun, is the Trail of Life. They symbolize this concept in their beadwork and basketry designs. So I walk from east to west, envisioning my own trail of life and pause to place another prayer stone on the central

Before I visit my medicine wheel garden to work or plant, I place about a half cup each of cornmeal and tobacco in separate small bags. I pray over each of these, offering my gratitude and asking that they be energized to honor everything for which they are used. Sometimes I offer a pinch of cornmeal, and at other times I feel that a pinch of tobacco is more appropriate. To energize the cornmeal and make it sacred, I softly sing or speak this prayer:

O spirit of sun reborn in spirit of corn, guide and protect us.

O spirit of rain reborn in spirit of corn, cleanse and inform us.

O spirit of earth reborn in spirit of corn, nurture and feed us.

I use the same prayer for the tobacco blessing, substituting the word *tobacco* for *corn*. This blessing can be modified for each plant set out in the medicine wheel garden.

My prayer for peace often changes to address the areas of greatest need, but it always begins: "Peace, blessed peace, is honored here and spreads with love and understanding throughout our world. Peace embraces the Americas and each continent, every people through every season. Peace and love are the great equalizers balancing the needs of all global life. May it always be so. Peace and understanding. Peace, blessed peace."

cairn around the peace pole. I sing and talk to the plants and the healing spirits as I walk.

Choosing another small stone from the garden soil, I rub it with my prayers for the day and place it on the cairn surrounding the western cardinal direction pole. I look to the western sky and offer a prayer of gratitude and renewal. Then I retrace my steps along the central crosswalk back to the peace pole and walk first to the south and then back to the north cardinal direction poles and cairns, again placing prayer stones and prayers at each. If I am going through a particularly difficult personal time, I may offer additional cornmeal blessings at the peace pole, asking for clarity and guidance.

As I walk the wheel, I offer a blessing to the larger sacred Stone People I have created in my garden. Each time I offer them prayers, I feel a more personal connection with Mother Earth, Father Sky, Sister Day, Brother Night, Grandmother Moon, and Grandfather Sun. Finally, I return to the central peace pole with a daily prayer for world peace.

I try to repeat my daily medicine wheel garden walk, rain or shine. In really bad weather I chant my prayers over my little indoor medicine wheel altar. I also do a special silent meditation, sitting and imagining the medicine wheel garden as I perform the rituals. This is usually done within the medicine wheel garden and is enormously helpful during stressful times. My rituals are not rigid, however. I am continually adapting them to my changing needs, and I work to mirror them when I travel to far-flung locations.

DRUMMING AND PRAYER TIES

The drum is the Great Spirit's favorite instrument. That's why we were all given a heartbeat.

—Mano, Navajo elder

The medicine wheel is the ultimate space in which to drum for world peace at full moons and new moons, as other people do around the world. This is a good way to honor the medicine wheel garden and bless any space wherein you drum. The rhythmic drumming of the heartbeat is what usually sets the pace of synchronous drumming in many groups.

Talk with a circle of your friends or work colleagues about starting a drumming circle. When you find interest in this idea, discuss where, when, and how often you might conveniently meet to drum. Consider where the best, most central gathering place might be. When you gather together five or more people to drum, the noise and vibrations can be considerable and wonderful. Keep this point in mind and alert the neighbors to what you are planning so that they don't become alarmed.

Several years ago, I formed a drumming circle to meet at the Institute of American Indian Studies after visiting hours. Most of the people had come to make a drum in my workshops there or had bought nice drums and simply wanted the opportunity to use them. Basically, we all wanted a comfortable, nonthreatening environment in which to drum together and learn more about this age-old art. We have been meeting regularly, once a month at seven o'clock in the evening, for more than four years. New people are always welcome to join us. Every kind of drum is welcome, although we have a majority of single-faced hand drums. We make a nominal donation to the institute for the two hours that we drum together, and someone offers to bring "circle food" each month.

We have learned that our drumming circle is a fine indoor/outdoor way to honor the medicine wheel garden and receive its benefits. If drumming indoors, we create an altar in the center of the room around a candle. Chairs are set in a large circle; some people prefer to sit on the floor. Many people bring extra rattles and drums to place around the altar. We smudge the room, each other, and our drums with sacred sage and cedar. We take time to center ourselves, breathing deeply, releasing all tensions, and feeling very grounded and happy in this special space. More than thirty people come to the drumming circle each month, creating sounds that seem to raise the roof right off the building! Our group drumming is very tribal.

As we begin slow, rhythmic drumming to the pulse, or heartbeat, we can all feel the energies building within the room. We drum together for a solid hour, speeding up to rapid drumbeats and slowing to slightly more mellow beats and occasional synco-

When beginning spiritual circle activities, we invoke this blessing:

The doors and gates and paths
of the kind and guiding
spirits are open to us.
And the doors and gates and
paths of anyone who
means to harm us or
Any of our loved ones are
forever closed.

pated beats. Many folks exchange their drums for rattles at the altar during the hour and try different drums. It is a rich time of open explorations of sounds and creativities. We often get up and continue drumming as we move around the room or walk outside to the medicine wheel garden.

When weather permits, we enjoy doing all our drumming outside. Drumming within and around the medicine wheel garden is an incredibly special experience, and the plants seem to love it, too. Plants thrive when they are "drummed" and seem to grow stronger than their counterparts outside the medicine wheel. For the people taking part, these walking, drumming meditations are quite insightful. Some experience unique visions and hear voices.

The drumming circle has developed a strong bond among all participants. Once a year we renew our drums with tiny prayer ties. To make a prayer tie, each person gives a prayer of silent gratitude, takes a small pinch of tobacco and other herbs, places this within a small circle of red cloth, and ties it snugly with red thread, all the while thinking of the prayer in silent meditation. Finally, the tiny prayer tie is securely attached inside the back opening of each person's drum. (See Chapter 14, where ceremonial items are discussed in greater depth.) Sometimes we make many prayer ties together and fasten them on one long cord. The Native American Spirituality Circle, which also meets at the institute, creates prayer ties at the beginning and end of each year, renewing our commitment to the land. These prayer ties are carried outside and placed in the branches of the white pine and hemlock trees around the buildings.

When hiking in some of the holy places out west, such as Bear Butte in the Black Hills or the Big Horn Mountains Medicine Wheel area, you will often see various prayer ties fastened onto the vegetation or fences along the pathways. These mark the places where people have paused to give thanks and prayer offerings. Prayer ties are considered sacred and should not be touched or removed.

The time is almost here. The season of the deep blue sea . . . Bringing good things from the deep blue sea. Whale of distant ocean . . . May there be a whale. May it indeed come. . . . Within the waves.
—Lincoln Blassi, St. Lawrence Island Yupik from Gambell, Alaska; fragment from "Prayer Song Asking for a Whale"

Seasonal Earth-Based Rituals

The medicine wheel garden inspires activities, ceremonies, and healing rituals for every season of the year. Seasonal events from a new moon in the sky to a new crop ready to harvest from the earth provide wonderful and varied opportunities to develop your own personal medicine wheel rites.

The solstices and equinoxes were and are especially important times for celebration. These four events in our calendar year have their roots in sacred ceremonies of many cultures.

My natural associations for these major turning points are based upon years of observation. I honor the wild turkeys congregating and mating through the spring equinox. The first young bluebirds are usually fledging by the summer solstice, along with many other songbird populations. I honor the wild mushrooms and fullness of wild and garden harvests during the autumnal equinox. Deer are rutting and wild geese are clustering and migrating during the winter solstice.

You might plan a special gathering at each solstice and equinox. Prepare long white prayer ribbons on which each person will write a prayer or brief thought. Then tie each ribbon into a suit-

A tree is our most intimate contact with nature.
—George Nakashima, author of *The Soul of a Tree*

Leading a Fire Ceremony

Major seasonal celebrations are splendid times for a fire ceremony. Make a small fire pit near your medicine wheel garden. Dig out the sod to about one foot deep and two feet across; line this little hole with small stones to create a safe fire pit. (In many areas you will need permission from a fire marshal to have an open fire.) With friends you have invited for an evening ritual of renewal, build and light a small fire in your fire pit.

Give each person a piece of paper and a pencil to write three key messages.

What three things do you most want to clear out of your life?
What three things do you most desire to have in your life?
What three things do you wish so that our group, our country, our world will have a better future?

Take ten minutes or so to accomplish this quietly. Some may want to do a sharing time to say what they have written. When everyone is ready, fold the papers and gather in a circle around the glowing fire. Begin drumming. One at a time, each person commits his or her paper to the fire while everyone else cheers. Follow around the circle in sequence until everyone has placed their paper in the fire and watched it burn up. Don't rush. This is a fine ceremony for a drumming group, as you can each drum as well as cheer for one another, heightening the supportive energies and providing a wonderful bonding experience for families and other groups.

able bush or tree where it will flutter in every breeze and whip wildly in strong winds. I have a tall prayer tree near my medicine wheel garden on which I tie a long, slim banner with new prayers for each quarter of the year. Over time I have dressed this young wild cherry tree with a number of fluttering banners, and I know that my prayers have flown around the world many times.

Each full moon and each new moon throughout the year also merits a small ritual celebration. Perhaps a potluck dinner and meditation for world peace with close friends would please you. Many of us take out our drums and drum for fifteen minutes on the morning or evening of new and full moons. One of my friends hosts a monthly full moon breakfast for a few close friends. These "power" breakfasts begin early and are a great way to start the day with chanting, drumming, and dancing.

Some families like to have meetings, "teachings," and celebrations in their medicine wheel garden once or twice a week. The "teaching" comes from a family member or friend who has something new to share with the group that may improve their outlook or life. This activity can rotate from one to another, each one choosing what they want to bring to the next medicine wheel meeting. The medicine wheel garden is also a fine place for storytelling. Storytelling is one of the oldest forms of teaching. These occasions are fine times to serve "circle food" to everyone at the end of the gathering. Any favorite food that is circular and can be eaten by the whole group fills the bill, from cake or cookies to carrots, oranges, apples, apricots, or crackers and a round of cheese.

Perhaps you wish to pattern a new personal ritual after a traditional tribal practice, with thoughtful respect. It is best not to copy but to create your own ritual based upon a specific tribal celebration. These seasonal rites and rituals, from winter festivities to harvests, were invariably keyed to giving thanks to the Creator and Mother Earth for abundance shared. Here are a few examples to inspire you.

■ *Zuni Deshqway rites* are observed over four days at both the winter and summer solstices. During the four days, no business of any kind can be transacted, and all outside fires are extinguished. This is a time of forgiveness, contemplation, prayer, fasting, and understanding. At the end of the fourth day, the Zuni priests go from house to house and relight new fires so that everything begins new again. The winter solstice generally calls for ten days of traditional observance. During these cold days, families bond more closely and look at their lives in deeper detail.

■ *Midwinter renewal,* celebrated among Iroquois and Cherokee people, was and is often their new year and a time for naming newborns and healing serious illnesses within the tribe. This is also the time when people (and debts) are forgiven and old grudges released. This is the time of dream sharing and dream guessing rites. This period embraced days of celebrations during which prayers and songs were performed for all the people. New hearth fires are kindled after a time of darkness and prayer. Everyone feasts, after a period of fasting, and gives thanks.

■ *The Great Lakes Algonquian celebration of Grandmother Maple* coincided with the late winter "sugaring-off" festivities and storytelling. Late January, February, and March is the time to tap the maple trees for their rich, delicious sap and render it into syrup and then sugar. This is an especially exciting period, as the maple sugaring cycle signals the end of winter. For many communities and families, it still means steady hard work to obtain and prepare the year's maple syrup crop before the maple trees put out their buds, ending the time for sapping. Various songs, chants, and games make the work time pass more interestingly.

■ *Native rites of spring* often embraced the days just before and after the vernal equinox in March. In some regions, ceremonies of blessing the seeds with prayers for abundant crops would be hosted over a four- or five-day period. These rites varied among the Pueblo tribes in the desert Southwest, where kachina dances and lengthy ceremonies petitioned Mother Earth and Father Sky to provide for a new, successful growing season followed by a plentiful harvest. Everyone in the farming and gardening communities knows the importance of celebrating this vital spring renewal and asking for the seasons ahead to be bountiful and kind. These rituals have evolved from ancient practices that also influence favorable hunting, human fertility, and family health.

■ *Iroquois strawberry festivals* celebrate the first ripe fruits in the wild. This event has long been, and continues to be, a great reason for spring festivals. Many different groups now host strawberry festivals in honor of these ancient Native American rites. The strawberry is a symbol of renewal and healing medicine, and it is also central to many tribal creation stories. The Delaware tell about how the first wild strawberries sprang from the mastodon's tears as these impressive animals marched toward extinction. The Iroquois tell of an argument between a loving couple long ago who split up but were prevented from hurrying away from each other because fresh, ripe strawberries covered the meadow. Hungry and sad, they stooped to pick the strawberries, and soon they realized their love could overcome their differences.

■ *Pueblo corn-planting rituals and earth renewal rites* each spring still vary from one pueblo to another. Among the nineteen pueblos in New Mexico and the Hopi in Arizona, this is a time of great celebration. At most pueblos, people proudly perform the Corn Dance, and many special corn foods are prepared to feed each family. The Zuni and the Hopi, through their kachina rites, petition the mountain spirits and the earth forces to bring forth a good growing season. They perform a traditional sequence of rituals to bless the first seeds and planting rites. Dances, chants, prayers, and beautiful objects reassure all life forces that the people's hearts are good and their families' needs are great. Imagine how our gardens would fare if we honored them this way.

■ *Navajo herb-gathering rites and songs* mark celebrations throughout the growing seasons. Special attention is given to gathering medicine plants in a sacred manner so that their spirits will work the maximum benefits of healing. Early in the growing season, the herb gatherers begin to pick young leaves of diverse herbs to make healing formulas. Healing roots are gathered in

Spring is the time to perform the age-old renewal ceremonies of the people. Medicine bundles will be opened and renewed with the first thunderstorms of the season, and many other ceremonies will be performed to petition the Creator for a healthy and prosperous year for the tribe.

—Curtis Yarlott, Cheyenne, St. Labre Indian School executive director, Ashland, Montana

late fall, winter, and early spring. Individual herbalists have their own favorite herb, and some may know as many as two or three hundred different plants and mushrooms. There is always a gift to the plant's spirit before it is harvested: a pinch of pollen or tobacco, along with a silent prayer, a petition for the plant's sacred help.

■ *The Plains Indians consecration of thunder* reflects upon the awareness of changing seasons and the need for rain, and welcomes the first thunderstorms. Each tribe has its own special traditional rituals embraced by this valuable renewal ceremony. This is the time to open and renew many aspects of hearth and home, healing and creativity. As gardeners, we can prosper by celebrating the rain and welcoming the thunder that renews our gardens and ourselves with life-giving resources. Lightning fixes nitrogen, and nitrogen enhances plant and leaf growth. Welcome the lightning into the garden and watch the plants flourish and the Stone People dance!

■ *The Algonquian cranberry festival* celebrates the autumn harvests of our native cranberries, which have become a major economic crop, fueling both the commercial food and beverage industries and the herbal healing networks. In these traditions, the Little People needed to be acknowledged and thanked.

■ *Ojibwa herb-gathering rites and prayers* are offered by herbalists who gather the seasonal herbs, wild rice, and fungi. Very special prayers are given during the Indian summer gathering times of wild mushrooms and late roots. Every type of healing organism has its own special time of harvest. Members of the Grand Medicine Society, the Midewiwin or Mide, who could read the sacred birch bark scrolls and carved wooden prescription sticks, would lead the seasonal gathering rites. This is one of the oldest medicine societies in North America. Like the Pueblo kachina societies and Iroquois false-face societies, Navajo Chant Ways, and Apache Mountain Gods, these medicine people can perform amazing curing rituals. But one must commit a lifetime of devoted study and work to walk these pathways.

He explained that Little People lived in the woods and along the beaches and that in early times it was customary for groups going out to gather food plants, herbs for medicine, fishing, or hunting to put some cornbread and meat in a small basket and leave it for the Little People. He added, "That was for good luck," Also while he made baskets, Eben told me about some herbal remedies as well as legends.

—Gladys Tantaquidgeon, Mohegan medicine woman, recalling Eben Queppish, Mashpee Wampanoag basketmaker, herbalist, and storyteller

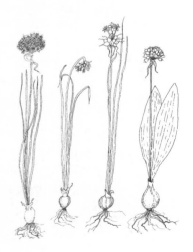

*The Medicine Wheel . . . as
the traditional map . . . to the
journey of the Four Winds,
would be our guide. The
sacred places of power that the
legends spoke of would be our
rest stops, our places of
communion.*

—Alberto Villoldo, 1990, author
of *Dancing the Four Winds*

Many of us are content to be herbalists, and this, too, is a life-time career. We each develop our own independent rituals, which help us know the plants deeply and communicate with their spirits. Often, sitting quietly by a plant or colony of chosen plants can clear your busy mind. As in a meditation, you can tune in to the plant's vibrations and hear its wisdom. This intuitive exchange can be quite profound. Those who believe in garden fairies and plant devas know the wealth of communication here. Your mind opens to a congress of voices and healing.

Grey Wolf is a Lakota medicine wheel teacher who learned his traditional teaching from his grandfather. He develops his own unique teachings and his spiritual philosophies are shared with a circle of special friends who seek to learn more about their life paths. Like many of his predecessors, his teachings wrap them-

Going Deeper with the Medicine Wheel

There are a number of approaches for "walking the wheel" that you may want to explore. The teachings of Hyemeyohsts Storm describe many of the traditional Cheyenne Indian medicine wheel concepts and give us a framework for incorporating these practices from the Plains Indian perspectives. The old Indian stories resonate with important visions and signs that tribal ancestors experienced. These were teaching tools that provided the framework for Plains Indian spiritual practices involving the medicine wheel. Legends tell of wheels within wheels in a multilayered constellation of healing energies. The medicine wheel is set according to the four main cardinal directions. At the end of each spoke there is another wheel, and this pattern is repeated on and on.

Sun Bear, the late Chippewa medicine man, created his own vision of a medicine wheel and incorporated a New Age approach to astrology within it. His books, gatherings, and practices have influenced many people to look more closely at self-reliance and achieving balance with oneself and Mother Earth.

American psychologist Alberto Villoldo takes participants deeper into the ancient realms of shamanic journeywork and explores the secrets of the Inca medicine wheel. The sacred places of power described in the old legends are seen as places created in the medicine wheel, where one can visit with them and be enlightened by them on an ongoing basis. Many ancient sites throughout South America come alive through medicine wheel and shamanic associations.

selves closely within the natural world, helping us to become more sensitive to all living things.

The British authority Kenneth Meadows has written extensively on the "hidden teachings" of the Native American medicine wheel. He has developed his own detailed interpretations as a way of understanding "earth medicine." Shamanic principles are applied within this work as a pathway toward self-discovery and wholeness.

There are also individual American Indians across the country teaching their own unique forms of medicine wheel concepts, from Cheyenne to Crow to Cherokee. Some take students and develop rich programs of medicine wheelwork. Each teacher has his or her own special vision about what the medicine wheel means. These teachings appeal to people who are seeking a deeper spiritual reality and feel drawn to Native American traditions. Invariably these practices lead each practitioner into a deeper relationship with nature and within themselves. (See Appendix 4 for more information.)

Nothing I have ever seen with my eyes was so clear and bright as what my vision showed me; and no words that I have ever heard with my ears were like the words I heard. I did not have to remember these things; they have remembered themselves all these years.

—Black Elk, Lakota Sioux holy man, speaking about his great vision

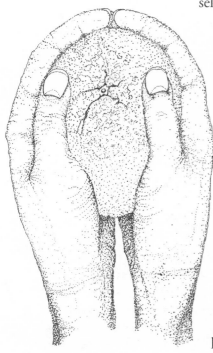

Orange ceremony

THE ORANGE CEREMONY

We gather in a small circle within or beside the medicine wheel garden or a large circle surrounding it, each person holding a single fresh orange. This simple ceremony is born from Native American and Zen Buddhist wisdom. It was given to me many years ago, and I have regularly enjoyed giving it away. Each time we perform this it becomes a gift to each one gathered in the circle. You can do this alone with a single orange, but the real dynamics come from sharing this in a circle. This can be done anytime, but its greatest symbolism is achieved when we assemble in a predawn circle, about fifteen minutes before the sunrise. As we perform this ceremony we "sing the sun up" in a circle of sharing. This is a meaning-filled salute to the sun, as well as a salute to the self.

We stand in a comfortable circle where we can see the sunrise. Each person warms an orange in his or her two hands, enjoying its fragrance. The orange symbolizes wholeness, the self, the universe, the sun and the sunrise, the family, and whatever else you need it to symbolize at this time. Holding the orange to your heart and then your nose, give it your prayers for cleansing and gratitude. This becomes a brief morning meditation. Together sing this morning chant in a singsong voice:

> *Dawn spirit, come dance in me,*
> *Day spirit, come warm me,*
> *Orange spirit, please feed me,*
> *Peel away my discomfort, and*
> *All nurture me home, and All nurture me home.*

With the emerging dawn, slowly begin to peel the orange. Inhale the fragrance; feel it nurture you. Each of you in this circle is

Walking Meditation

Direct your thoughts inward, clear your mind, breathe deeply, and extend your awareness to everything around you. Really notice all that is going on around you. As you walk slowly along, pick up two small stones; they will find you. Rub the first one with your prayers for something you presently want to have in your life. Rub the other one with your prayers for something you really want to eliminate. Walk along this way until you find the right place to release the two stones, and with them, give your prayers to the universe.

focused on completeness and honoring your wholeness. As you peel the orange you are consciously peeling away anything unwanted and releasing all disease and disorder from your healthy life. (Save the collected peels for composting.)

Cradle the whole naked orange in your hands and enjoy its fragrance. Now carefully open the orange into two equal halves. Section the first half into two quarters. Turn to the person on your right and offer the first quarter to her, and receive with gratitude her first quarter of orange in exchange. Slowly eat this first "taste of the morning" and savor its flavor and fragrance in a meditative manner. Now turn to the person on your left and offer the second quarter to him, and receive with gratitude his quarter of orange. Again, slowly eat this in a meditative manner.

Section your remaining half into two quarters. Step across the circle and offer your third quarter of orange to the person opposite you, while accepting with gratitude his or her third quarter of orange. Return to the circle and slowly eat this, noticing the slight differences in taste. Finally, slowly eat the last quarter of your own orange with gratitude. Feel the nurturing and sharing of various tastes, energies, and feelings within this circle. Hold these moments as long as seems comfortable in silence. Sometimes I take a pocketful of wet wipes along for everyone to clean their hands. Other times we just rub in the "orange perfume" and continue our morning meditation. It is important to ask for what has come up for individuals who want to share. Some folks simply want to be quiet and process all this, and others are deeply moved by their own personal issues. Following a brief period of sharing, we conclude with a twenty-minute "walking meditation" envisioned by my daughter Kimberlee from a beautiful dream she had in the Shawangunk Mountains.

SHAMANIC JOURNEYWORK

Perhaps one of the oldest and most unusual methods of medicine wheel visionary work is through shamanic use. Shamanic

There were those shamans who made magical flights, the very first people to fly through the air, before the white men began to fly. Llima.tuat, they called those who could fly.
—Frank Ellanna, Inupiat from King Island, Alaska

practitioners use the medicine wheel and prayer cairns as journey points to enter and leave the present world for the otherworld. This allows them to access sacred space in healing and other specialized work. Suppose that a shaman must journey, in a trance, to the underworld to meet with spirits to divine the cause of someone's illness. The shaman can visualize the medicine wheel garden as the journey point for departure and reentry. (A shamanic journey is like an out-of-body experience in that the shaman's spirit leaves, in a deep meditative trance, to find hidden information in nonordinary reality. This work is always used for peaceful, healing needs.)

Because shamanic journeywork does not require the shaman actually to leave a set place, s/he is free to pick any power spot. The medicine wheel is an amazing power spot for this work. As a shamanic practitioner, I use my own medicine wheel garden with great results. My journeys are much more powerful when I journey down through the medicine wheel garden than when I depart from any of my other favorite places. My end results are always amazingly rich and filled with more particular details. I can journey from one medicine wheel site to another in shamanic trance; I can visit sacred sites that I have never physically seen and would have difficulty getting to in ordinary reality.

Some authorities believe that the ancient medicine wheels were used in shamanic journeywork. This idea actually makes good sense. Many of the old medicine wheel locations are difficult to get to, and yet easy for the shaman to access and visit in trance. Shamans can travel in trance state, through nonordinary reality, around the world, and beyond this world and back. Shamans have been adept at doing this since earliest time. Shamanism is a part of every culture's past, present, and future. It is not a religion; rather, it is a pathway for discovery and healing.

You understand that there are certain things one should not talk about, things that must remain hidden. If all was told . . . there would be no mysteries left, and that would be very bad. Man cannot live without mystery. He has a great need of it.

—John Fire Lame Deer, *Lame Deer: Seeker of Visions,* 1972

Herbs for the Medicine Wheel Garden

If all the plants and beasts were gone, we would die from loneliness of spirit, for whatever happens to the plants and beasts happens to us. All things are connected. Whatever befalls the earth befalls the sons of the earth.

—Chief Seattle, Duwamish, 1854

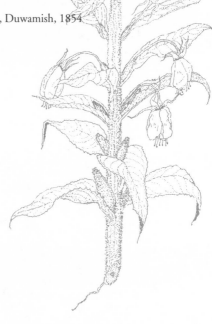

CHAPTER NINE

Healing Herbs from Angelica to Yucca

Fifty Key Plants, with Illustrations and Profiles

IMAGINE YOUR OWN SACRED space, filled with just the right plants for your needs. You are the creative designer for this garden retreat. In designing your medicine wheel garden, perhaps you want it to be sparsely filled with just a few select healing herbs so that other creative accents can be enjoyed. You may want a low, lush alpine or rock garden of bearberry, ginger, pennyroyal, partridgeberry, pipsissewa, purslane, heal-all, hepatica, strawberry, and wintergreen growing around special standing rocks, a stone bench, and a small fountain or fish pool. If you choose a shaded woodland site, you might select ferns and herbs such as maidenhair, ginseng, hepatica, goldthread, bloodroot, birthroot, wintergreen, pipsissewa, and partridgeberry, which thrive in this environment.

When I was planning my first medicine wheel garden years ago, I began by watching the site for months to find out what plants flourished there. I had chosen a space beyond the meadow's edge, below our apple orchard, now frequented by a growing herd

The earth does not belong to us; we belong to the earth, and we have a sacred duty to protect her and return thanks for the gifts of life.

—Oren Lyons, Onondaga
faith keeper

*In the Beginning of all things,
wisdom and knowledge were
with the animals;
for "Tirawa," the One Above,
did not speak directly to man.
He sent certain animals to tell
man
that he showed himself
through the beasts,
and that from them,
and from the stars and the sun
and the moon,
man should learn.
Tirawa spoke to man through
his works.*
    —Chief Letakotys, Lesa
        Pawnee

of deer. The sweetgrass is very fragrant in the hot sun. Stepping into the shady hedgerow requires effort to push through the tangle of dogwood and alder shrubs supporting bittersweet vines. Farther into this green jungle a few maple and hickory trees support wild grapes and Virginia creeper vines above an understory of barberry, cinquefoil, jewelweed, and goldenrod. Jack-in-the-pulpit (Indian turnip) peeks out of the dark, moist areas, and speedwell trails over the ground where sun filters into the rich soil.

Gradually I brought in a selection of favorite herbs and mosses to accentuate the plants already at home here that I wanted to continue to grow. Each year I add more sweetgrass and black cohosh, two of my favorite herbs. I believe that it is important, too, to choose plants that draw the hummingbirds, bees, and butterflies. Many gardeners also want to see a balance of wildlife around and within their property. The animals are important residents, especially the rabbits, foxes, skunks, and deer. Fortunately, they are not usual predators on most of these native herbs.

Whatever your site—woodland, meadow, or rocks—some combination of plants described in this chapter will suit your garden preferences. Each entry identifies the herb, its closest relatives and family, and describes the history of its uses and how to grow the plant and harvest specific parts in the proper season. Included

An Early Compendium of Native Plants

The earliest written and illustrated work on North American plants used in medicine is the 1552 Badianus Manuscript (Codex Barberini) in the collection of the Vatican Library. This manuscript, written in Nahuatl and Latin, bears illustrations of 184 Mesoamerican plants and trees on sixty-three painted folios, each accompanied by detailed descriptions of the illnesses for which the plants were used and their curative properties. The codex is divided into thirteen chapters devoted to either a group of maladies similar in type or collections of ailments that affect certain portions of the body. Two Aztec scribes painted and lettered this work: Marinus de la Cruz, a traditional healer, and Juan Badianus, who translated the text from Nahuatl into Latin.

are many appealing choices of herbs for different climates and elevations, and special attention is given to drought-hardy plants suitable for xeriscaping.

Plants have very special growth needs, and some plant associations work better than others. Because of this, you would not find all the plants described here together in one garden. Each entry notes appropriate plant companions that might work well together in your medicine wheel garden.

WHAT'S IN A PLANT NAME?

Plants, like people, have immediate relatives forming a closely knit group as well as a larger extended family. In classifying plants into these related groups, the Latin binomial (two identifying names) given to each plant species provides useful clues to identity. The first Latin name, which is capitalized, refers to the genus to which a plant belongs. A genus embraces closely related individual species. The second Latin name, not capitalized, designates the species itself. For example, American ginseng has the Latin name, *Panax quinquefolius*. *Panax* identifies the genus including various ginseng species, and *quinquefolius* alludes to a distinguishing feature of American ginseng: its five-part leaves. Scientific and sometimes common plant names may also embody remarkable information and history, useful to gardeners as well as to herbalists and healers. American ginger's Latin name, *Asarum canadense,* suggests that this lovely low native herb with heart-shaped leaves was first identified in regions of Canada and eastern North America. Sometimes this history borders on the magical and mystical, as with the angel-like angelica, which was long believed to protect those who wore it or ate it from the plague or witchcraft.

Some of our native plant names may seem musty and old-fashioned, and some are even misnomers, yet they reveal much about how the system of observing and learning plants has

Many plants were given their Latin binomials by Carolus Linnaeus (1707–1778), the Swedish plantsman who originated the system of taxonomic classification. Linnaeus never visited North America but relied heavily on pressed plant specimens and careful notes sent to him from "the colonies."

evolved. Most important, this two-hundred-year-old system of identifying plants holds up well today and helps to banish confusion. As you shall see and read, most of these plants have many colorful English and Indian names, reflecting their long history of use on this continent. For example, poke may be called pokeweed, scoke, poocan, pigeon berry, or cancer root—among other names—in different regions. And yet it is universally identifiable by its Latin name, *Phytolacca americana*. This helps when ordering and buying specific species for your medicine wheel garden.

Just as each species belongs to a genus, every genus belongs to a much larger family, indicated by the Latin endings *-ae* or *-aceae*. The family names help us to see plants not just as individuals but as members of a network of relationships that share common characteristics. Their similarities and differences can be intriguing and useful tools for gardeners. For example, one vital plant family, the Solanaceae (nightshade family), includes some of our most delicious vegetables (tomatoes, potatoes, eggplant) and some striking poisons. Chili peppers, jimson weed, and tobacco are among the Solanaceae in the medicine wheel garden. As you will see, each has special merit. Most nightshades are "heavy feeders"; they take a lot of nutrients from the soil, and so they prosper with additional feeding and top dressing around the plants during the height of the growing season. Each nightshade member also exhibits some degree of toxicity in its foliage, and many bear toxic fruits. In the case of tobacco, native people used the somewhat toxic foliage as a powerful substance for ritual use, prayer, and offerings.

Plant family names are capitalized, but unlike species and genus names, they are not written in italics. While more than three hundred plant families have been recorded, most gardeners need concern themselves only with some twenty-four. Among these, the main plant families focused on here are the Compositae (daisy), Labiatae (mint), Liliaceae (lily), Ericaceae (heath), Solanaceae (nightshade), and Ranunculaceae (buttercup). You also will get to know more than a dozen other plant families that encompass some of the key healing herbs important for the medicine wheel garden.

LIFE STORIES

Each of the special plants pictured and discussed here has its unique history of human use. The profiles trace patterns from past to present, bringing together traditional American Indian medicinal plant uses with other historical herbal practices and finishing with how the plant is used today. For example, in both North America and Europe, arnica has a long, illustrious history of serving people's needs for pain relief, for which it continues to be quite valuable. Some other plants that now serve for one or two needs have a background of many more varied uses. American Indian herbal uses were often quite diverse. Many of these traditional uses continue to be modern American Indian uses and valuable to other health care practitioners. Where possible, profiles include related species that show how you can widen your choices for your medicine wheel garden.

Each plant profile includes:

Plant name and classification
Background and plant "personality"
Size and distinguishing features
American Indian traditional uses
Plant part(s) and uses for healing
How this herb is used today
Cautions (if any)
Growth needs and propagation methods
Garden companions

THE IMPORTANCE OF ROOTS

The more we nurture and encourage the plants growing in our gardens, the more we enrich our own spiritual and aesthetic life. Propagation, the different means we employ as gardeners to promote the growth of plants and to increase their numbers, is a fascinating aspect of gardening. The underground parts of a plant,

The tidy cabin and the familiar smell of herbs and roots and wood-smoke, and the rabbit soup simmering on the stove, all made me feel like I had come home again.
—Maria Campbell, Canadian Métis, from her autobiography *Halfbreed,* 1973

central to its vitality, are also commonly the key to propagation. As you will notice in the following illustrations and plant profiles, what we usually refer to as a plant's "roots" or "root system" may vary considerably. The form that the root system takes determines the best way to propagate the plant successfully. Botanists and gardeners have specific names for different root forms: rootstock (found in, for example, angelica), runners (strawberry), corms (jack-in-the-pulpit), bulbs (onion), rhizomes (iris and ferns), tubers (groundnut), and stolons (wintergreen).

Understanding how to deal with different kinds of roots is particularly important because some of our native herbs have diminishing populations in the wild yet thrive under propagation. American ginseng, bearberry, cardinal flower, butterflyweed, maidenhair fern, and lady's slipper are all on this list. Your medicine wheel garden has a secondary benefit of possibly replenishing native herbs in other gardens and surrounding areas.

An easy way to propagate perennials, such as ginger, ginseng, bloodroot, and mayapple, is by digging up and dividing their rootstocks, as most gardeners call them. This work is best done while the plant is dormant, usually in late fall, winter, or early spring—also the time when herbalists seek the rootstocks for medicinal uses. Cut the rootstock with a sharp, clean knife and make sure that each new piece has at least one bud, or "eye," and roots (depending upon the species) attached. Corms and bulbs of plants such as wild onion and garlic, jack-in-the-pulpit, and trillium usually develop small offsets on the side of the main growth as it matures. These little cormlets and bulblets can also be removed with a sharp knife when the plant is dormant. Each will develop into a new plant.

There's nothing new about propagating and transferring plant populations. Native Americans have been moving key plants around this continent for millennia, especially since they began to establish permanent settlements. Particularly valuable medicine plants such as pennyroyal, wintergreen, ginseng, bee balm, blueberry, blue cohosh, and black cohosh could be readily established in some areas of settlement. Herbalists have always gone into the meadows and woods to seek other wild plants that could not easily be managed closer to dwelling sites.

Ours is a nation inextricably linked to the histories of the many peoples who first inhabited this great land. Everywhere around us are reminders of the legacy of America's first inhabitants. Their history speaks to us through the names of our cities, lakes, and rivers; the food on our tables; the magnificent ruins of ancient communities; and most important, the lives of the people who retain the cultural, spiritual, linguistic, and kinship bonds that have existed for millennia.

—President William Jefferson Clinton, Proclamation 7247 for National American Indian Heritage Month, 1999

Should You Be Your Own Herbalist?

Certainly natural is good, but your own garden may not always be as reliable as the local health food store for larger amounts of healing herbs. Rather than digging up your own echinacea and black cohosh roots to prepare healing remedies, simply working among these healthy plants may strengthen your appreciation of the herbal supplements you purchase and use. On the other hand, you can enjoy years of happy harvesting from your medicine wheel garden for simple herbal teas, tisanes, potpourris, and other herbal foods and products if you gather carefully, giving plants ample time to replenish. In Part III you will find additional recipes and harvest details for your garden, along with more practical health care suggestions and ceremonial items you might create.

This continent's earliest gardeners must have felt a deep kinship with the earth. Some of the ritual objects found by scientists working at sacred sites reflect a desire to give beautiful works of craftsmanship to the earth. Perhaps these offerings were meant to ensure greater harvests. The sense of ceremony and respect reminds everyone that plants and harvesting are much more than chores. They are direct communion with the earth and the Creator.

AMERICAN ANGELICA

Angelica atropurpurea
Umbelliferae (parsley family)

Angelica has a long history of uses around the world, from practical to magical. Its name, meaning "of angels; angel like," comes from Latin *herba angelica* (angelic herb), reflecting the importance of angelica as a perceived preventive to plague, witchcraft, and poison. The deeply cut compound leaves of the tall, graceful plants can sometimes look like "wings" fluttering in the summer breeze. The species designation *atropurpurea* means "dark purple"; it certainly describes the round ruby stems of this herb.

As the family name suggests, angelica grows like parsley, producing flowers in big compound umbels—multiple flowers on stalks that branch from a central stem and grow to a uniform height. The small, greenish-white flowers cluster at the top of sturdy, hollow stems during the summer months, ripening into clustered aromatic seeds by late summer. Robust in form, angelica will grow up to six feet tall.

About fifty species of aromatic herbs in this genus are native to the Northern Hemisphere. Angelica grows wild from Labrador south to Maryland and west to Indiana, Minnesota, and Iowa. In the wild it appears to grow prolifically one year and then disappear for a year or two before it resumes growing in healthy profusion.

American angelica
Angelica atropurpurea

Traditional uses: The Missouri River Indians highly prized this plant, which they called *lagoni-hah*. Young leaves were eaten to relieve digestive problems and also used as a hunting lure. During the late 1600s, the Virginia Indians were known to eat so much angelica that they smelled of it. These eastern Algonquians apparently planted the seeds and unused portions of the root to ensure that they would have more, as they also used this herb for healing, hunting, and fishing. Some tribes used the pounded roots and dried powdered stems to reduce skin tumors.

Great Lakes Indians valued angelica as a poultice on swellings and tumors. The roots were cooked and then pounded into a pulp and applied to the surface of the skin where pain and swelling persisted. The poultice was noted for pain relief. The Canadian Malecite Indians used angelica roots to treat colds, flu, coughs, and sore throat. It was also said to promote mental clarity and a sense of well-being. Many tribes used the dried leaves mixed into their tobacco to enhance the fragrance and taste. Iroquois traditional healers used this herb as a preventative for the wrath of ghosts and on the "spirit plate" for certain ceremonies.

Modern uses: Today, herbalists recommend angelica for many needs. Both American and European angelica, *A. archangelica*, are used to aid digestion and to improve circulation, and as a general tonic. Chinese angelica, *A. sinensis (dang gui),* is a valued blood tonic and is often used in cooking. The whole plant strengthens the liver and has an antibiotic effect in the body. The rhizome is the part most valued for its medicinal properties. Angelica stems and roots are also useful in cooking, especially for winter vegetables and condiments.

Extensive commercial uses for angelica range from flavoring liqueurs, such as Benedictine and Chartreuse, to gin and vermouth. The young leaves and shoots may be eaten in salads; the greenish-red stems are candied or preserved in syrup and used as condiments. The essential oil is added to perfumes, shampoos, ointments, creams, and soaps.

Cautions: Be careful to avoid angelica's harmful relatives, poison hemlock and water hemlock. These plants lack angelica's aromatic quality.

Growth needs and propagation: Favoring ditches, stream banks, and bottomlands in the wild, angelica prefers rich, moist, well-drained soil and partial shade. The best way to propagate angelica is by its seeds, which have a short viability. Sow them as early as possible where you want the plants to grow. Do not cover them, as they need light to germinate. Our native angelica is basically an annual herb, which must self-sow in order to regenerate. If you cut the bloom stalk early, the plant might live for another year. Work to establish a small colony of angelica plants in the medicine wheel garden, as they are tall, strikingly attractive, and almost insect-proof.

Companions: Angelica will grow fairly well in the company of hellebore, jack-in-the-pulpit, sweetgrass, cardinal flower, blue flag, and sweet flag. Elderberry shrubs are also good companions.

For flu, as used in the epidemic of 1924, pulverize angelica root and boil. . . . Drink ½ glassful.

—Kate Debeau, Mohawk herbalist, Caughnawaga Reserve, 1939

The patient must be in a certain frame of mind—it must be flexible. He must work in conjunction with the medicine. He must have faith in its power in order to help it. In the Indian philosophy of sickness, it is thought that one's mind must be freed of worry and distrust in order that the patient may get well.

—Jesse Cornplanter, Seneca herbalist and storyteller, 1933

Arnica mollis and other species
Compositae (daisy family)

These dwarf sunflowers with downy opposite leaves produce their yellow daisylike blossoms from June through August in flower heads two to three inches across. They thrive in sandy, rocky soils and tend to colonize entire areas, especially old fields. This naturalizing habit enables the various species of arnica to be gardened and farmed with excellent results. They seem to prosper in the medicine wheel garden and will spread over an entire area without choking out other plants.

Arnica is modified Latin of unknown origin. The species name, *mollis,* means "soft, flexible, and mild." Other well-known species names in the closely related arnica group include *A. montana,* "of the mountains," and our native western species, *A. cordifolia,* "with heart-shaped leaves," an attractive, distinguishing feature.

Thirty or so species of arnica grow worldwide, favoring higher elevations in both woodsy and open places. They include nine native species, which greatly resemble their European cousin *A. montana.* There are also several East Asian species and the alpine arnica, *A. alpina,* which grows around the world's northernmost regions and stays close to the ground, rarely reaching more than fifteen inches in height.

Both *A. amplexicaulis* and *A. chamissonis* are native across the western United States into Canada and southern Alaska, where subspecies grow. Much the same is true for *A. latifolia,* which can grow to two feet tall, and the diminutive *A. lessingii,* which rarely grows to more than ten inches. The arnicas flourish in northern mountain states and southern Canadian provinces up into the Yukon and Alaska.

Traditional uses: Native to Europe, *A. montana* is widely distributed in our western regions and is planted in many herb gardens. Also called leopard's bane and mountain tobacco, this species was officially listed in the USP (United States Pharmacopeia) from 1820 to 1851, when doctors prescribed it for external pain relief. Flowers and roots of arnica have been used in medicinal preparations for centuries. The Catawba Indians used *A. acaulis,* which they called "water root," in a tea that was applied like a liniment to relieve back pain. Catawba herbalist Carlos Westez (Red Thunder Cloud) often advised the use of this root tea as a rub for sore back, leg, and arm muscles. Scientists credit American Indians with discovering the medicinal healing values of their native species of arnica. According to Virgil Vogel in his book *American Indian Medicine,* the four major native species used by various tribes are *A. fulgens, A. sororia, A. cordifolia,* and *A. caulis.* Presumably, tribal Indians knew the use of other species of arnica as well.

Modern uses: Flowers of heartleaf arnica, *A. cordifolia,* and broadleaf arnica, *A. latifolia,* are harvested during early blooming, as they ripen and turn to fluff with maturity. The rhizomes are harvested after the plant has died back to the ground in autumn. All plant parts are active and used medicinally.

Today, commercial interests in arnica continue to increase. Many western acres are sown in arnica to meet growing international market demands. Farming arnica as a subcrop on some western ranches and reserves provide extra annual income for some ranchers.

American arnica
Arnica mollis

Arnica ointment and compresses are effective treatments for bruises, muscle pain, sprains, and backaches. Arnica speeds healing by locally improving the blood supply and functions as a powerful antiinflammatory agent, increasing the reabsorption of internal bleeding. Homeopathic dilutions (taken internally in minuscule amounts) are generally for shock and pain. Trained herbalists and naturopaths treat angina and stimulate circulation with small doses of arnica tincture or decoction, internally and externally.

Cautions: *Arnica preparations should not be taken internally or used on broken skin.* Arnica is poisonous. The only safe internal use is in the minute homeopathic dose. Dermatitis can result from external use for those who have sensitive skin. It is best to have use of arnica monitored by a health care professional.

Growth needs and propagation: Arnica will grow in most soils but prefers a slightly acidic, well-drained soil in full sun. Plants will tolerate light shade. This herb can be easily propagated from seeds and cuttings. Spread the seeds sparsely over prepared ground in late summer and cover them with barely an inch of fine soil. Pat this area down gently and cover it with a light layer of leaf mulch. Plants should sprout in late spring. Allow them to grow and develop some vigor before transplanting them to the desired location. Root cuttings can be made in late summer. Each two-inch piece of root, planted two inches deep, should produce a new plant by the following spring.

Companions: These diminutive sunflowers grow handsomely under angelica plants, rudbeckias, and elderberry shrubs in the medicine wheel garden. Allow arnicas to colonize their own small area in your garden and enjoy their golden blossoms throughout summer.

Grandmother Moon and the Earth and all those things . . . They are very dear to me, and I respect them. But I also respect God through my Christian belief. And to me God and the Great Spirit are the same.

—Hannah Averett, Mashpee
Wampanoag historian, 1977

AMERICAN GINGER

Asarum canadense
Aristolochiaceae (birthwort family)

Known as Canada snakeroot, colicroot, and Indian ginger, this beautiful native wildflower and medicinal herb grows from southern Canada south to North Carolina and Tennessee, and as far west as Kansas and Missouri. The species name, *canadense*, suggests Canada, the region where the plant was originally identified. The Latin genus name, *Asarum,* means "heart-shaped," referring to the leaves.

The soft leaves, two to seven inches broad, top seven- to ten-inch velvety stems that divide just above the ground. In spring, a single, low reddish-brown tubular blossom with a slightly creamy interior develops in the notch of the stem division. These spring blooms lie almost on the ground and are pollinated by carrion beetles and ground insects drawn to the slightly rank odor.

Traditional uses: Native Americans used ginger as a primary digestive aid and valuable heart medicine. Ojibwa Indians of Lake Huron regions called it *pegamagabow* and seasoned many different foods with the roots. It was also considered a powerful protection against unseen forces or illness. Ginger roots were worn and carried as charms as well as used to treat certain heart conditions, headache, colds, sore throat, coughs, and cramps.

The Illinois and Miami Indians used wild ginger roots to ease childbirth and relieve pain. They called the plant *akiskiouaraoui,* "herb of the rattlesnake," and applied pieces of the root to snakebite injuries and also chewed it. Throughout the tribal northeast American ginger, also called wild ginger, had many special applications and added its strength to vital formulas.

Modern uses: Wild ginger roots contain the antitumor compound aristolochic acid, which also has antimicrobial properties. This herb substitutes for oriental ginger in many medicinal preparations and continues to be used in ways similar to those traditionally favored by American Indians.

Today we are much more familiar with the commercial oriental ginger, *Zingiber officinale* (Zingiberaceae), known as *sheng jian*

American ginger
Asarum canadense

in Chinese medicine. It is a close relative of turmeric, *Curcuma longa*. This aromatic rhizome contains high levels of a volatile oil that is warming and stimulating. It acts as a circulatory stimulant given to relieve headache, fever, and aching muscles and also relieves nausea, morning sickness, and motion sickness.

Growth needs and propagation: American ginger is an easily cultivated perennial. It prefers rich, moist woodland earth, and thrives in shade or dappled shade. The low-growing, aromatic plants are often set in shaded show gardens, interspersed with clumps of European ginger, *A. europaeum*. Sometimes growing in dense colonies in the areas they favor, these creeping, slender plants also form a lovely ground cover along wooded pathways and foundation areas.

It is easiest to increase American ginger by taking root cuttings with buds and roots in the late fall. These should be planted in rich, moist soil at a depth of about two inches. It is best to mulch ginger plants with generous layers of leaves for the winter.

Companions: American ginger grows well with maidenhair fern, goldenseal, goldthread, hepatica, and Indian turnip, and underneath bayberry and elderberry shrubs.

AMERICAN GINSENG

Panax quinquefolius
Araliaceae (ginseng family)

The name *ginseng*, of Chinese origin, means "essence of earth in the form of a man," referring to the almost humanlike shape of this plant's taproot. Ginseng has been a traditional Chinese tonic medicine for more than two thousand years. The genus name *Panax* comes from the Greek *pan* (all) and *akos* (ills)—when ginseng was formally named in 1753, it was considered to be a plant that cured all ills. Ginseng leaves, carried in whorls, are toothed and usually palmate, cut like the fingers on a hand—*quinque-folius* simply means "with five leaves," the hallmark of these herbs.

The *Panax* genus has some six species of herbs with thick roots and simple stems, native to North America and East Asia. American ginseng grows about one to two feet tall and bears small clusters of up to forty whitish flowers in late spring. Bright red berries, each with two or three whitish seeds inside, cluster above the leaves in fall. Our other native species, dwarf ginseng, *P. trifolius,* has roots that are more globelike. Both these native perennials are found in rich eastern woodlands, especially mountainous regions from Nova Scotia south to Georgia and west to Indiana, Iowa, Oklahoma, and Minnesota.

Some of the earliest botanical exports from North America were the carrotlike taproots of wild American ginseng, which were shipped to China in the early 1700s. French Jesuit missionaries working among the Iroquois Indians north of Montreal recognized the native species as similar to the highly valued Chinese ginseng.

American ginseng
Panax quinquefolius

Traditional uses: Native Americans used both native ginseng species extensively throughout their range. They stewed the whole plant and drank the water to treat colic, indigestion, rheumatism, and other skin and circulatory problems. The flowers and later seeds were chewed to treat breathing difficulties. The roots were the most important part for healing; they were chewed or otherwise used in many medicinal and tonic applications.

To treat sore eyes in a two-year-old child (ulcerated cornea): Slightly steep one small root in one cup of water. Bottle it. Wash eyes every hour with a clean rag, squeezing drops into the eye. Keep up treatment after cure for two months.

—Herb Johnson, Seneca herbalist, Tonawanda Reserve, 1912

Lacrosse medicine. When a rival is trying to get the ball, the captain shouts "djitgaye" and that makes the other lose the ball for sure. A decoction [of dwarf ginseng roots] is rubbed on the arms and legs [before the lacrosse game.]

—Peter John, Onondaga herbalist, Six Nations Reserve, 1914

Modern uses: Another ginseng species highly valued in health care is the Chinese or Korean Ginseng, *P. ginseng,* noted for its warming properties. It is yang (hot) in nature and used by people who are yin (cool). The Chinese favor the American ginseng because it is a yin tonic for those who are yang in nature. Tien chi ginseng, *P. notoginseng,* which grows in southern China, is traditionally used to lower blood pressure and reduce cholesterol levels. Siberian ginseng, *Eleutherococcus senticosus,* is a close botanical cousin valuable in helping people adapt to stress. It also strengthens the immune system.

Today ginseng is a multibillion-dollar business, and the number of ginseng growers is continually increasing. The ginsengs are considered *adaptogenic,* helping to normalize body functions by enabling them to utilize other substances more efficiently, and also helping to eliminate toxic substances from the body. Ginseng is considered a whole-body tonic. It tones the organs and enhances their functions, while helping to strengthen all of the body's systems.

Cautions: Large doses of ginseng are said to raise blood pressure. This tonic should be used with caution and respect. Many people are wolfing down ginseng extracts, teas, roots, and tonics for their many benefits and energy boosts. Some care must be exercised not to overdo a good thing.

Growth needs and propagation: Ginseng has very special growth needs and profits from being pampered. Plants prefer a humus-rich, well-drained, loamy soil and partial shade. Principally a woodland crop, they thrive in dappled shade and with a winter mulch. The seeds need a good four months of cold stratification to germinate, and they require five to seven years to produce mature plants. It is best to start with young plants and cluster them in a cool, rich setting in the medicine wheel garden.

Companions: Ginseng grows beneath elderberry, bayberry, hellebore, or angelica. It will also be a companion to hepatica, pennyroyal, bloodroot, strawberry, and bearberry in the garden.

Veratrum viride
Liliaceae (lily family)

These ancient medicinal plants take their genus name, *Veratrum*, from the Latin word for "hellebore." The species name, *viride*, means "green." A stout perennial plant of moist, rich bottomlands that can grow seven feet tall, American hellebore is also known as white hellebore, Indian poke, itchweed, and devil's tobacco.

There are about forty-five species of *Veratrum* native to North America, Europe, and Asia. All favor wet soil. Most are cultivated for specialty gardens and have important medicinal qualities. *V. californicum* is the strikingly attractive corn lily that may grow to six feet tall in regions from Baja California to Washington State and eastward to Colorado, Montana, and New Mexico. It is favored in wildflower gardens, as is *V. woodii*, a more slender, shorter species native to the central United States from Ohio to eastern Oklahoma.

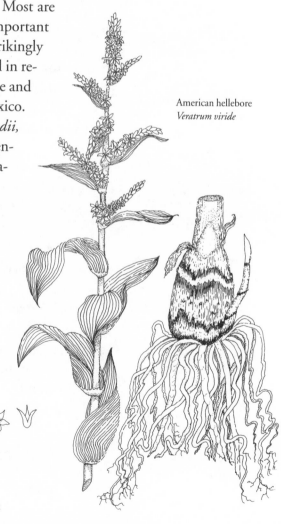

American hellebore
Veratrum viride

The typically robust, ovate leaves of American hellebore, reaching one foot long, are strongly ribbed, a help in distinguishing this species from any look-alikes. Branched clusters of yellowish-green star-shaped flowers bloom from April through July in many places. The seed pods ripen in late fall, producing many seeds. In the wild, this species grows in swamps and woodland streamsides from Labrador, New Brunswick, Quebec, and Ontario to Minnesota, Georgia, and Tennessee.

Traditional uses: Historically, Indians used these toxic medicinals wisely to treat epilepsy, convulsions, and pneumonia, as well as for pain relief. The Cherokee used hellebore root extracts to treat rheumatism. Some tribes made heart sedatives from *Veratrum,* and weak teas were used to treat sore throats and chronic rheumatism. The Iroquois used the root to treat congestion. Indian women used decoctions to treat head lice and other vermin; the dried, powdered root served to heal wounds and also as an insecticide. Some accounts say that the eastern Indians used the root as a suicide drug. It was also used to treat toothaches and skin tumors. Shoshone women used the western species as a female contraceptive, and it was said to produce sterility if taken for three weeks.

Modern uses: Extracts (tinctures) from American hellebore are used in homeopathy to treat fever, flu, headache, measles, and pneumonia. Scientists have discovered that the alkaloids and steroids from this plant lower blood pressure and dilate the peripheral blood vessels. Extracts have been used to treat gout. Though highly respected, American hellebore is rarely used by herbalists today because of its toxicity.

Cautions: All plant parts, especially the roots, are highly or fatally toxic. Contact can cause mild dermatitis to those with sensitive skin.

Growth needs and propagation: Hellebore prefers rich, wet earth, open to partial shade. It is readily propagated from root division and seed. Handle rootstock carefully (wear gloves), and plant each piece six to eight inches deep in moist, rich earth. Tamp down the area well and mulch with fallen leaves over the winter for fine spring growth in the garden. Seeds need to be spread thinly in moist soil, covered with two inches of fine soil, and kept moist. It may take several years for plants to mature from seeds and bloom.

Companions: Hellebore grows well with Indian turnip, birthroot trillium, cardinal flower, elderberry, sweet flag, goldthread, boneset, and jewelweed.

Hedeoma pulegioides
Labiatae (Lamiaceae) (mint family)

Hedeoma's original meaning is obscure. The species name comes from the Middle English meaning "mock pennyroyal"; *pulegium* comes from the Latin for "flea," referring to this herb's traditional use as a flea and bug repellent. Squawbalm, squawmint, and pudding-grass are folk names for our diminutive yet powerful native pennyroyal.

Ongnehem was the Huron name for this fragrant, self-sowing annual mint. They put it in their soup of corn and gourds, along with wild onions, to give a wholesome flavor, as was recorded in the 1600s by early explorers in southern Canada. Many other native uses have been noted, primarily for healing and medicinal needs.

Pennyroyal favors dry woodlands from Quebec to Georgia and westward to Oklahoma, Nebraska, and Michigan. Tiny bluish flowers appear in the leaf axils throughout late summer. The small lace-shaped leaves can be toothed or smooth-edged along these slender, branching plants, which rarely stand more than twelve to eighteen inches tall. Pennyroyal often grows in clusters along old wagon trails and footpaths where its highly aromatic qualities can surprise travelers even in the dead of winter.

Traditional uses: Like the European pennyroyal, *Mentha pulegium,* our native species, *H. pulegioides,* was greatly respected as an herbal medicine and used with caution, as both could be toxic and abortive. Many tribes made a soothing tea of this native herb to relieve headaches and cramps and used it as a skin wash to treat rashes and irritating itching. The fresh or dried plant (whole) also served as a valuable insect repellent.

American pennyroyal
Hedeoma pulegioides

Modern uses: Pennyroyal tea has been a reliable cold remedy for centuries. Even a mild tea will promote sweating, relieve fevers, and soothe coughs, flu symptoms, headaches, and indigestion. Herbalists continue to use these teas or tinctures to induce menstruation and for late-onset, crampy menses. Some midwives use pennyroyal in late-term pregnancy to assist in childbirth.

Tickweed is yet another name for this remarkable herb, as it is a valued tick repellent. Many hunters and hikers rub their boots and socks with these plants before setting off through the woods.

Many of us simply place a little pennyroyal in our socks, pockets, and bandanas in order to be "bug-free" while outside.

Cautions: Do not use during pregnancy. Pennyroyal can be very toxic. The essential oil can cause dermatitis for some people, and pennyroyal tea or tincture should only be used with great caution, as it can cause liver damage.

Growth needs and propagation: Pennyroyal likes dry shaded ground in woodland settings. Once it settles into a place it likes, it will self-sow annually.

Companions: Pennyroyal grows well with goldenseal, hepatica, Indian turnip, moccasin flower, and bayberry.

ANGEL'S TRUMPET

Datura stramonium
Solanaceae (nightshade family)

Indian apple, locoweed, thorn apple, and sacred datura are some of the regional names for this striking plant. Two other popular names, jimsonweed and Jamestown weed, go back to Jamestown, Virginia, where early colonists once mistakenly ate some of the greens and became quite silly. The large white trumpet-shaped blossoms inspire the idea of trumpeting angels, though considering the plant's possible effects, some might call its flowers "devil's trumpets." The genus name, *Datura*, comes from the early Hindi and Sanskrit word *dhatura,* meaning "trumpetlike," *stramonium* from the Tatar word *turman,* "horse medicine."

The eight species of *Datura,* all annuals or short-lived perennials, are native to the tropics and warm temperate regions of the Americas. The irregularly toothed alternate leaves, dark green on top and lighter green underneath, are slightly hairy and sticky. Notable for their strong, rank odor, the leaves can grow five to six inches long. The solitary white flowers arise from points where the leaf stems grow from the stalk and may reach a length of six inches, resembling giant morning glories. The single large green, spiny seedpod usually has four chambers filled with small, flattish seeds. The plant can grow up to five feet tall in some locations.

The downy angel's trumpet, *D. inoxia (D. meteloides),* which spreads more readily, grows to about three feet tall in waste places across the southern United States and northern Mexico. You see this species especially along roadways and arroyos in the Southwest. The stunning *Brugmansia* species and other tree daturas are exciting to greenhouse growers and gardeners across America. All had early tribal uses as respected hallucinogens, "plants of the gods."

A beautiful Zuni legend tells of the divine origin of *aneglakya,* *D. inoxia,* their most sacred plant, which is named for a young Zuni boy who lived in earliest times. He and his sister lived in the earth's interior, yet they could easily go and come from the outer

Angel's trumpet
Datura stramonium

The original plant has many children scattered over the earth; some of the blossoms are tinged with yellow, some with blue, some with red, some are all white—the colors belonging to the four cardinal points.

The Zunis believe that the plant belongs to the Rain Priest Fraternity and rain priests alone may collect its roots. These priests put the powdered root into their eyes to commune with the Feathered Kingdom at night, and they chew the roots to ask the dead to intercede with the spirits for rain. These priests further use D. inoxia *for its analgesic effects, to deaden pain during simple operations, bone-setting, and cleaning ulcerated wounds.*

—Richard Evans Schultes and Albert Hofmann, *Plants of the Gods: Origins of Hallucinogenic Use,* 1979

world, where they would walk around observing many things closely. Eventually the Divine Ones (twin sons of the Sun Father) banished the brother and sister from the outer world because they knew too much. Large flowers sprang up from the spot where the two descended into the underworld.

Traditional uses: Angel's trumpet is a noted folk remedy for cancer, and the leaves were once smoked as an antispasmodic for asthma. South American Indians used these plant extracts as anesthetics for setting bones after injuries and as part of some puberty rites. It was said to be an aphrodisiac for women. Indians in the Southwest used these botanicals in shamanic ceremonies and curing rites. The Yokut Indians called it *tanayin* and gave it to their adolescents only in the spring to ensure a long life. The Yuman Indians called it *toloache* and used it to foretell the future in sacred ceremonies. The Pima Indians sang about this plant in hunting songs. The Huichol Indians created beautiful yarn paintings of this plant. The Navajo Indians used it for visionary diagnosis to effect healing. The eastern Algonquian Indians called it *wysoccan* and used it in initiatory rites for the *huskanawing* ceremony, which was a two- or three-week-long puberty ceremony.

Modern uses: This whole plant contains atropine and other alkaloids, used to treat eye diseases; atropine dilates the pupils. Extracts from the plant serve in treating Parkinson's disease. Angel's trumpet also yields scopolamine, used in skin patches placed behind the ear to treat vertigo. The plant is widely grown commercially for research as a source for the alkaloidal drug hyposcamine and other properties.

Cautions: Eating any plant parts causes severe hallucinations and may be fatal. Excessive handling can cause eye irritations and swollen eyelids.

Growth needs and propagation: Despite the fact that many people view angel's trumpet as a rank weed, gardeners love its attractive blooms and seedpods and increasingly grow it. The blossoms attract hummingbirds and butterflies, as well as the hummingbird moth. Angel's trumpet will grow in a range of conditions, from poor soil to improved garden soil, and from the desert Southwest to southern New England. These showy plants are easily propagated from seeds, sown indoors in early spring, then planted in the garden in early summer. However, it is easiest to purchase healthy plants from your garden center for setting in the medicine wheel garden.

Companions: Angel's trumpet grows well with yarrow, prickly pear, sage, and yucca. It will also accompany American angelica in the event that you want to group your "angels" together.

The earth was now dry and there grew a tree in the middle of the earth. The root of this tree sent forth a sprout beside it and there grew upon it a man, who was the first male. This man would have remained alone. But the tree bent over until its top touched the earth, and there shot another root, from which came forth another sprout. There grew upon it a woman, and from these two are all people produced.
—Traditional Lenape creation story, 1679

BAYBERRY

Myrica pennsylvanica
Myricaceae (wax myrtle family)

The genus name *Myrica* comes from the Greek prefix *myri-*, meaning "very many," as in "myriad." This many-branched shrub puts forth a profusion of small blossoms, which mature into waxy gray berries (actually nutlets). The species name *pennsylvanica* refers to the region in eastern America where this shrub was first identified. Bayberry flourishes in sandy, sterile soils from eastern coastal regions and inland meadows extending from southern Canada to Virginia and parts of North Carolina.

Stout and aromatic, bayberry grows from three to twelve feet tall, with numerous grayish-white branches, supporting many glossy leaves. The male catkins appear in early spring, generally before the new leaves. Tiny yellowish flower clusters are closely spaced along the downy stems below the outer leaves, blooming from April through July; the hairy, green berrylike fruits, clustered along the midbranches, ripen to a downy, waxy grayish white in late fall and winter. Many people collect the waxy berries to make aromatic candles.

Bayberry leaves, bark, twigs, and fruits have diverse medicinal uses, as do its close relatives candleberry, *M. cerifera* (wax myrtle), and sweet gale, *M. gale*. All have aromatic qualities, especially in their leaves, which have tiny oil glands on the underside. It is sometimes difficult to tell the species apart because the leaves and growth habits are very similar.

Traditional uses: Creek and Seminole Indians used bayberry in some of their "spirit ceremonies" and carried the fragrant leaves and twigs as preventive medicine to ward off disease. Louisiana Choctaws decocted the leaves and twigs in water to lower fevers, as did the Houma; many tribes also used similar fragrant bayberry decoctions to bathe skin irritations and to sprinkle inside their houses to counteract sadness. Besides valuing bayberry leaf decoctions for skin irritations, Lumbees chewed the fresh roots to relieve stomach pains and ulcers. Micmacs and other northern Algonquian peoples used dried, powdered bayberry leaves as snuff to treat headache and nosebleeds.

Astringent, aromatic bayberry leaf tea served as a stimulant and to treat afterbirth pains. Pounded root bark was boiled and made into a poultice to treat toothaches and applied to wounds and bruises to reduce infection and inflammation. Many tribal groups used the fresh aromatic twigs as chew sticks and dentifrices to massage their gums and clean their teeth. Some Great Lakes Indians used the fresh branches as insect repellents, and dried the branches to burn as an insecticidal smudge.

Modern uses: Today bayberry root bark infusions are used to increase circulation, stimulate perspiration, relieve sores, and fight bacterial infections. Bayberry's astringent qualities help ease

Bayberry
Myrica pennsylvanica

intestinal problems and ulcers and, in a gargle, help relieve sore throat. The leaves, fresh or dried, make enjoyable teas and food seasonings. The leaves are also used as insect repellents.

Cautions: The wax and essential oil can be toxic for people with skin sensitivities. *Do not use during pregnancy.*

Growth needs and propagation: Bayberry will grow well in poor sandy soil and sun to open shade. It will tolerate moist, peaty soil. It flourishes in full sun. The plants can be grown from seed, but best results come from root cuttings and young slips that grow from the mother plant.

Plant new bayberry plants, or their roots or seeds, in the early spring or fall. Young shrubs should be cut back after planting and watering, because the new root systems often have difficulty sustaining all the foliage and branches. Bayberry shrubs require very little attention or maintenance after this early stage. Their rugged, classic form and fragrance make them desirable garden plants, widely cultivated and used in herb gardens.

Companions: Bayberry will grow well with yarrow, plantain, betony, strawberry, and blue flag, among many other herbs. Ferns also grow well beneath or near bayberry shrubs, especially the sensitive and royal ferns. Various mosses also grow well beneath bayberry, especially hair cap moss.

Once a man dreamed of seeing a plant, called by the Delaware "frost" or "ice weed." He heard a voice, which said to him, "I am strong and great. Stronger than any other plant because I stay green longer in the fall. Use me and I will make you strong." The man then went out and obtained a specimen of the plant for his medicine bundle.

—Gladys Tantaquidgeon
Mohegan medicine woman

BEARBERRY

Arctostaphylos uva-ursi
Ericaceae (heath family)

Both the common and scientific names for this attractive evergreen shrub make clear that its fruit appeals to bears. The Latin species name, *uva-ursi,* means "bear's grape." By coincidence, the

Arcto- in the genus name, indicating northern regions, comes originally from the Greek word for "bear," referring to the Great Bear constellation in the north. And *staphylos* means "bunch" or "cluster"—most commonly a cluster of grapes. Both this species and the related alpine bearberry, *A. alpina,* grow across the northern United States, from the coastal regions up into the mountains.

These diminutive shrubs grow on exposed rocky and sandy sites from subarctic regions south to Virginia and down into Mexico, and west to Indiana and northern Illinois. They are a welcome ground cover in sandy areas of the Northeast, especially on Cape Cod, the Shinnecock Reservation in Southampton, New York, and in the New Jersey pine barrens.

Low and trailing, bearberry has small, glossy, oval leaves that are smooth, leathery, and dark green. Long-running branches can reach out for two feet or more. The pale, fragrant blossoms that in most regions appear from May through July produce terminal clusters of white to pale pink bell-shaped flowers, which ripen to glossy red berries during late summer and autumn. Appealing at any season, bearberry makes a stunning evergreen addition to the winter garden.

Traditional uses: Bearberry is a sacred plant to many Native Americans, who know it as an ingredient in *kinnikinnik,* an Algonquian Indian word for botanical mixtures used for smoking or smudging. Most native kinnikinniks were blends of bearberry, sumac leaves, bark, and berries, and the bark of silky dogwood, *Cornus sericea,* along with more than thirty other botanicals. These were prepared and combined into seasonal mixtures that varied in composition from region to region. Though often favored over native tobacco, kinnikinniks could also include mixtures of tobacco species. Some tribes, especially Great Lakes and Eastern Algonquians, esteemed bearberry so highly as a fragrant smoking substance that they used it alone as their favored kinnikinnik. Canadian Algonquians called it *sagakomi,* which means "smoking leaf berry." A certain number of inner leaves darken and fall off each year, and these can be easily gathered for kinnikinnik, particularly in spring. The leaves and berries were also consumed in therapeutic teas.

The Chippewa carefully cleaned and aged the leaves of bearberry for smoking along with tobacco and red willow as a headache remedy, and also as a means to attract game animals. Bearberry was primarily smoked for medicine ceremonies and in tribal meetings in carved catlinite (pipestone) pipes. These distinctive red Calumet pipes have become a symbol of peace making and are often called peace pipes.

Besides praying and offering sacrifices of tobacco and bearberry before they started out, Delaware (Lenape) hunters prepared special medicine lures—good-luck amulets for hunting—that included bearberry. Bear meat and fat, both highly prized, were often preserved with dried bearberries and pressed or pounded into ceremonial pemmican (dried meat and fruit mixture).

Modern uses: Bearberry is organically grown for the herbal health care industry. Both the leaves and berries have been tested by centuries of dependable therapeutic use, assuring this herb an enduring place of contemporary value.

Today bearberry leaf teas and tinctures rank as primary treatments for urinary tract infections, especially cystitis and kidney stones. The leaves are highly astringent and diuretic. Bearberry is also one of the most useful tea herbs for diabetics to treat excessive blood sugar and help the body's natural insulin production. Bearberry products are usually labeled uva-ursi in health food stores.

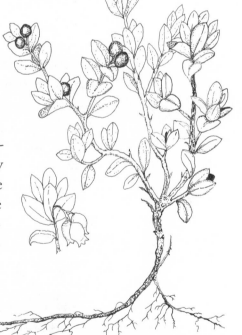

Bearberry
Arctostaphylos uva-ursi

Bearberry fruits, cousin of the native blueberry and cranberry, are somewhat mealy and become tastier after being "kissed" by hard frost. Like the leaves, the berries are medicinal and astringent, best used by working them into foods or other botanical formulas. Scientific research shows that extracts of this herb are antibacterial.

Other fine medicinal botanicals in the heath family include the evergreen leatherleaf, *Chamaedaphne calyculata;* trailing arbutus, *Epigaea repens;* and wintergreen, *Gaultheria procumbens,* whose leaves were valued as external astringents, along with the prized Labrador tea, *Ledum groenlandicum,* long valued as a herbal tea, fumigant, herbal salve ingredient, and insecticide.

Cautions: Do not take during pregnancy. Limit your dosage and use of uva-ursi to just a week to ten days at a time if needed to treat bladder or kidney complaints. Many of us keep a tincture of uva-ursi or the capsules on hand as a safeguard, in hopes it will not be needed.

Growing conditions and propagation: Bearberry and related medicinal plants of the heath family are excellent choices for inclusion in the medicine wheel garden. Cultivated for use in landscape plantings, the thick, weblike growth of this evergreen makes it a valuable plant to check wind and water erosion and hold in ground moisture, especially along slopes. It also creates an excellent low edging texture along paths and walkways.

Bearberry flourishes in loose, sandy, loamy soil with stones and rocks to help anchor its root system. It prefers a slightly acidic soil and prospers beneath evergreen shrubs and laurels where it can receive open shade. It thrives underneath bayberry, black currant, blueberry, and elderberry. The plants grow well in rock garden settings and along ledges, from coastal gardens to alpine settings. Root and stem cuttings root readily and help increase these plantings. When you have a long, trailing branch, place a large stone on the middle of it and cover with a little soil. The part in contact with the soil should root readily and produce another plant.

Bearberry is relatively slow-growing and low-growing, making it vulnerable to disturbance. Give it special attention and protection against predators and erosion until it develops a strong foothold in your garden. It is ruggedly enduring when it likes where it is growing.

BEE BALM

Monarda didyma
Labiatae (mint family)

Bee balm is also known as Oswego tea, for the Oswego Indians of western New York State, who used this plant extensively for beverages, medicines, foods, and smoking mixtures. Indian plume is another popular name. The more official genus name, *Monarda,* for this showy perennial mint pays respects to Nicholas Monardes, a noted Spanish physician in sixteenth-century Seville. The paired flower stamens perhaps inspired the species name *didyma,* meaning "in pairs." The species name for the closely related plant *M. fistulosa* means "tubular," calling attention to this family's characteristic tubular flowers, which lure the hummingbirds and butterflies. Some twelve species of perennial, aromatic *Monarda* are native to North America.

Native to the Northeast, bee balm produces bright red flowers throughout the summer, and its citrus-minty fragrance makes it most desirable. Overharvested from the wild, it is an endangered species in some eastern states. Yet you will see it in almost every wildflower and perennial garden, adding color and elegance.

As its name suggests, bee balm is a plant attractive to bees and a fine source of honey. Leaves of this herb are often used as a caffeine-free substitute for Earl Grey tea, as its fragrance so closely resembles that of orange bergamot, *Citrus aurantium.* Because of this association, our native herb also bears the common name bergamot.

Traditional uses: Native herbalists used all parts of bee balm plants to treat colic, gas, PMS, insomnia, stomachache, and heart troubles. The Delaware Indians favored bee balm and wild bergamot as perfume and used the dried blossoms and

Bee balm
Monarda didyma

The late Delaware herbalist Nora Thompson Dean, Touching Leaves Woman, recalled that pink bee balm was their favorite medicinal plant as well as perfume. They dried the whole herb (above-ground parts) to pack with ceremonial clothing, masks, and sacred rattles. I once bought a large packet of this herb from her, which she called "Delaware Perfume."

leaves to pack among their most valuable belongings, especially masks and leather clothing. The various Great Lakes tribes used these herbs for treating colds and as burn remedies. They ate the fresh leaves to help clear the mind and settle the stomach. The Meskwaki Indians used the powdered dried leaves as snuff to treat headache.

Pink or lavender bergamot, *M. fistulosa,* also gives off a spicy, minty odor and in most ways has exactly the same uses as the royal red bergamot. Native people used both species: stems for dentifrices, leaves and blossoms for headache and cold remedies (in strong teas and steamed), and in foods, teas, seasonings, smoking mixtures, insecticides, preservatives, and in the sweat lodge. The bergamots were also used to treat measles by inducing sweating. The slightly more diminutive pink bee balm, or wild bergamot, grows across the country in dry, open soil, ranging as far as Texas and Oklahoma and up to British Columbia, where it is appreciated as a valuable wildflower. Both red and pink bergamot are extensively cultivated as ornamentals and hybridized in an array of vivid colors ranging from bright magenta to white.

Horsemint, *M. punctata,* is another strongly aromatic member of this striking family. Favoring dry soil from southern New England to Florida and westward to Texas, Arkansas, and Kansas, it puts forth yellowish-purple blooms with lilac bracts throughout summer. Native herbalists used this strong mint to treat cramps, PMS, coughs, colds, fevers, and digestive problems. Horsemint is also a commercial source of thymol, a highly aromatic and antiseptic substance. Today it is chiefly manufactured synthetically. Dotted horsemint, *M. punctata,* another choice wildflower that was used extensively, is a species of the Plains and Southwest.

Modern uses: Herbalists today recommend bee balm infusions for nausea, sore throats, coughs, colds, and menstrual cramps. The infusions are also a digestive aid and help to relieve gas and colic. Besides its value as an attractive ornamental, bee balm is also readily used in cooking and beverages. The blossoms and leaves are delicious in raw salads and summer soups. The leaves may be cut up and steamed with various vegetables and breads to enhance their aroma and taste.

Growth needs and propagation: Bee balm prefers moist rich soil with humus and will grow from two to three feet tall. The aromatic paired leaves seem to radiate north-south and east-west along the square stem, topped with the vibrant red tubular flowers in a crowded head. One of this plant's many virtues is that it will readily adapt to either full sun or partial shade. Although bee balm can be propagated from seeds, the colors might not be uniform because of cross-pollination. The best method is to make root divisions from healthy plants in the fall or spring. Dig the new growth into the garden and water it well.

Companions: Bee balm is a good companion for blue flag and bloodroot and will grow well with bearberry and strawberry. It is also known to enhance the growth of tomatoes by hastening pollenation.

BIRTHROOT TRILLIUM

Trillium erectum
Liliaceae (lily family)

Bethroot, wakerobin, squawroot, purple trillium, red trillium, Indian balm, and stinking Benjamin are just a few of the common names for this striking plant. The common and genus name, from the Swedish *trilling*, refers to the plant's most conspicuous feature: its three large leaves. The species name, *erectum*, reflects its habit of shooting straight up. By any name these lovely wildflowers are welcome harbingers of spring.

Birthroot trillium, which can grow two feet tall, is one of about thirty species of low, perennial, woodland herbs in this

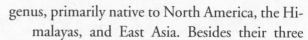

genus, primarily native to North America, the Himalayas, and East Asia. Besides their three wavy leaves, these unusual plants have a single deep-red flower with three sepals and three petals that ripens in late summer to a deep-red three-celled berry. The flowers are usually visited and pollinated by flies.

In the wild, birthroot trillium grows in rich woodlands from Ontario and Nova Scotia south to Florida, and west to Michigan. Among its relatives, painted white trillium, *Trillium undulatum,* grows almost twenty inches tall, is found in the same areas, and favors the same soil. Dwarf white trillium, *T. nivale,* has a more southerly range, and generally grows about six inches tall. Toadshade trillium, *T. sessile,* with purplish-brown flowers, grows about a foot tall and is found across the southern part of the United States. Another southerner is whippoorwill flower, *T. cuneatum,* which grows about ten inches tall and has a mottled dark maroon flower.

Traditional uses: Native peoples used each of these trillium species medicinally for menstrual problems, to induce childbirth and aid labor, for menopause, and as a general uterine tonic. The whole plant was poulticed on wounds, inflammations, ulcers, and tumors. Root decoctions were used by the Menomini to reduce eye swellings and irritation and by the Chippewa to treat rheumatism. Canadian tribes chewed the roots to relieve the pain of snakebite. Trillium roots were noted antiseptics and astringents, used for centuries to treat menstrual problems, diarrhea, coughs, asthma, and night sweats. Early physicians used these trusted botanicals to treat difficult breathing and chronic lung disorders, skin irritations, snakebite, and poisonous stings. Trillium teas were once included in formulas to treat diabetes.

Birthroot trillium
Trillium erectum

Modern uses: The roots of birthroot trillium contain a steroid saponoside, trillarine, used by modern herbalists to treat heavy menstrual and intermenstrual bleeding, helping to reduce the flow. It continues to be a valuable tonic in facilitating childbirth and for treating uterine fibroids. A douche of birthroot is helpful in treating excessive vaginal discharge and yeast infections.

Cautions: Do not take during pregnancy except under professional supervision. The trilliums are on the protected-species list in many states and should not be dug from the wild. As responsible gardeners, we can work to increase these native plant populations by cultivating and propagating them and buying plants from reliable nurseries.

Growth needs and propagation: Trilliums require fertile, moist soil and partial shade to prosper. Following standard practices, root divisions and seeds easily propagate them. It is easiest to purchase healthy young plants from growers or nurseries specializing in cultivating native species.

Companions: This striking trillium accompanies most of the shade-loving plants in the medicine wheel garden, especially Indian turnip, blue cohosh, bloodroot, and ginseng.

BLACK COHOSH

Cimicifuga racemosa
Ranunculaceae (buttercup family)

In the insect world, the Cimicidae are a small family of bloodsucking bugs, including bedbugs. *Cimicifuga,* the Latin genus name for the stately giant black cohosh, suggests putting these bugs to flight. The species name, *racemosa*—literally, "growing in racemes"—describes flowers opening along a central stalk from the bottom to the top, such as lily-of-the-valley. *Cohosh* is an old Algonquian word meaning "rough root" or "medicine root," as the large, distinctive roots of cohosh plants of this and related species were highly esteemed for medicinal needs.

Black snakeroot, squawroot, and bugbane are some of the regional names for this attractive native perennial herb. Like the bug-chasing scientific name, "bugbane" is accurate, as the strong odor of the crushed leaves does indeed repel insects—but perhaps only certain kinds. Every type of insect pollinator seems to buzz to the tall, stately spires of white flowers, rising like delicate candelabra with a host of tiny fragrant white blossoms. These summer-bloom spires, up to eight feet tall, make black cohosh a stunning choice for the garden.

Black cohosh grows in rich woodlands from southern Ontario to Georgia and Tennessee, and westward to Arkansas, Missouri, and Wisconsin. Its large, dark rhizome and roots send up tall, graceful deep green stalks that support three-part, three-lobed, sharply toothed featherlike leaflets. The spires of flowers rise high above the leaves from June until September.

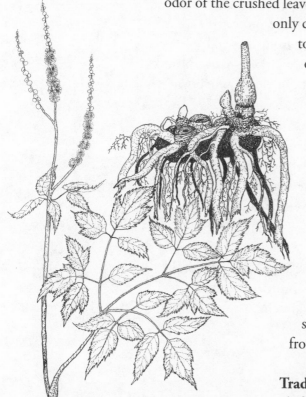

Black cohosh
Cimicifuga racemosa

Traditional uses: Indian tribes in the Northeast used four different species of cohosh herbs. Along with black, there are also blue, red, and white cohosh perennial plants. Each is toxic, even poisonous, yet native herbalists knew how to use them successfully to relieve numerous health problems. The large, dark roots of black cohosh have served for centuries to treat a wide variety of human needs. This herb was a staple of Native American gynecological treatments. Root decoctions were a primary aid to ease childbirth, relieve menstrual cramps, and treat nervous disorders and rheumatism. Pounded, boiled, and poulticed on snakebite, the roots served as an antiseptic.

Modern uses: Continuing research has verified the anti-inflammatory, sedative, estrogenic, and hypoglycemic properties of black cohosh. Not soluble in water, its roots are best tinctured in alcohol. The plant's sedative properties make it valuable for treating conditions ranging from high blood pressure and asthma to whooping cough and tinnitus (ringing in the ears). Today this valued herb is highly regarded as a treatment for symptoms of menopause, especially depression, hot flashes, and debility. Black cohosh has long been a treatment for menstrual pain. Contemporary research proves that it is also effective, in combination with St. John's wort, in relieving hot flashes and other related problems where progesterone production in the female body is too high. Its

Lydia Pinkham's Vegetable Compound

Black cohosh roots were an important mainstay in Lydia Pinkham's Vegetable Compound, which was first marketed in 1875 and is still used today. This famous "restorative" tonic (and patent medicine) also contained butterfly weed (pleurisy root) and three other botanicals in an 18 percent alcohol solution. Lydia Pinkham's tonic works to ease menopausal and post-menopausal symptoms. These vital phytomedicines fell out of favor in the United States during the twentieth century's focus on pharmaceuticals, yet they remain popular abroad. There is intense modern interest in the healing role of phytoestrogens such as those found in black cohosh roots and soy, which do not exert estrogenlike effects in women's ovarian and breast tissues. Today a variety of black cohosh preparations are available alternatives for women who are unwilling or unable to take hormone replacement therapy.

Lydia Pinkham's Vegetable Compound

12 ounces fenugreek seeds, *Trigonella foenum graecum*
6 ounces black cohosh roots, *Cimicifuga racemosa*
6 ounces pleurisy root, *Asclepias tuberosa*
6 ounces life root, *Senecio aureus*
6 ounces unicorn root, *Aletris farinosa*

estrogenic properties can reduce levels of pituitary hormones, thus decreasing the ovaries' production of progesterone. There are numerous black cohosh preparations on the market.

Several related Asian species of cohosh, such as *C. dahurica* and *C. foetida,* are used in Chinese medicine as *sheng ma.* This medicine works to relieve toxicity, treat asthma, headaches, measles, and to "clear heat." The rhizomes and roots are dug in late fall for maximum medicinal potency.

Cautions: In large doses black cohosh can be poisonous.

Growth needs and propagation: Black cohosh will thrive in rich, moist, humus-enriched earth that is well drained. It loves both sun and shade. Because it is unusually tall, it provides an appealing background for other garden plants and can take over a large area. This herb can be propagated from seeds or root division. Seeds should be planted outdoors as soon as they are ripe, after the first frost. Divide roots in early fall or spring and dig them in to their new location.

Companions: Besides black cohosh, there are blue, red, and white cohosh species. (See the entry on blue cohosh for more information.) The four cohoshes make interesting companions in a shade garden. Black cohosh also grows well with yarrow, maidenhair fern, American ginger, and ginseng.

BLOODROOT

Sanguinaria canadensis
Papaveraceae (poppy family)

In early spring, the white daisylike flowers of bloodroot often bloom in cheerful colonies, welcoming winter's retreat. Orange-red juice spurts from freshly broken parts of this perennial plant, accounting for its common name and the genus name, *Sanguinaria*. The species name, *canadensis,* designates Canada and also the northeastern regions of America, the areas where this plant was first collected. The names of many native herbs go back to astute naturalists, who journeyed from Europe in the 1600s and 1700s to see what they could discover in the "New World." They often worked for wealthy patrons wishing to collect new specimens.

Also called red puccoon, Indian paint, redroot, or war paint, this native poppy, the sole North American species of its genus, favors wet banks and open woodlands ranging from Quebec south to Florida and west to Texas and Kansas. This is a powerful herb and stunning wildflower. The white blossoms usually appear before the distinctive basal leaves unfurl from March until May. They typically have eight petals spreading two to three inches across the flower, which stands, solitary, above the deeply lobed, veined (seemingly quilted) leaf. A single palm-shaped leaf, pale gray-green underneath and darker green on top, envelops each spring bloom. After flowering, the leaves enlarge. By midsummer the slim green pods stand erect six to ten inches tall with ripening seeds, which are flung about when the ripe pods finally burst open. Thus, you will find dense clusters of bloodroot colonies in undisturbed areas.

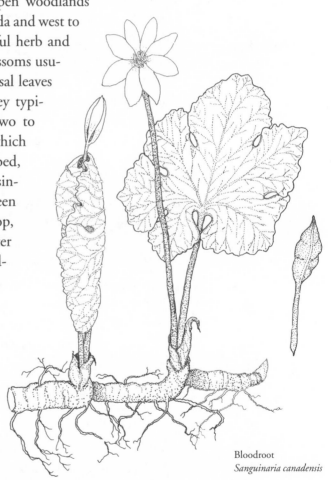

Bloodroot
Sanguinaria canadensis

Traditional uses: A widely used medicine, this small native poppy was called *musquaspenne* by the Powhatan

I heard the story of an Indian woman who lived on Green Pond Mountain. . . . She was called Granny Cudjo and was known for her remedies and for her helpfulness to all who lived in the Hollow.

For her work, she collected supplies of bloodroot, butternut bark, snakeroot, and spice woods. And it was said that she knew all the cures . . .

—A. H. Giddings, New England historian, 1976

Indians in the Virginia Tidewater regions in the early 1600s, and also known to many native peoples as *puccoon,* one of its popular names today. Captain John Smith noted in 1612, in Jamestown, Virginia, "they use [the bloodroot] for swellings, aches, anointing their joints, painting their heads and garments." He also added that "they set a woman fresh painted red" to entertain the colonists. Many different tribes used the roots and colored juice as love charms.

For generations, early doctors studied with the Indians; during the 1800s, they often called themselves "Indian doctors" because of their increased awareness of healing plants. They learned that the bright orange-red sap from the stout, prominent bloodroot rhizomes can be caustic, yet it was particularly well used by diverse native peoples. Medicinal uses of the perennial roots by the Indians spanned the health spectrum, treating skin tumors, internal cancers, eczema, fungal growths, warts, and hemorrhoids. It was also used as an insecticide, as a dye, and as a face paint—even for the lips and teeth and gums. The root juice was once used in cough medicines; in treatments for bronchitis, asthma, lung problems, rheumatism, and fevers; as an emetic; and as a digestive stimulant. Prepared as a dried powder, bloodroot was sniffed to treat nose polyps.

Modern uses: Chemists have identified the isoquinoline alkaloids sanguinarine and berberine, among others, and an extract, sanguinaria, which shows anticancer activities. They are also antiseptic and act as local anesthetics. Development of the commercial product Viadent has brought to the market toothpastes, mouthwashes, and rinses that contain plaque-inhibiting sanguinaria extract. It is fascinating to contemplate what future products will come, in part, from our native plants and indigenous herbalism.

Cautions: Each plant is a complex "chemical factory" and should be respected as such and approached with caution. Bloodroot sap is caustic.

Growth needs and propagation: Easily cultivated in the garden, bloodroot is quite rewarding for its beauty and resilience. This perennial herb does most of its growing in early spring, when it prospers in full sun. Otherwise it can grow in sun or shade. Rich, moist, well-drained soil is best, and a thin mulch covering of leaves is best in winter.

Bloodroot can be readily propagated from seeds and root division in late summer and fall. Wear gloves. Collect the fresh, ripe seeds from the swollen pods and spread and plant immediately before they dry out. Plant them thinly, directly where you want them to grow next year. Cover them with about an inch of humus-enriched compost. Dig up mature roots and break or cut off pieces with a bud and roots attached. Plant these at least an inch deep, covering them with topsoil containing humus, well patted down. Top-dress with well-rotted leaf mulch. Plants from rhizome divisions may flower the following year; plants from seeds may take three years to flower. Wash hands well after planting bloodroot.

Companions: American wild ginger, ginseng, purple trillium, hepatica, foamflower, false Solomon's seal, eastern columbine, and Dutchman's breeches are all favorable companions for bloodroot.

BLUEBERRY

Vaccinium angustifolium
Ericaceae (heath family)

The genus *Vaccinium* includes blueberries, cranberries, huckleberries, and bilberries—in all, perhaps 150 species of deciduous and evergreen shrubs or vines native to the Northern Hemisphere. *Vaccinium,* like "vaccine," seems to derive from the Latin word for "cow," but the reason for its choice remains unclear. Many are grown for their prized edible fruits and medicinal

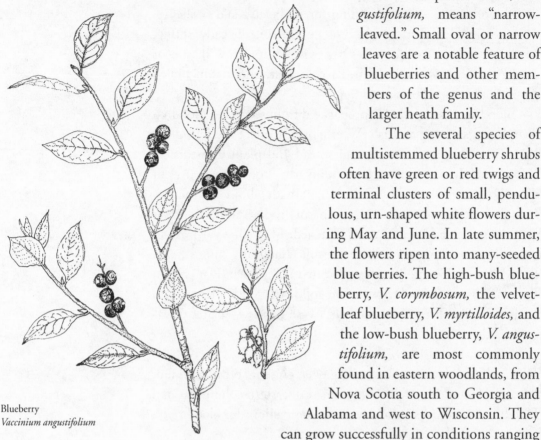

Blueberry
Vaccinium angustifolium

leaves. The species name, *angustifolium,* means "narrow-leaved." Small oval or narrow leaves are a notable feature of blueberries and other members of the genus and the larger heath family.

The several species of multistemmed blueberry shrubs often have green or red twigs and terminal clusters of small, pendulous, urn-shaped white flowers during May and June. In late summer, the flowers ripen into many-seeded blue berries. The high-bush blueberry, *V. corymbosum,* the velvet-leaf blueberry, *V. myrtilloides,* and the low-bush blueberry, *V. angustifolium,* are most commonly found in eastern woodlands, from Nova Scotia south to Georgia and Alabama and west to Wisconsin. They can grow successfully in conditions ranging from swamps to dry upland woods. All three have been cultivated for garden enjoyment, and hybrids from these species are some of the best-bearing, winter-hardy blueberry shrubs offered for gardeners across the country.

Traditional uses: *Uwada'hio'ni'*—"plenty of berries"—is the Cayuga term for late summer when ripe berries abound, especially the delicious blueberries. The Oneida called blueberries and huckleberries "the early berries," *uhia'dji' niyuhu'ndagwaha,* and picked them in great numbers, collecting them in berry baskets. To help preserve the tart wild fruits, they lined their wood-splint baskets and bark buckets with large basswood leaves or fern fronds. Tribal people in the Northeast also used aromatic sweet-fern leaves and hay-scented fern fronds for this purpose. In years of abundance, berries were dried, and even smoked, to preserve them. Some were mashed into berry cakes and dried on large basswood and sycamore leaves in the sun or beside the fire, to be rehydrated later in soups, stews, or hot maple syrup water.

Native people drew benefits from blueberry shrubs well beyond the season of ripe fruits, collecting the small mature blueberry leaves before they reddened and fell from their shrubs in autumn. Blueberry leaf teas are mineral-rich astringents that were used to wash the skin and hair. They were also drunk to prevent the formation of bladder or kidney stones. Many tribes considered the blueberry leaf teas to be "blood purifiers" because of the tonic effect on the general digestive system. Algonquian Indians used blueberry leaves in teas to treat colic and stomach cramps and painful menstruation, as well as to aid uterine contractions during childbirth. Dried leaves were smudged and burned in kinnikinnik mixtures (and alone), and the smoke inhaled to clear congestion and treat nosebleed.

Modern uses: Blueberry leaf tea continues in use as a diabetes treatment, esteemed by many native herbalists, and also to treat bladder and kidney complaints. Its diuretic and astringent benefits make it a valuable choice for relieving urinary tract infections. This tea is also a helpful gargle to soothe swollen glands, sore throats, or mouth sores, and strong blueberry leaf teas (decoctions) are valued as antiseptic skin washes and to treat everything from poison ivy rashes to muscle cramps and insect and spider bites.

Along with huckleberries and bilberries, blueberries contain valuable compounds called anthocyanosides and arbutin. The first helps to treat, and even prevent, cataracts as well as aiding general eyesight; and the second helps to treat yeast infections. Some studies show that eating these berries in moderation helps to protect the stomach against ulcers by strengthening the stomach lining. Blueberries' compound oligomeric procyanidins (OPCs) have anti-inflammatory benefits that may relieve some symptoms of multiple sclerosis. The dried fruits have concentrations of their inherent tannins and pectin, making them valuable treatments for diarrhea.

Blueberries are high in vitamin C and are favored as healing antioxidants.

Growth needs and propagation: Most blueberry shrubs thrive in sandy or peaty, acidic soils, though some will do well in moist rich earth. As acid-loving perennials, most varieties will perform best if fed a soil acidifier. They prefer full sun or open shade for healthiest growth.

It is best to have at least two or three blueberry shrubs in the medicine wheel garden to assure good cross-pollination for maximum fruits. Plant them two or three feet apart, depending upon size and species, and set them in a small triangle. Excellent new hybrid varieties that bloom and bear fruits early to late in the season are available, as well as fine dwarf low-bush (about eight inches tall) and stunning high-bush varieties (about three to four feet tall).

Velvetleaf blueberry, *V. myrtilloides,* makes a colorful show in the garden in autumn, when its oval, velvety leaves, which can grow two inches long, turn vibrant red. This low shrub favors moist, acid soil and will grow up to three feet tall and develop a dense root system. If allowed to, it can generate a colony of numerous additional shrubs.

BLUE COHOSH

Caulophyllum thalictroides
Ranunculaceae (buttercup family)

Blue cohosh, a much less toxic plant than red or white cohosh, favors moist, rich woodlands from New Brunswick to Manitoba and southward to Alabama and Arkansas. It can grow two to three feet tall. A bluish stem bearing a single bluish-green, fine-cut leaf emerges in spring and divides into three small, oval, three-lobed, notched leaflets. Large blue berrylike seeds follow spires of clustered tiny greenish-yellow flowers in spring to late summer. Native people sometimes roasted these berries to make a coffeelike beverage, while the large powerful rhizomes and roots were and are sought in early spring and late fall for specific herbal medicines.

Traditional uses: The Omaha-Ponca called blue cohosh *zhu-nakada-tanga-maka,* meaning "great fever medicine," as they considered it the most effective treatment for fever. They made a strong decoction of the root to sip for colds, flu, and other illnesses accompanied by high fever. The thick, knotty rhizome and roots were dug in late fall after a killing frost, then dried and ground into a fine powder. The root tea also served to treat profuse menstruation, abdominal cramps, and urinary tract infections.

Today, blue cohosh is also called blue ginseng, squaw-root, and papoose root—names that indicate its strengthening properties as a parturient (an aid in childbirth), especially during the last two weeks of pregnancy.

Modern uses: Contemporary herbalists use blue cohosh root teas and tinctures to treat rheumatism and bronchitis. Tests showing antispasmodic properties in the roots confirm its beneficial effect. Root glycosides (steroidal saponins) are also responsible for the uterine-stimulant activity—this is the reason why this herb should be taken only during labor or the last two weeks of pregnancy, never earlier. Indeed, current medical uses for blue cohosh are remarkably similar to Native American traditional uses. Taken as a contraceptive and to treat genitourinary conditions, its key actions are diuretic, anti-inflammatory, anti-

Blue cohosh
Caulophyllum thalictroides

spasmodic, to promote menstrual flow, and as a uterine tonic and antirheumatic.

Cautions: This plant should be avoided during the first thirty-eight weeks of pregnancy because it can cause abortion. The plant can be a skin irritant to those with sensitive skin. The root powder can be caustic and irritating to the mucous membranes.

Growth needs and propagation: Blue cohosh prefers rich, moist, well-drained soil improved with humus. It will grow well in shade and dappled shade. New plants can be easily started from seed by planting the seeds as they become fully ripe, in the late summer. Plant them outdoors or layered in cold propagation trays (propagation trays kept in a refrigerator or cold cellar). Most take a year to germinate. Cultivation is easiest from root division. Divide healthy rhizomes in the fall or early spring, planting each new division about six inches deep in rich, moist earth and firming the earth well over them. New plants should appear and bloom the following year.

Companions: Blue cohosh provides good company for elder-berry, bayberry, bearberry, maidenhair fern, and hellebore. This perennial will mature to make handsome colonies with attractive foliage, spring blooms, and pale-blue summer berries. It thrives in various shade garden settings.

BLUE FLAG

Iris versicolor
Iridaceae (iris family)

These tall, beautiful irises are also known as flags because of their long, narrow leaves—like the banners carried by medieval knights. Their intricate multicolored blossoms explain the name iris: in Greek mythology, Iris was the goddess of the rainbow and served as a messenger to the gods. *Versicolor* means "variously colored." The mature long leaves of this plant were collected and dried to be woven into baskets and rush seats and backs for chairs. The iris blossom, sometimes called fleur-de-lis, served as the model for the emblem of French royalty.

What an incredible repertoire of beauty and meaning come together in our native flags! In many northeastern towns and villages there is a Flag Swamp Road, indicating an old region where they grew.

The iris family embraces about fifteen hundred species in almost sixty genera, distributed in temperate and tropical regions, and more than two hundred species native to northern temperate zones. Many gardeners grow colorful iris varieties. These were my grandmother's favorite flowers in Tennessee.

Blue flag is also called water flag, poison flag, and liver lily. In Middle English, the word *flagge* referred to a rush or reed, and this attractive native wildflower flourishes in marshes and wet meadows as well as in drier meadows. It grows from Labrador to Manitoba; James Bay, Ontario, south to Virginia; and west through Ohio to Wisconsin and Minnesota. The coastal slender blue flag, *Iris prismatica,* has very narrow, grasslike leaves only a quarter inch wide. A smaller southern blue flag, *I. virginica,* which rarely reaches two feet tall, grows from Virginia to Florida and west to Texas in wetlands. These irises can grow in ever-enlarging, cosmopolitan groups. White varieties also occur near blue colonies.

Close relatives are the more diminutive blue-eyed grass, *Sisyrinchium angustifolium* and *S. montanum.* These ancient American Indian medicinals are widespread across North Amer-

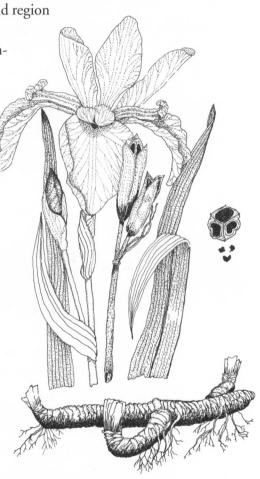

Blue flag
Iris versicolor

ica. The tall, rugged yellow flag, *I. pseudacorus,* introduced from Europe, escaped cultivation and also spread widely. It, too, has native medicinal uses.

The tall, swordlike grayish-green leaves of blue flags arise from sturdy, creeping rootstocks. From May to July, these irises flaunt their violet to pale blue blossoms with attractive yellow, green, or white veins and markings on the large recurved petals (sepals). The flowers can be two to four inches wide, sometimes branched, atop sturdy stalks. In late summer the flowers ripen into erect three-lobed green capsules filled with dark seeds. These woody iris pods mature to dark brown, with shiny interior chambers (exposed when they open), and stand tall through winter snowstorms to mark the thick rhizomes underground. The woody pods are considered "climax flowers," or final flowers, and are often gathered for winter bouquets.

Traditional uses: Blue flag has a long history of healing uses among the many Native American tribes throughout its range. The rhizomes, though extremely poisonous, were valued root medicines among Eastern Woodland Indians and many others. They were dried and used in small amounts both topically or internally, very diluted, and were included in compounds and formulas to treat a variety of disorders from indigestion to rheumatism.

Some tribes planted blue flag near their dwellings and villages among other important medicinals. For example, William Bartram (1791) recorded the cultivation of "little plantations" of blue flag near the Creek Indian town of Attasse. The Delaware made a root medicine from blue flag for treating rheumatism, scrofula (glandular, lymphatic, and respiratory infections), and liver and kidney disorders. The Mohegans pulverized the root for an external pain-relief poultice, bound by mixing it with flour. The Seneca used the rhizomes for a physic, to treat problems of menses, and to help induce labor, and Creek Indians used them in decoctions taken as strong cathartics during times of fasting and grieving.

Modern uses: Today, herbalists recommend blue flag as a blood purifier and to treat skin problems. The dried rhizome, tinctured for use in dilute formulas, also aids digestion. Decoctions of the rhizome are worked into healing salves and creams for skin care. In small doses, blue flag works to detoxify the body by increasing urination and bile production. It acts with a mild laxative effect as well as the internal cleansing action, helping to treat chronic skin diseases such as acne and eczema. It especially treats gallbladder problems and constipation, which contribute to these skin conditions. Blue flag in small doses will relieve nausea and vomiting, but in large doses it causes these reactions. Many cautions are attached to the use of this powerful healing herb.

Cautions: Blue flag is toxic and should not be used for self-medication. People with skin sensitivities may develop a rash after touching the rootstocks, so wear gloves and wash your hands immediately after handling the rhizomes. *Do not take during pregnancy.*

Growth needs and propagation: The foliage and blooms of blue flag are very desirable in the medicine wheel garden, especially in the blue section. The winter forms, too, are quite attractive and tantalize the songbirds that come for the seeds. After the plants have finished flowering in late summer, cut the leaves back to about four to eight inches and divide the rhizomes with a sharp knife or shovel. Plant each piece of rhizome, with attached leaf clump, horizontally just beneath the soil and pat it down well. The healthiest divisions will flower the next year.

Seeds can easily be collected from the dried, mature pods as soon as they split open. Sow the seeds immediately about one-third of an inch deep in the desired location outdoors where they can overwinter and germinate in the spring. It will take about three years for plants to mature and flower from seeds. Once established, blue flag will spread and self-seed naturally until you get a large colony.

Companions: Blue flag grows well in most locations and keeps good company with cardinal flower and jack-in-the-pulpit and yarrow, as they seem to strengthen one another. This combination gives you a flowery red, white, and blue.

Eupatorium perfoliatum
Asteraceae (sunflower or aster family)

Infusions of this native perennial herb were widely used in past centuries to treat influenza (flu), then known as "breakbone fever" because of its debilitating effects—hence the common name boneset. White settlers on the continent learned of its uses very early from Native Americans.

Mithridates Eupator (134–63 B.C.), Greek king of Pontus, inspired the genus name; he was the first person noted to have used a plant of this genus to treat liver complaints. Our plants continue to bring ancient history to life. The species name, *perfoliatum,* meaning "through the leaf," reflects an interesting feature of this species: clasping leaves joined around the plant stem, which appears to pierce right through them.

Boneset is an erect, attractive herb growing from one to five feet tall. The unique opposite leaves are long, slender, spear-shaped blades that radiate north-south and east-west up the fuzzy stems. Atop the main stem, dense, flat-topped clusters of small white flowers bloom from July until October in many regions. This native of North America grows from Quebec to Manitoba, south to Florida and Texas, and west into Minnesota, Oklahoma, and Nebraska. Other North American natives in this family of five hundred or more species of perennial herbs include white snakeroot, *Eupatorium rugosum,* and sweet joe-pye weed, *E. purpureum,* along with joe-pye weed or smoke weed, *E. maculatum.* Each of these species is fairly common in the eastern United States and adapts well to the garden. Many other species are native to tropical America.

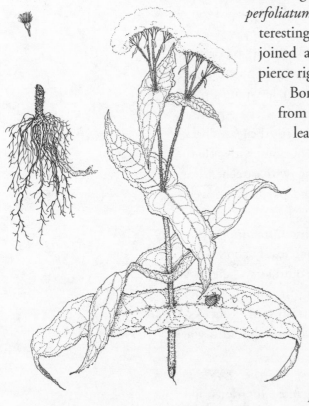

Boneset
Eupatorium perfoliatum

Traditional uses: Boneset is also known as wild sage, Indian sage, feverwort, thoroughwort, and agueweed. Indians must have had many different names for it, too, as various tribes used it to treat numerous common problems. They used the entire plant as a tonic and stimulant, and the leaves and blossoms as emetics and to kill parasites.

A strong boneset tea served the Meskwaki Indians as a snakebite cure; the Seneca and Mohegans used it as a tonic. For many years, physicians used boneset tea as a substitute for quinine to treat fever. Zuni Indians in New Mexico use the related species *E. occidentale* to treat rheumatism and arthritis as well as other joint pains. Many American Indian tribes used boneset infusions to treat cold, flu, fever, rheumatism, and arthritic problems.

Modern uses: Boneset shows valuable immune system stimulation. A hot infusion of boneset will relieve symptoms of the common cold and helps to reduce a fever. Boneset tea has been used as a tonic and laxative; it also relieves rheumatism, as well as some skin conditions. Boneset's upper plant parts, principally blossoms, stems, and leaves, are the choice botanicals used medicinally. A bitter drink, boneset has antibiotic properties and is being explored for anticancer activities.

Cautions: Boneset can be toxic if taken in excessive doses. It can be emetic and laxative in large doses and could be harmful to the liver.

Growth needs and propagation: Boneset prefers moist, rich earth and open sun to partial shade. It will accommodate well to most garden situations. It is best propagated by cuttings and root divisions in late summer and fall. These can be started in a greenhouse or indoors and then moved outside into the garden. Many species in this family have been cultivated for show gardens, especially the lovely ageratums and stevia, the Mexican sweet herb.

Companions: Boneset grows well with cardinal flower, maidenhair fern, sweet flag, goldthread, hepatica, and Indian turnip. It will also accompany elderberry, hellebore, and angelica in the medicine wheel garden.

There is probably no plant in American domestic practice that has more extensive or frequent use than this. The attic, or woodshed, of almost every country farmhouse has its bunch of dried herbs hanging, tops downward from the rafters during the whole year, ready for immediate use should some member of the family, or that of a neighbor, be taken with a cold.

—Charles Millspaugh, author of *American Medicinal Plants,* 1892

BUTTERFLY WEED

Asclepias tuberosa
Asclepiadaceae (milkweed family)

Both the family and genus of this stunning herb are named for the Greek god of medicine, Asklepios. The species name, *tuberosa*, means "full of swellings or knobs" and describes the enlarged root system characteristic of this plant. The milkweed family is noted for both toxic and healing properties. The distinguishing feature of many members of this family is a milky sap that oozes out when plant parts are broken.

Each of the two hundred or so species of perennial herbs in this family, mostly native to North America and Africa, draws most butterflies and some hummingbirds to their blossoms, as well as many other insect pollinators. Some very distinctive species are found throughout the Americas, and many of these make beautiful additions to the medicine wheel garden.

Also known as pleurisy root, Choctaw root, Indian paintbrush, and orange swallowwort, butterfly weed will grow up to three feet tall from its stout, woody rootstock. This herb prospers in dry, sandy earth and grows naturally from southern Ontario through New England south to Florida and west to Texas, Arizona, and Colorado. Its lance-shaped leaves crowd along a slightly hairy stalk. Clusters of showy, bright yellow-orange flowers bloom from May through September in most of these areas. The vibrant flowers draw many butterflies for the nectar.

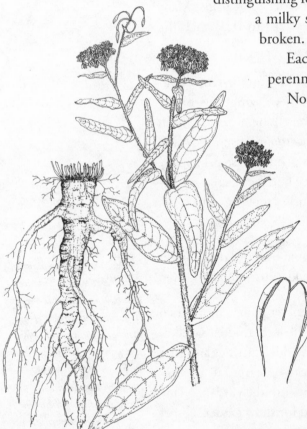

Butterfly Weed
Asclepias tuberosa

Common milkweed, *Asclepias syriaca,* has an equally broad range and grows up to six feet tall. The dense cluster of white to pale pink flowers emits a heavenly fragrance. All plant parts are poisonous except for the very young spears, blossoms, and very young pods. The toxic substances are cardiotonic glycosides. The monarch butterfly, which depends completely on the milkweeds for food, is protected by these toxins because they render it inedible by predators. Native Americans used these properties to treat heart problems and numerous other health needs.

Horsetail milkweed, *A. verticillata,* grows to almost three feet tall through the central and eastern United States, and the southern antelope milkweed, *A. viridifolia,* grows up to five feet tall from Massachusetts to Georgia and west to Arizona and New Mexico. The striking blossoms of these plants, pale green to whitish gold, make them most appealing for cultivation in the medicine wheel garden.

Traditional uses: Butterfly weed was one of the most important Menomini medicines. They used the roots as wound dressings and for many other remedies, often mixing the roots with other botanicals in particular formulas. Penobscot Indians used them as cold medicines and as a dressing for sores. The Omaha Indians used this plant as one of their sacred medicines in the Shell Society. Special ceremonies accompanied the digging, consecration, and preparation of the roots over a four-day period. Many tribes gathered and steamed the blossoms to eat for food and medicines. This was a special plant for dreaming and magic.

Modern uses: Herbalists rarely use butterfly weed today because of its highly toxic properties. It is on the endangered species list in many states and is being widely propagated as a showy ornamental.

Cautions: Poisonous if taken in large doses.

Growth needs and propagation: Butterfly weed grows well in most soils and propagates readily from seed and root divisions. Follow traditional methods for each.

We are ruled by the examples set for us by all our relations of the Creator. Our leaders take responsibility for the care and well-being of all the people. They are to see that no one is hungry when others are well-fed, and no one is cold when others are warm. The strong ones are to protect the weak ones, and all are to respect the wisdom and experience of the elders.

—Nanepashemet, the late Wampanoag artist and historian, 1983

Companions: Chili peppers, blue flag, bayberry, and evening primrose are good companions for butterfly weed.

CARDINAL FLOWER AND OTHER LOBELIAS

Lobelia cardinalis

Campanulaceae (bellflower family), subfamily Lobeliaceae (lobelias)

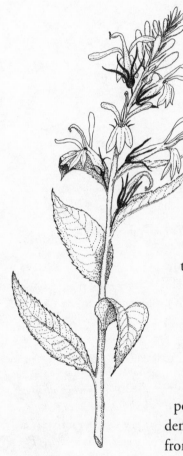

Cardinal flower
Lobelia cardinalis

With its spires of brilliant crimson tubular flowers waving in the breeze, like the flash of a male cardinal in flight, the cardinal flower is aptly named. Hummingbirds and swallowtail butterflies frequently visit these vivid flowers, the most striking blooms of our native lobelias. The name lobelia honors a Flemish physician and herbalist, Mathieu de Lobel (1538–1616). The Latin *cardinalis,* meaning "principal," was first extended to describe the principal dignitaries of the Catholic Church and then the distinctive red color that cardinals wear. Applying the same word to a brilliant red bird and flower was only another short step.

Indian red is another common name for this striking perennial, which can grow three feet tall. These plants, with handsome dark green foliage beneath their regal bloom spires, are happy in moist soil, especially around ponds and marshes, yet the species adapts well to normal garden conditions. Cardinal flower is found growing in the wild from New Brunswick south to Florida and East Texas, and west as far as California.

The genus *Lobelia* includes about 375 species native to warm, temperate, and tropical regions. Most are native perennials and annuals, extensively cultivated, with distinctive flowers attractive to butterflies and hummingbirds seeking nectar. Several species are noted drug plants today, and Native Americans probably used most of the lobelias throughout their range for healing purposes.

Traditional uses: Cherokee and Iroquois Indians used strong teas made from cardinal flower roots to treat syphilis, typhoid fever, and stomach problems. Many tribal medicine people also used leaf teas from this herb as nerve tonics and to treat cramps. The leaves and blossoms were dried for use in medicinal smoking mixtures to stimulate the heart. The herb was also extensively included in "love medicines" and "love potions" employed by many different tribes. The intense red was held sacred and symbolic of the heart and love.

Indians smoked the dried leaves of the related Indian tobacco, *L. inflata,* to treat asthma, bronchitis, and sore throat and to enhance the actions of other herbs. This finely hairy native annual blooms with white to pale blue flowers in spires that can reach six to eight inches high and ripen into small, inflated seedpods after summer. Self-sowing, it is widespread across eastern fields and open woods from Nova Scotia to Saskatchewan and south to Georgia, Louisiana, and Arkansas.

Great lobelia, or blue cardinal flower, *L. siphilitica,* is another related herb long used by Indians for medicinal purposes. Centuries ago, they made herbal root decoctions (strong teas) to treat syphilis, while leaf teas served to treat colds, headaches, and stomach problems. Leaves were poulticed on sores and used as wound dressings and smoked to treat respiratory ailments. The slim, attractive perennial herb, which can top five feet tall, puts forth blue-lavender flowers tightly clustered along the bloom spire. It favors stream banks and open meadows from Maine to North Carolina and westward into Mississippi, Arkansas, and Minnesota.

As with other lobelia relatives, the leaves, stems, and blossoms of pale-spike lobelia, *L. spicata,* were dried and smoked to treat respiratory and circulatory problems. Indians also used the whole plant to make medicinal skin washes to treat sores and wounds, and it was drunk as an emetic. This perennial herb with pale blue to whitish flowers grows to almost four feet tall in fields and meadows throughout the region from New Brunswick to Minnesota and southeast to Georgia. Lobelias' pale blue flowers were believed to have magical properties, such as the ability to ward off ghosts.

Modern uses: Contemporary herbalists continue to use lobelias in many of the traditional Native American applications. Upper parts of Indian tobacco, *L. inflata,* the primary medicinal herb, are used in tinctures, tablets, and infusions. It yields several substances similar to nicotine, which has led herbalists to use lobelia to help patients give up smoking. Lobeline, one of fourteen alkaloids present in *L. inflata,* goes into commercial antismoking lozenges, chewing gums, and patches. Lobelia is also valued as a respiratory treatment, especially for bronchial asthma and chronic bronchitis. It relaxes the muscles of the smaller bronchial tubes, opening the airways and stimulating breathing. Combined with cayenne pepper, lobelia has been used as a chest and sinus rub.

Cautions: Lobelias are toxic and can act as strong emetics. Do not use them to self-medicate.

A person who is suffering sleeps on lobelia to learn the cause of his suffering. Put it under your pillow at night and dream about your sickness during the night to discover what is wrong with you. Only the sick person does this and the next morning he will know what medicine to use.

—Jemima Gibson, Cayuga herbalist, Six Nations Reserve, Canada, 1914

Growth needs and propagation: Cardinal flower thrives in rich, moist soils and full to partial sun. It prefers slightly acidic to neutral soil and should be mulched in winter, especially in northern areas. The other species of lobelia will tolerate mixed soil types and dry conditions, and they like full sun. They are remarkably enduring and rugged. All, cardinal flower included, are hardy plants that flower from midsummer into early fall, when they set seeds. Sow the tiny seeds in humus-rich soil and cover them with a thin layer of mulch. They need to overwinter outdoors for maximum hardiness. Carefully remove the mulch in spring. Plants from seed will usually flower in the second year.

Easy propagation by stem layering and root division is also possible, the latter best done in early spring. Set the roots almost a foot apart with the new buds just at the soil surface. Keep the soil moist. Stem layering is easiest to accomplish in midsummer. Carefully bend the stem over until it touches the ground. Stake it, cover a portion of the upper stem with a half inch of soil, and keep this moist. New shoots will form and emerge; the stem can be cut between the new shoots in the fall.

Companions: Great companion plants are blue flag and sweet flag as well as elderberry shrubs. Angelica and heal-all also go well with lobelias in the garden.

CHILI PEPPER

Capsicum frutescens
Solanaceae (nightshade family)

Called cayenne and Tabasco pepper, this hot pepper plant is the kissing cousin of the sweet, or bell, peppers, *Capsicum annuum.* The genus name comes from Latin *capsa,* meaning "box," for the podlike fruits. The species name, also from Latin, means "bearing fruit." Yielding some of the world's best-known spices, *Capsicum* embraces about twenty species, all native to tropical America.

The chili originated more than three thousand years ago, yet its exact birthplace is still a mystery. Prehistoric people greatly predating these cultures first began cultivating wild chili peppers in regions of today's Mexico and Central America. The Spanish "discovery" of these amazing New World plants led to revolutionizing foods and medicines worldwide. Now more chilis are produced and eaten than any other seasoning in the world.

Long before the Spanish arrived, Mayan and Aztec Indians and their ancestors were growing diverse peppers for myriad uses,

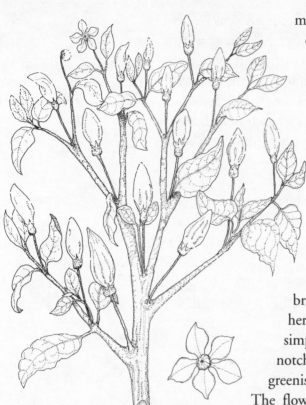

Chili pepper
Capsicum frutescens var. *tabasco*

many noted in pictures and glyphs of Mayan codices. After Diego Alvarez Chanca, a physician accompanying Columbus's second voyage in 1494, first described these spice-laden fruits for Europeans, they were carried on Spanish and Portuguese voyages of trade and exploration and became essential plants from Europe and Africa to eastern Asia. Chili peppers are grown in warm climates around the world and the majority of the world's capsaicin now comes from Japan and India.

The simple leaves of these multi-branched, shrubby perennial (and annual) herbs are alternate, oval, and smooth. The simple flowers, which appear in the forked notches of the plants' stems, are usually white or greenish-white, and some are tinged with violet. The flowers can appear as solitary blooms or in groups of two or three. Behind the pollinated flowers, the ovary swells into a shiny green, podlike, many-seeded berry, which ripens to become red, orange, yellow, or purple. This fruit varies in size, shape, and pungency with each different species and variety. Chili pepper plants can grow up to two or three feet tall, though many are much smaller. Some are grown as ornamentals with purple blossoms and purple chili pods.

Traditional uses: Early South and Central American cultures used chilis medicinally to treat toothaches, and to cure colic and colds (and as a preventative). Chilis, like cocoa beans, were also used as currency among many southern tribes. The Aztec mixed chili peppers with wild honey, spirulina (a blue-green alga), and cornmeal to make ceremonial foods. Throughout the desert Southwest, these chilis were favored native foods and medicines. Many tribes used chili peppers to stimulate circulation and ease headaches, reduce inflammation from swollen joints, and in countless ceremonial items.

Modern uses: Modern herbalists and physicians continue to recognize the virtues of chili peppers and their principal ingredient, capsaicin (also capsicine). The peppery, reddish-brown liquid obtained from the genus *Capsicum* is used in topical preparations for relief from pain (as an irritant, it blocks the transmission of other pain signals). It is also widely used in flavoring vinegars, oil, and other foods. Cayenne is so popular in Mexico, where it originated, that it even serves to flavor ice cream!

A pinch of ground cayenne in water is an excellent gargle for sore throats, and drinking this mixture can relieve both diarrhea and headaches. Taken internally, cayenne and chili pepper can help relieve gas, stimulate digestion, and relieve/prevent some stomach and intestinal infections. They also stimulate the body's metabolism. Extracts of these peppers applied to the skin provide mild pain relief and improve the blood flow to the affected parts. This virtue makes capsaicin a key ingredient in many liniments and creams. Red-hot chili peppers and cayenne are inhospitable environments for bacteria, so their extracts have been used as antibacterial agents with great success.

Cautions: When handling these plants, take care not to rub your eyes or any sensitive areas of your body, as you could experience mild to caustic irritations. Be especially careful if you have any open cuts on your hands.

Growth needs and propagation: Chili peppers grow well in full sun and enriched soil. They are grown easily from seed and are usually treated as annuals in most regions. You can also purchase healthy young plants from a nearby nursery.

Companions: Chili peppers are good company for many of the sun-loving plants in the medicine wheel garden. Chilis grow well alongside yarrow, arnica, butterfly weed, and angel's trumpet.

Echinacea angustifolia
Compositae (daisy family)

The Greek word *echinos* described two spiny animals, the hedgehog and the sea urchin. The genus name, *echinacea,* retains the "spiny" idea of this word, which early naturalists thought accurately described the plant's ripe, rounded spiny seed head. The species name *angustifolia* simply means "narrow-leaved."

There are four species in the genus *Echinacea* of large, coarse, rough-hairy perennial herbs native to North America. Now rarely found in the wild, the easternmost plant in this group, *E. tennesseeiensis,* is on the endangered-species list because of overharvesting. The three remaining species are fairly widespread in the wild and even more so among perennial gardeners and herbalists.

Prairie coneflower or narrow-leaved coneflower, *E. angustifolia,* is a deep-taprooted wildflower found across the prairies from Manitoba and Saskatchewan south to Oklahoma and Texas. Pale to deep magenta-purple daisylike flowers with narrow rays surround a prominent cone-shaped disk, rising above stiff, hairy, lance-shaped leaves. At maturity this plant can reach two feet in height.

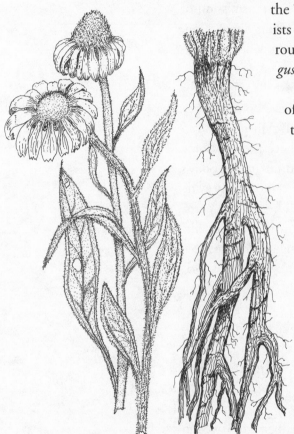

Echinacea
Echinacea angustifolia

Purple coneflower, *E. purpurea,* shares many of these same attributes, and when mature can stand two to three feet tall, blooming throughout the summer. It grows in the wild across the middle prairie regions from Michigan south to Oklahoma and Texas. These two species are cultivated broadly as showy wildflowers in many states and farmed to supply the growing health care industry. Very similar to these species, the pale purple coneflower, *E. pallida,* often hybridizes with the narrow-leaved cone-flower, and has much the same uses medicinally. Found across the midprairie regions from Wisconsin and Minnesota to Arkansas and eastern Oklahoma, this stout perennial can reach three feet tall with maturity and, like the other species, is widely cultivated. Each species also has hybrid white flower varieties.

Traditional uses: Indians used all plant parts of narrow-leaved coneflower for foods and medicines, and it was and is one of their most often used wild herbs for treating colds, flu, cancers, toothache, spider bites, and snakebite. They also used the chewed roots of purple coneflower to treat chronic inflammations and infections. Root and leaf teas and decoctions have long proven popular and reliable treatments for weakened immune systems.

Modern uses: Following traditional practices, many of us take some form of echinacea preparations periodically to boost or strengthen our immune system. Modern herbalists and health care practitioners consider echinacea the most important immune stimulant in Western herbal medicine. It helps fight infections of all kinds, particularly colds, flu, respiratory problems, and skin disorders. Especially valuable for chronic fatigue syndrome (CFS) and viral illnesses, it is also a useful remedy for asthma and other types of allergies. Scientific research confirms the remarkable health benefits of these plants. More than two hundred pharmaceutical preparations are made from them in Germany, including extracts, salves, tinctures, and pills.

Cautions: Do not take this herb if you suffer with MS (multiple sclerosis) or other autoimmune disorders. Do not take it regularly in any case; use echinacea supplements only when the need arises, or your immune system might grow dependent upon this additional assistance.

Growth needs and propagation: The purple and narrow-leaved coneflower species are perhaps the most distinctive and recognizable native healing herbs. These rugged perennials like most soil types and

In every region of the Americas the people tell the story of the other worlds which came and went, which were swallowed up by misfortune and catastrophe, from which the four-legged and two-legged beings fled. These tales of beginnings are at the core of all Indian rituals—they tell of other suns and other moons and of a long and difficult migration.
—Jamake Highwater, 1983, author of American Indian Art

full sun. They will increase by division and by seeds sown in the garden in late summer and fall. Start with healthy plants purchased from a nursery or grower who is cultivating native wildflowers.

Companions: Echinacea grows well with other sun-loving herbs in the medicine wheel garden, especially heal-all, chili peppers, evening primrose, and yarrow.

ELDERBERRY

Sambucus canadensis
Caprifoliaceae (honeysuckle family)

Elderberry
Sambucus canadensis

American elderberry, sweet elderberry, and elder are some common names for this native deciduous shrub. The genus name may come from the Greek word *sambuke,* for a musical instrument that was once made of elder wood. For centuries elderberry has been used to heal the body, mind, and spirit through its gifts of medicines and charms. The species name, *canadensis,* denotes Canada or the Northeast, where this plant was first identified.

Sambucus embraces about twenty species of shrubs and small trees with pithy stems that grow mainly in temperate and subtropical regions. In North America there are perhaps four species, which native populations used extensively for foods and medicines.

Elderberry grows from three to twelve feet tall in moist, rich soil and ranges from Nova Scotia to Georgia, west to Texas, and north to Manitoba. It has opposite toothed, feather-like leaves and creamy white spring flowers that form broad wheel-like, flat-topped clusters. The flowers ripen in late summer to clusters of juicy blue-black berries.

The American red elderberry, *S. pubens,* grows in the East, and the Pacific coast red elderberry, *S. callicarpa,* is found in the West along with the larger blue elderberry, *S. caerulea,* which can grow to twenty feet tall. All are attractive ornamentals, frequently cultivated in mass plantings for their spring blossoms and autumn fruits. All were also important American Indian medicinals. The red-berried elders are more toxic than the blue elderberry.

Traditional uses: Indians ate the elderberries ripe and dried, and the spring blossoms were used in foods and steeped into restorative teas and salves. Teas made from the inner bark served as a strong laxative, emetic, headache remedy, and diuretic; on the skin it was a valuable treatment for eczema, swellings, and skin eruptions. The Onondaga used the inner bark as an emetic to counter poisoning; it was also used to treat toothaches. The inner bark was also pounded and poulticed on cuts, burns, and sores, and on newborns' navels, as it provided pain relief and reduced swelling. The Illinois and Miami Indians used strong root-bark decoctions to treat people with debilities and general weakness. Elderberry syrup was a treatment for coughs, colds, and flu.

Indians made hunting whistles and courting flutes from the dense, creamy white wood; the stems have a fibrous pith that can be easily hollowed out. Some tribes carved spiles for tapping sugar maple trees from elderberry, as well as from sumac wood. Indian boys fashioned blowguns from elderberry stems.

As they moved to the New World, our European ancestors brought the European elder, *S. nigra,* because of its vital importance in their traditional lifeways. Many believed that the elderberry was imbued with special spirits and powers. Planting an elderberry shrub touching the house was considered a deterrent to witches and ghosts, preventing them from appearing or harming the inhabitants. Our Scandinavian forebears thought that tying a cross of elderberry sticks to the head of the bed would prevent bad dreams and nightmares. They used the fresh and dried leaves in the garden around vegetables to keep away mice and insects and prevent fungal damage to their garden crops, and they made wines and vinegars from the ripe fruits and blossoms and salves from the inner bark and flowers.

Modern uses: Modern herbalists continue to recommend the virtues of elderberry. The spring flowers and ripe berries are used as foods, flavorings, wines, tisanes (of blossoms), and teas (of leaves). They are worked into a variety of syrups, infusions, tinctures, and teas to treat coughs, colds, arthritis, congestion, and allergies. People take elderberry syrup and capsules to strengthen the eyes.

Cautions: The bark, roots, leaves, and unripe fruits of elderberry are toxic. Only the blossoms and ripe berries are edible.

Growth needs and propagation: Elderberry thrives in rich, moist soil with good mulch. It is easily cultivated from seed, cuttings, and some sucker growth, which can be cut off and rooted. For success, follow traditional methods. It is easiest to purchase healthy young specimens from nursery stock.

The well-developed root of the mature elderberry shrub can spread underground, sending up new shoots nearby. This habit allows the elderberry to establish groves in likely areas. Using a sharp shovel, you can dig out these "new starts" and create an elderberry grove elsewhere on your property, or give new plants to friends for their medicine wheel gardens.

Companions: Elderberry grows happily with shade-loving herbs in the medicine wheel garden, as it provides the shade. Blue cohosh, bearberry, pennyroyal, and goldenseal are good companions.

EVENING PRIMROSE

Oenothera biennis
Onagraceae (evening primrose family)

Oenothera is named for an herb to induce sleep described in *Historia Naturalis,* a work compiled by the Roman scholar Pliny the Elder (A.D. 23–79) that remained a standard reference for many centuries. The common name, evening primrose, reflects this plant's habit of blooming just at sundown, as evening begins. Its species name, *biennis,* means "lasting for two years"—another habit of this herb.

The genus *Oenothera* embraces about eighty species of herbs, mostly sun-loving, widely distributed throughout the Western Hemisphere. Evening primrose favors dry, sunny soils of meadows, roadside edges, and other waste places from Newfoundland to British Columbia, south to Florida and Texas, and west to Idaho. It grows erect, up to eight feet tall, on sturdy, hairy, pithy stems bearing numerous alternate lance-shaped leaves.

The familiar four-petaled yellow flowers of this biennial plant appear in the second year of growth, blooming from June through October in the Northeast. The large and often showy blooms with their drooping sepals and X-shaped stigmas open on cloudy days or just before or at sunset for the evening pollinators. The blossoms have slight phosphorescence acquired from absorbing and storing up sunlight during the day; on a dark night the petals emit their own faint light. This unique attribute was well noticed by our ancestors.

A medley of common names from different regions speaks of multiple uses for this trusted healing plant. Sometimes called night willow herb, sundrops, coffee or fever plant, scurvish or scabbish, evening primrose is also known as tree primrose, large rampion, four o'clock, and king's cure-all.

Evening primrose
Oenothera biennis

Traditional uses: All plant parts were used, in their specific seasons, for a wide variety of healing purposes. The Great Lakes Ojibwa and Potawatomi Indians bruised and soaked the plant for wound dressings and to relieve bruises and other skin problems. They used the fine black seeds as food and a healing medicine. Roots steamed as vegetables and made into teas were used to treat obesity and aid digestion, as well as to treat skin disorders and to promote clear skin.

Modern uses: Today many people take EPO (evening primrose oil), usually in soft gel caplets. Made from the plant's seeds, it is particularly popular among active people, especially women, seeking natural nutritional support. EPO is a rich source of linoleic acid and gamma-linoleic acid, important essential fatty acids that aid proper cellular metabolism and that are not found in most common foods. EPO has been used to treat multiple sclerosis and schizophrenia, and to aid stabilization of kidney transplant patients, especially in Britain and Europe. Research shows that EPO is also useful for treating eczema, asthma, migraines, PMS, breast problems, diabetes, alcoholism, and arthritis.

Cautions: Do not take evening primrose oil if you suffer from epilepsy.

Evening primrose provides athletes with great strength—for lacrosse, Snowsnake, wrestling. Chew roots and spit on hands and rub on arms and all over muscles.
—Chauncy Johnny-John, Seneca/Cayuga herbalist, Allegany Reserve, 1938

Growth needs and propagation: Evening primrose grows well in dry, open, sunny locations. Seeds can be sown directly in the garden where you want this plant to grow. It generally takes two years for seedlings to bloom, so you will want to continue sowing the seeds in your chosen location, as it will self-sow elsewhere. The seeds are also excellent to eat and very worth collecting in late summer: a few for the garden, most for the kitchen.

Companions: Evening primrose grows happily with many sun-loving herbs in the medicine wheel garden, especially bee balm, coneflower, and chili peppers.

Chamaelirium luteum
Liliaceae (lily family)

Blazing star, false unicorn root, colicroot, and devil's-bit are some of the common names descriptive of this perennial native herb. The Greek terms *chamai,* "on the ground," and *leirion,* "lily," lie behind its genus name, possibly referring to its small size and delicacy compared to showier lilies. The species name comes from the Latin *luteus,* "yellowish." Actually, the flowers are first white and gradually turn yellow.

The only species in its genus, fairywand is native to eastern North America, favoring meadows and moist woodlands from Ontario to Florida and west to Mississippi, Arkansas, and Illinois. It grows from one to four feet tall from the tuberous underground stem (rhizome), producing broad basal leaves in early spring, then a slender stalk tipped with tight clusters of small flowers. The female plants are slightly taller and leafier than the male plants.

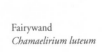

Fairywand
Chamaelirium luteum

Traditional uses: American Indian herbalists chose fairywand for a uterine tonic, and women also chewed the roots to prevent miscarriage. Later in their pregnancy, they used the tea as a tonic to aid childbirth by stimulating the muscles of the womb. Fairywand was also a useful treatment for nausea, especially in early pregnancy. The dried roots served medicinally for their tonic, astringent actions, both internally and as a skin wash. Some tribal herbalists worked the dried powdered roots into a salve to massage the womb.

Modern uses: Modern herbalists continue to rely on fairywand tonics to treat uterine disorders, for pain relief, and as a diuretic. It is also valued as a digestive tonic. All plant parts are

When collecting plants for curing an individual, tell the person's name and the disease first. If the medicine is for curing of a private person, the prayer would be recited beside the first of each plant taken. When a lot of medicine is taken and the person taking it is not known to the one collecting it, one prayer is said for the whole thing. Do not pick the first plant of the first species sought, but put tobacco beside it.

—Kate Debeau, Mohawk herbalist, Caughnawaga, 1933

useful, but the roots that are tinctured in alcohol offer the widest use. The dried roots are sometimes carried in a medicine bag and chewed on to relieve indigestion and headache. These roots are also considered important "love medicines."

Cautions: Avoid using fairywand during pregnancy unless prescribed by a health care specialist.

Growth needs and propagation: Fairywand favors moist, shady soils enriched with humus and decayed leaves. It can be started from seed and root divisions. This herb is so unusual that it is best to start with healthy plants purchased from a responsible nursery and cultivate your own small colony of fairywands.

Companions: Fairywand grows well with other shade-loving herbs in the medicine wheel garden. It especially appreciates ginseng, pipsisesswa, wintergreen, hepatica, and goldenseal as companions.

GOLDENSEAL

Hydrastis canadensis
Ranunculaceae (buttercup family)

Yellow bud scars left on the rhizome by the new stem this herb produces each year reminded observers in past centuries of letter seals then commonly used, hence the name *goldenseal.* In various regions, this distinctive native perennial is also known as orangeroot, yellow puccoon, or turmeric. The genus name, *Hydrastis,* relates to the Greek word for water, and also probably comes from the hydra, the many-headed monster of Greek mythology that grew back two heads for each one cut off—here referring to the two distinct leaves, and multistamen flowers. The family name Ranunculaceae—meaning "little frog"—goes back to Latin, referring to the moisture-loving quality of the typical genus in the buttercup family, as we see with *Actaea* (baneberry) and *Hepatica* (red and white cohosh).

Besides goldenseal, native to eastern North America, the *Hydrastis* genus includes only one other species, native to Japan. The low-growing goldenseal, hairy and delicate, can stand six to eighteen inches tall. Usually only two leaves, one larger than the other, develop at the top of the forked, slender stem. These palmate leaves are broad and double-toothed. A single cluster of greenish-white flowers appears in April and May and ripens to a cluster of red raspberry-like berries in early fall. Each red berry contains two shiny black seeds. Goldenseal grows in the wild from Vermont to Georgia and Alabama, west to Arkansas and Minnesota. It was once very common throughout these regions, but wild-crafting and overharvesting for commercial markets have put goldenseal on the endangered-species list. The medicine wheel garden is a perfect habitat for generating new colonies of this attractive little herb.

Goldenseal
Hydrastis canadensis

Traditional uses: Few wild medicines were as valuable to the Indians as this versatile botanical. The Cherokee mixed the powdered root with animal fat to wear as an insect repellent and to treat ulcers. A root tea was effectively used as an eyewash to treat eye infections. The roots were also used in teas, poultices, or tinctures to treat mouth and throat problems and jaundice, as well as uterine and digestive disorders. The dried, powdered roots served to treat infected wounds and relieve skin problems, and also for some cancers and tumors and to stop bleeding.

Indians also fancied the brilliant yellow dye made from these roots for face paint and adornment for their clothing, baskets, mats, and tools. The Algonquian word *puccoon* refers to this dye, and also signified the plant's importance. Goldenseal seemed a virtual panacea; it could help with almost everything.

Modern uses: Today goldenseal is commercially grown and harvested for its medicinal roots. Modern investigations indicate that the berberine contained in the roots is antibacterial, with beneficial effects on the kidneys and intestines. It is a digestive tonic. Goldenseal eyewash is mildly antibiotic and can reduce inflammations. Goldenseal extracts also seem to lower blood sugar levels. As a mild sedative, it helps lower blood pressure, and relieves stress and anxiety.

Tea made from the roots has been used as a douche for vaginal inflammations and to treat yeast infections. It also helps reduce heavy menstrual bleeding, and is used following childbirth to check postpartum hemorrhage. Root infusions are a valuable remedy for psoriasis. Goldenseal roots have a bitter taste and are slightly sweet, with a distinctively licorice odor. The dried, powdered roots are snuffed (with caution) up the nose to relieve chronic sinus problems.

[As a tuberculosis treatment,] take a small one-inch piece of goldenseal root, with a one-half-inch piece of ginseng root, and a one-inch piece of bloodroot root, and a three-inch piece of ginger root; steep long in water and drink this.
—Josephine Jimmerson, Seneca herbalist, Allegany Reserve, 1939

Cautions: Avoid all use during pregnancy. The goldenseal plant alkaloids are very caustic and are poisonous in large doses. Do not take goldenseal without medical supervision.

Growth needs and propagation: A challenging plant to cultivate, goldenseal takes about five years to mature from seed and demands just the right growth environment of moist, rich soil and a shady plot. A number of specialty native plant growers offer plants for the shade garden. Set the young plants about one inch deep in rich, moist earth and space them about eight inches apart. Mulch these plants well in early winter. This plant is a beauty in the medicine wheel garden, well worth the time and trouble to cultivate.

Companions: Goldenseal will grow well with sweet flag, ginseng, goldthread, hellebore, cardinal flower, boneset, and angelica.

GOLDTHREAD

Coptis groenlandica
Ranunculaceae (buttercup family)

This small, shiny evergreen plant greatly resembles the wild strawberry. Each leaf actually consists of three leaflets united at the end of the leaf stem. The genus name, *Coptis,* from a Greek verb meaning "cut off," seems to relate to this leaf division, as if each leaf had been cut apart. The species name *groenlandica* means "of Greenland," as this diminutive plant was thought to be native to northern, colder regions.

Also called cankerroot, yellow root, and mouth root, goldthread puts forth its solitary white flowers on slender, leafless stalks from May through July. Its shallow root systems resemble masses of gold threads, explaining the popular name. Hugging moist fertile ground, like strawberry plants, this lush perennial makes a dense carpet of growth in shady environments on the edge of swamps, bogs, and woods from Greenland to Alaska, south to Iowa, and southeast into North Carolina. It is one of some ten species in this genus of small perennial herbs spread across northern temperate regions. Several are cultivated in gardens as a border plant and for their medicinal qualities.

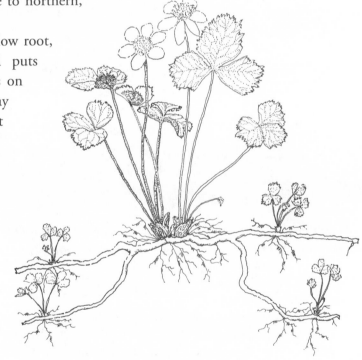

Goldthread
Coptis groenlandica

Because of ever-shrinking environments and overharvesting by wildcrafters to meet the growing demand from the health care market, goldthread is on the endangered-species list in many states. Fortunately it grows readily in moist, shady soil and prospers under cultivation, so that more gardeners and herbalists are farming goldthread.

Traditional uses: Penobscot Indians chewed the bitter roots of goldthread to relieve "smoker's mouth" and soothe sore throats and coughs. They used a strong tea of goldthread rhizomes to treat ulcers and mouth, throat, and eye problems. This tea was also applied to babies' gums as a topical anesthetic while teething problems persisted. The Montagnais used root decoctions to treat problems of the mouth and eyes, and the Menomini used them as gargles for children's throat problems and to treat canker sores and tumors.

Modern uses: Highly astringent roots of goldthread are chewed to relieve canker sores, fever blisters, sore throats, and indigestion. The inherent alkaloid berberine (in the roots) is a mild sedative, which also has anti-inflammatory and antibacterial properties. Some health care practitioners recommend a decoction of goldthread and goldenseal in equal parts to relieve the craving for alcohol.

Cautions: Do not use goldthread during pregnancy. At any time, use it only with professional supervision.

Use goldthread roots to treat sore mouth in baby. Put warm water over a few dry roots. Steep. Apply to inside of mouth with a small teaspoon, a little at a time.
—Albert Jonas, Seneca herbalist, Allegany Reserve, 1938

Growth needs and propagation: This herb prefers cool, rich, shady areas for growth. It is often cultivated as a ground cover in woody areas and around bog gardens in dappled sunlight. Goldthread is readily propagated from seed and division of root clumps. These want to be thinly covered with humus-enriched earth and well mulched with decayed leaf mold. A slightly more acid soil is perfect for goldthread.

Companions: Goldthread will grow well among hellebore plants, as well as American ginger, ginseng, and maidenhair fern.

HEAL-ALL

Prunella vulgaris
Labiatae (mint family)

In the mid-1500s, soldiers in Germany suffered from a rampant outbreak of quinsy, commonly known there as "the browns." Translated into Latin, the German *Braun* became *Prunella,* the name chosen for this genus of plants believed to cure the "brown" infection. The common name, heal-all, says much about how this plant has been viewed across time. Our European ancestors brought heal-all to America as one of their most vital medicines. The species name, *vulgaris*—Latin for "common"—is certainly the hallmark of this resilient herb, which seems to grow everywhere and adapts to prevailing conditions.

An early Eurasian introduction to North America, this rugged perennial mint has naturalized widely throughout the continent. Heal-all, or self-heal, can be found growing in dense, matlike forms in our lawns and meadows, roadside edges, woodland borders, and waste places. Its purple flowers crown a dense terminal conelike head atop distinctive square stems throughout the summer. Opposite oval to lance-shaped leaves surround the creeping stems in almost compasslike symmetry of north-south and east-west. It grows from three inches to one foot tall. There are perhaps seven species of perennials in the genus *Prunella* found across North America. Heal-all is also closely related to ground ivy, or gill-over-the-ground, *Glechoma hederacea,* as well as to our native downy wood mint, *Elephilia ciliata,* and lyre-leaved sage or cancerweed, *Salvia lyrata.* All are members of the great mint family and were

Heal-all
Prunella vulgaris

used by American Indian herbalists in many special applications from headache treatments to backache relief. *S. lyrata* has long been a valuable folk remedy for certain cancers and for removing warts.

Traditional uses: Native American and Eurasian traditions trained herbalists to use the leaves and blossoms of heal-all to treat sores, wounds, bruises, and ulcers when poulticed on top of the problem areas. Leaf and blossom teas were also used to treat mouth sores, relieve sore throats, reduce fevers, and relieve diarrhea. A tea made from the flowering plant in China is considered cooling and tonic for the liver, as well as an aid for circulation.

Modern uses: Modern research bears out the healing benefits of heal-all, which contains the antitumor and diuretic compound ursolic acid. This plant possesses antibiotic and hypotensive qualities and has antimutagenic action. Many contemporary herbalists prescribe heal-all, and clinical herbalists provide tinctures as well as dried herbs for teas and poultices. How fortunate we are that this natural resource prospers throughout our region.

Growth needs and propagation: Heal-all thrives in almost any type of earth. Several other members of this hardy genus have been propagated and hybridized for rock gardens and shade gardens and are highly prized for their rugged endurance, especially in the medicine wheel garden. Like many mints, heal-all grows readily from root and stem cuttings. Follow normal procedures of snipping ample stem or root cuttings and covering them with two inches of good earth. Tamp it down well and water. These perennials overwinter very well and regenerate themselves, almost without need of any help.

Make a small bundle of the whole heal-all plants, steep to a good strength in two quarts of water. Take a cup at a time when you want to cure stomach cramps.
—Mrs. Reuben, Seneca herbalist, Tonawanda Reservation, 1912

Companions: Heal-all grows favorably with hepatica, elderberry, bayberry, Indian turnip, and bee balm. Actually, it could accompany every herb in the medicine wheel garden! It is best planted around the center prayer cairn surrounding the peace pole. Low-growing plants accentuate the peace pole and allow you to move around it easily.

Hepatica americana
Ranunculaceae (buttercup family)

Hepatica takes its common and genus names from the supposed resemblance of its lobed leaves to the shape of the liver—in Latin, *hepaticus* means "liver." As its important earlier uses include treatment for liver problems, that connection may also have influenced the choice of name. Earlier observers watched nature closely for useful healing medicines. Hepatica's species name affirms that it is a native American plant, as is the sharp-lobed hepatica, *H. acutiloba,* whose species name literally means "sharp leaf," from the Latin *acus,* "needle."

These two native species favor moist rich woodland soil and grow from Nova Scotia to Georgia, Alabama, and Louisiana, west to Missouri and Minnesota. Their diminutive daisylike flowers with five to seven pastel petals range from lavender and blue to white or pink. The genus embraces about ten Northern Hemisphere species of small, hardy perennials. These ephemeral wildflowers are slightly downy (hairy) and bloom in early spring, after which their distinctive shiny green leaves dominate. They stand about four to eight inches tall.

Hepatica
Hepatica americana

Traditional uses: Indians used hepatica leaf teas and decoctions to treat liver ailments, as a laxative, as a digestive aid, and to wash sore, swollen breasts. This mildly astringent botanical also served as a diuretic and a treatment for colds, coughs, and fevers and, for the Seneca, as a tonic. The Cherokee chewed the roots to relieve coughs and sore throat, and the Delaware used them as hunting charms. The Forest Potawatomi used the root and leaves in a sweet tea to relieve vertigo. For the Meskwaki, the root provided decoctions to drink to treat various ailments, and the Menomini combined the hepatica roots with the roots of maidenhair fern in decoctions to treat female disorders.

During the late nineteenth century, hepatica leaves were consumed by the hundreds of thousands of pounds in various "liver tonics." Numerous root decoctions were used as treatments for stomachaches and diarrhea and as laxatives.

Modern uses: Today herbalists use hepatica roots and leaves in some tonic preparations to treat liver and kidney problems. Hepatica also has virtue in treating indigestion, coughs, and fevers.

Growth needs and propagation: Hepatica thrives in rich, well-drained soil in mostly shade or open shade. The plants may be easily propagated from seed or root divisions or purchased from native plant nurseries.

[Sharp-lobed hepatica] prevents conception. Steep 3 plants in three quarts of water for a strong dose. Drink the quantity as soon as possible.
—David Jack, Cayuga herbalist, Six Nations Reserve, 1912

Companions: The hepaticas grow well with other members of the buttercup family in the medicine wheel garden. They also keep good company with hellebore, maidenhair fern, ginseng, goldthread, and goldenseal.

INDIAN TURNIP

Arisaema triphyllum
Araceae (arum family)

Very early European accounts detail how Indians living in Virginia in the 1500s dried the turniplike roots of this perennial plant and used them for bread and in soups, inspiring the name Indian turnip. Another popular name, jack-in-the-pulpit, reflects the plant's unusual form at flowering time in spring, when a hooded vaselike structure, the "pulpit," enclosing an upright fleshy-hollow spike, "Jack," appears at the top of the stem. Yet this is actually Jack and Jill together, as the tiny flowering portion rests at the base of the spike. It is Jill, when pollinated, who produces the stunning shiny red berries in late summer after the hood has withered away.

In various places, Indian turnip is also called marsh pepper, bog onion, dragonroot, wake-robin, and starchwort. The genus name, *Arisaema,* derives from the Greek for "arum," a plant type this species represents, and *haima,* Greek for "blood," apparently because some arums have redspotted leaves. Along with its importance as a healing herb, Indian turnip makes an attractive addition to shade gardens, especially a medicine wheel garden.

The hooded "pulpit" of this plant is actually a leaf called the spathe, which covers and conceals clusters of minute yellowish-green flowers pollinated by ants and other crawling insects. They form at the base of the tubular spike, known as a spadix, which can be dark green to brown. The spathe may vary from green-and-white stripes to green-and-purple stripes. Later in the year, flowers ripen into tightly clustered shiny green berries, which turn shiny red before frost. Although the species name, *triphyllum,* means "three leaves," Indian turnip usually has only two, but each is composed of three wavy leaflets.

The plants can grow up to two feet tall from their underground corms. These corms have the innocent look of a small turniplike potato, but they are fiery hot to the taste until boiled or roasted. Like the other plant parts, they contain irritating oxalate crystals, most unpleasant to eat uncooked, but when rubbed on swollen joints they provide relief for rheumatism and swelling.

Indian turnip
Arisaema triphyllum

Indian turnip is almost a loner in the *Arisaema* genus of about two hundred species, most native to Europe and Asia. The only other prominent North American species is green dragon, or dragonroot, *A. dracontium,* found from Quebec to Florida and west to Texas, Wisconsin, and Nebraska. It had medicinal uses among many native tribes, principally for women's needs.

Traditional uses: Documented accounts through the past four centuries report American Indian uses of Indian turnip in myriad medicinal treatments, both alone and in formula with other botanicals. For example, Indian herbalists used the dried, aged root (corm) to treat colds and coughs and to strengthen the blood. The corm and ripe berries, rubbed on or poulticed externally, served to ease rheumatic joints, sores, boils, abscesses, and ringworm.

Historically a tea from the roasted root was used as a purgative and treated asthma, colds, bronchitis, coughs, laryngitis, and headaches. The external applications treated snakebite, boils, and rheumatic pains.

Modern uses: Indian turnip's dried corm (rhizome) is used in a treatment for chest conditions, but only under professional supervision, as it is very toxic. The related Chinese species, *Arisaema consanguineum,* tian nan xing, is used also for respiratory chest conditions and always prescribed along with fresh ginger root, *Zingiber officinale,* internally. Each species continues to be used fresh externally for arthritic problems, ulcers, and other skin conditions.

Cautions: Do not eat or taste any fresh plant parts, which are intensely irritating. Calcium oxalate crystals found in the whole plant are especially concentrated in the berries and corm.

Growth needs and propagation: This hardy plant favors shady locations with rich, well-drained, humus-enriched soil. It grows readily from seeds and natural offsets from the main corm. The corm should be planted eight to twelve inches deep, as the

For baby when it lies still all day and night as if thinking about something . . . is lonesome, not satisfied with home (they know as much as old people). Smash 2 [Indian turnip] roots, put in one quart warm water. Do not let stand long. Wash whole body.
—John Jamieson Jr., Cayuga herbalist, Six Nations Reserve, 1914

roots come out of the upper portion. However, the corms will also grow in more shallow situations, and sometimes even over large stones.

Companions: Indian turnip grows well with other shade-loving wildflowers in the medicine wheel garden. It especially likes the company of hepatica, blue flag, ginseng, ginger, goldenseal, and goldthread.

JEWELWEED

Impatiens capensis
Balsaminaceae (touch-me-not family)

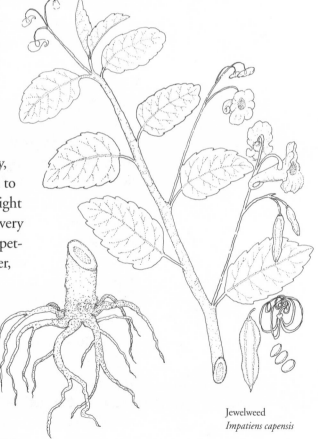

Jewelweed
Impatiens capensis

When you touch the ripe green seedpods of jewelweed, they immediately fly open, as if they couldn't wait even a moment to fling their turquoise seeds everywhere. That habit accounts for the genus name, *Impatiens,* and also for its other common name, touch-me-not. Be wary, especially for children's benefit, if you wish to pop a seedpod, as it could hurl a seed straight into your eye! These plants also grow very fast. Like little jewels, their bright trumpet-shaped flowers dangle from the slender, translucent stems through much of the summer, drawing hummingbirds. The Latin species name, *capensis,* refers to the Cape of Good Hope, where these plants were thought to originate.

Widespread across North America, jewelweed is among the most common native annuals. It grows in moist areas and shaded wetlands, often near (even in) poison ivy and stinging nettles. When crushed and rubbed on exposed skin, the succulent stems are a useful antidote (and preventive) for poison ivy and other types of skin irritations. These tall, multibranched herbs have smooth green ovate leaves, long with scalloped edges and pale and glaucous underneath. Slender bloom stalks emerge from the plant stem at upper leaf axils and ripen into the dangling, swollen green fruit capsules that explode and scatter their seeds so readily. This mechanism explains why you often see dense colonies of jewelweed dominating some wet areas. These tender annuals are quite sensitive to cold, and decline quickly with the first touch of frost in autumn.

Long considered herbs for special uses, three species of jewelweed grow wild in the Northeast, where American Indians used them in various topical medicines. In this region, they usually germinate from seeds in April and grow rapidly in favorable soils to reach heights of two to five feet by July.

The common jewelweed, *I. capensis* (previously known as *I. biflora* and *I. fulva*), is also called orange jewelweed, spotted touch-me-not, or lady's-earrings. In the summer months, it flashes its golden-orange flowers. The spurred blossoms, spotted with orange, resemble miniature cornucopias and are especially attractive to hummingbirds, bees, and butterflies. Pale or yellow jewelweed, *I. pallida,* has slightly larger blossoms: pale yellow, sometimes spotted with dots of orange-brown. Otherwise, this species is similar in most ways to the previous one and can often be found growing nearby. A large purple- to rose-flowered royal jewelweed, *I. glandulifera,* has been naturalized in areas of the Northeast, as well as in some areas of the Northwest coast. Introduced from the Himalayas, it is a striking beauty.

Traditional uses: Many American Indian medicine people used applications of common and yellow jewelweed to treat a broad range of internal and external problems. These botanicals have probably been valued medicinals for far longer than we could know. The young shoots and blossoms are esteemed wild edibles among many native peoples and foragers. Some Great Lakes and Plains tribes used these native herbs to treat colds, cramps, sprains, and much more. Jewelweed was both used alone, for its soothing analgesic benefits, and mixed in formulas and tinctures and poultices with other botanicals for broader therapeutic applications. The Nanticoke applied jewelweed leaves as a poultice to treat burns and also used jewelweed tea to wash, disinfect, and to soothe burns and other skin eruptions, as did the Mohegan, Delaware, and other eastern tribal peoples. Creek and Cherokee peoples used the crushed plant and its juice to rub on the skin to treat a number of skin eruptions, including hives, eczema, measles, insect stings, spider bites, and poison ivy rashes, as well as to heal bruises.

In dealing with poison ivy, the principal benefit of this herb comes from early treatment, as the soothing juice of jewelweed counteracts the more deleterious oils of poison ivy (and also the urtic acid of stinging nettles). Rub the jewelweed plant juices on the skin parts exposed to poison ivy as soon as possible. Once the poison ivy rash appears, the jewelweed juice (and tincture) can calm the inflammation, which invariably must run its course. Almost nothing can cure poison ivy, yet applications of jewelweed can usually prevent its most irritating skin eruptions.

Modern uses: Modern investigations show that jewelweed has a soothing fungicidal benefit useful in treating athlete's foot, ringworm, and other skin problems. It is used fresh or frozen, or in tinctures and liniments. It continues to be used as an early antidote to poison ivy rashes.

Growth needs and propagation: Jewelweed is a self-sowing annual that prefers to grow in moist, rich soil. It is easily grown from seed.

Companions: Jewelweed grows well with other moisture-loving plants in the medicine wheel garden. It is especially agreeable with yellow dock, mayapple, and maidenhair fern.

To induce childbirth and stop suffering, wash whole plant, including root, and put in water. Drink a panful, cease suffering—immediate delivery.

—Jonas and Josephine Snow, Seneca herbalists, Allegany Reserve, 1933

Eupatorium maculatum
Compositae (daisy family)

The name joe-pye weed supposedly comes from an Indian medicine man named Joe Pye who used this species successfully to treat typhus throughout New England in the late 1700s. Some say he was a Wampanoag Indian herbalist. *Eupatorium,* the genus name, also has a fascinating origin—see the entry on boneset for details. The Latin species name, *maculatum,* means "spotted": this species is often called spotted joe-pye weed, for its purple-spotted stems. *E. purpureum,* a closely related herb, is known as sweet joe-pye weed, or gravel root.

Also called trumpet weed, kidney root, queen of the meadow, and quillwort in various regions, spotted joe-pye weed ranges from Newfoundland to British Columbia south to Maryland, Ohio, Illinois, and New Mexico, favoring wet meadows and mountainous areas. This lanky, sturdy herb can grow from two to six feet tall. Long lance-shaped leaves emerge from its purple or purple-spotted stem in whorls of four to five, like collars. Large purple flower clusters appear atop the tall stems in July and bloom through September. Sweet joe-pye weed, *E. purpureum,* also called king-of-the-meadow, can grow up to twelve feet tall. Its sturdy stems, pithy and green with purple at the leaf nodes, are topped with pale pink to light purple flowers densely packed into a rounded blossom head.

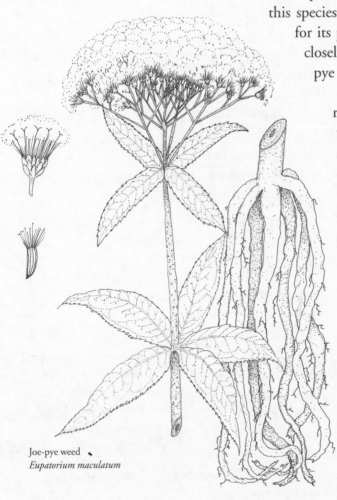

Joe-pye weed
Eupatorium maculatum

As with its "spotted" cousin, blooming continues from July through September. The whorls of long lance-shaped leaves surrounding the stem give off a fragrance like vanilla when stroked or lightly brushed.

Traditional uses: All parts of this perennial plant were used in various herbal preparations. American Indians made root and leaf teas and decoctions to treat gout and kidney infections as well as rheumatism. These teas also were used as a diuretic and to relieve bladder complaints. In addition, they served to treat fevers, colds, diarrhea, and liver ailments. The Ojibwa washed their children with a strong decoction of this plant to strengthen them and prevent illness. The Potawatomi used the leaves as a poultice on burns and the root medicine to clear and tone the uterus after childbirth. The flowers were considered a good-luck talisman. The Meskwaki used this plant as one of their love medicines.

Modern uses: Herbalists today use these herbs (both species) to treat colds, fevers, and support the immune system. The whole plant is considered a tonic, and the roots provide a laxative.

Cautions: Do not use while pregnant; at any time, use these plants only with a specialist's supervision.

Growth needs and propagation: Joe-pye weeds prefer moist, rich earth and full sun to partial shade. Both species adapt well to the garden, where they provide a tall, sturdy backdrop for shorter herbs. They are best propagated from root divisions in late summer and fall. Cut generous sections with enough bud and root to sustain new growth. Dig them into the medicine wheel garden, six to eight inches deep, water well, and tamp the earth over them, top-dressing them with leaf mulch.

Companions: Both species grow well with sweet flag, black cohosh, boneset, Indian turnip, and cardinal flower. They will also happily accompany angelica, jewelweed, sweetgrass, and hellebore.

[Joe-pye weed] heals soreness of womb and abdomen after childbirth. Also good for kidneys. Steep well three roots in four quarts of water. Drink a lot anytime until soreness goes away.
　　—Elijah David, Seneca herbalist, Tonawanda Reserve, 1912

MAIDENHAIR FERN

Adiantum pedatum
Polypodiaceae (fern family)

The fineness of the fan-shaped leaflets and stems of this dainty native fern were thought to inspire the common name, maidenhair, also reflecting its ephemeral, airy quality. The genus name derives from a Greek word meaning "drench"; together with the species name, a Latin word meaning "foot," it properly suggests a plant growing in moist places, capable of having wet feet.

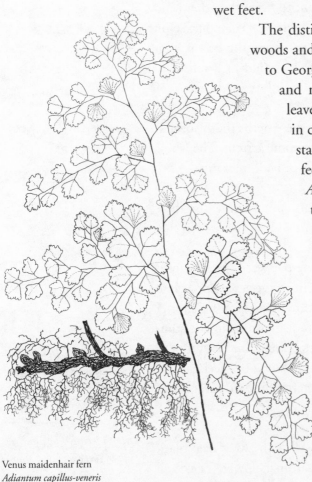

Venus maidenhair fern
Adiantum capillus-veneris

The distinctive maidenhair fern grows in rich woods and other moist, shady areas from Maine to Georgia, west to Louisiana and Oklahoma, and north to Minnesota. Its thin, simple leaves are delicate and fan-shaped, spread in curving fronds atop a slim, shiny black stalk. It can stand up to one and a half feet tall. The Venus maidenhair fern, *Adiantum capillus-veneris,* standing up to twenty inches tall, grows in moist limestone areas in more southerly regions from Virginia to Florida, west to Texas and California. It too prefers shaded locations. These two plants number among the few species of *Adiantum* ferns that grow in temperate North America. Most of the more than two hundred members of this genus are found in the American tropics, and a few in East Asia.

Traditional uses: Both North America's maidenhair fern species have considerable folk traditions of uses. American Indians used the maidenhair fern as an important medicine plant, brewing the whole plant into teas to treat asthma, nasal congestion, sore throats, hoarseness, flu, colds, and fevers. Many tribes considered maidenhair tea a valuable hair wash and scalp treatment. They also used both species to treat snakebite and poulticed them on wounds and swellings. Some tribal basket weavers used the shiny black stems and weaving elements to create striking basket designs.

Modern uses: Today, herbalists recognize the continuing virtues of maidenhair fern extracts in treating coughs, bronchitis, sore throat, excess mucus, and chronic nasal congestion. Many also use these fern extracts to treat hair and scalp conditions. A related species, *A. caudatum,* is an antispasmodic that is useful in treating asthma.

Cautions: Maidenhair fern is on the protected and endangered-species list in most states and should never be dug from wild habitats. It contains no known toxins.

Growth needs and propagation: Maidenhair ferns grow best in rich, moist, limestone soils in semishade to full shade. It is worthwhile to treat the soil where you wish to plant them with some additional powdered limestone if you feel it is necessary. They will thrive when protected against strong wind. Planting sturdy plants adjacent to the maidenhair, like an elderberry shrub, or positioning standing stones nearby on the windward side of delicate plants provides effective windbreaks. Although these ferns can be grown from spores and from root divisions, success is greatest when you purchase healthy plants from a nursery growing them for market.

[Use maidenhair fern] for excessive menstruation. Steep a handful of roots until water gets dark. Use two quarts of water. Take any amount, anytime.

—Mrs. Sundown, Seneca herbalist, Tonawanda Reserve, 1912

Companions: Maidenhair fern grows well with mayapple, moccasin flower, pipsissewa, and skullcap as well as other shade-loving plants, in the medicine wheel garden.

Podophyllum peltatum
Berberidaceae (barberry family)

Wild lemon, Indian apple, American mandrake, raccoon berry, goosefoot, and wild jalap are some of mayapple's common names. Each speaks to a part of this plant's personality. The genus name, *Podophyllum,* means "plant with footlike leaves"—a good description of this plant, which has large leaves with the stalk attached at the center of the surface, as well as footlike roots that lateral off at right angles an inch below the soil surface. The species name, *peltatum,* is derived from the Greek *peltatus,* meaning "having a shield." Indeed, the large, smooth leaves do shield the whole plant like an umbrella.

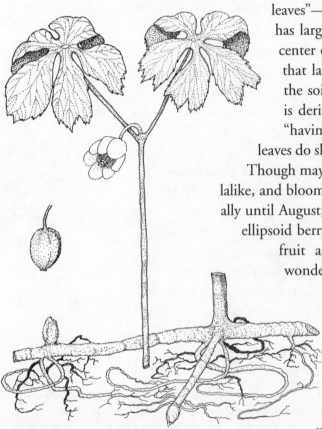

Mayapple
Podophyllum peltatum

Though mayapple emerges from the earth, umbrellalike, and blooms in May, it takes another season, usually until August, to set the apple, a small, single, green ellipsoid berry that ripens to a golden yellow fleshy fruit and becomes heavily fragrant. These wonderfully aromatic fruits smell almost tropical, the quality that draws the deer, fox, possum, raccoon, and wild turkey to eat them.

The small, unique *Podophyllum* genus has only two species, native to North America and Asia. Mayapple grows vigorously in the wild, in rich woodland environments, from Quebec to Florida and Texas. Each of its large, solitary leaves is deeply, palmately lobed. A single (occasionally double) white flower, daisylike with six waxy petals, appears in the fork between the leaves; this is a classic May bloom. The whole plant may stand one and a half feet tall and almost a foot across. It is a stunning plant in shade gardens.

Traditional uses: American Indians used mayapple roots as a strong purgative and liver cleanser. Some tribes used the pounded fresh or powdered dried roots to shrink skin tumors. The Cherokee used the juice of the roots dropped into the ear to cure deafness. Many tribes worked the root juices into syrup to take as a systemic cleanser and cathartic. The Meskwaki used these roots to treat rheumatism, and it was one of their nine herbs formulated to treat snakebite. Many different tribal groups knew of its poisonous qualities and used it to attempt suicide, and some tribes put it into their enemies' food. Most tribes enjoyed eating the fruits, which are not toxic when fully ripe.

Several tribes used decoctions of mayapple roots to treat corn kernels before planting to keep the birds and other predators from eating them. The Iroquois relied on the leaves as one of their important corn medicines, along with the flowers of elderberry. The same treatment was used for potatoes in the garden to kill potato beetles. It was considered sympathetic magic. Canadian research has found that mayapple grows on the sites of old Indian villages, and many authorities believe that Indians planted their most important medicine plants close to their dwellings in order to ensure ready supplies.

[Use mayapple, with caution,] as a cathartic. Bake roots until just quite dry—do not burn them. Make into a powder. Use a little (about the size of a dime) and pour over boiling water in a cup. Drink.

—Delia Carpenter, Onondaga herbalist, Onondaga Reservation, 1973

Modern uses: The active principle, podophyllin, is found throughout this plant but is intensively concentrated in the rhizome. Scientists are exploring this chemical as a possible treatment for skin cancers and some tumors. Some scientists have suggested that mayapple be grown on a commercial scale as a cash crop because of the growing interest in it as a cancer treatment.

Cautions: Mayapple is poisonous. Only the fully ripe fruits are edible, and they tend to be too aromatic for most people's palate. The powdered root can cause skin and eye problems.

Growth needs and propagation: Mayapple prefers the damp, rich earth of open woodlands and pastures. It accommodates very well to the medicine wheel garden, where it will create a stunning colony. As it begins to spread, you can dig out the extra plants and place them in another wildflower garden or at the edge of a meadow or woods, or give them to interested friends. Mayapple is easily divided by rootstocks in the fall, or sow the seeds in spring. As it likes partial shade and a moist soil high in organic matter, top-dressing with well-rotted compost is important for healthy plants.

Companions: Mayapple is a good companion for maidenhair fern, skullcap, cardinal flower, ginseng, goldthread, and goldenseal.

MOCCASIN FLOWER

Cypripedium calceolus
Orchidaceae (orchid family)

Said to have risen from the sea at the island of Cyprus, the Greek goddess Aphrodite (Roman: Venus) was also called Cypris. When the genus name *Cypripedium* and the species name *calceolus,* meaning "shaped like a slipper," are linked, they suggest that the form of this native orchid's flower resembles Venus's slipper or sandal. Early observers gave the stunning plant the more down-to-earth name moccasin flower because the flower reminded them of the gathered leather moccasins worn by American Indians. One way or the other, shoes seem to be part of the picture! Nerve root, American valerian, and whippoorwill-shoe are some of moccasin flower's other popular names.

Moccasin flower grows from Nova Scotia south to Alabama and west to Missouri and Minnesota, favoring moist woodlands, open meadows, and swampy banks. This showy perennial herb grows one to two feet tall. The large oval leaves can be up to eight inches long, clasping a solitary sturdy stem. A single yellow blossom appears in late spring, often tinged with purplish brown. The large lower petal transforms into a yellow pouchlike feature (the slipper), supported by more slender petals (sepals) twisting out around it.

The smaller related species *C. calceolus* var. *parviflora* tolerates a more northerly range but grows to only about eight inches tall. The robust pink moccasin flower, *C. acaule,* often called pink lady's slipper, grows to about fifteen inches tall in similar environments. The small white moccasin flowers, *C. candidum* and *C. passerinum,* are also worthy of consideration for the medicine wheel garden. The latter species ranges from Canada to Alaska, blooming in early summer.

Traditional uses: Each of these species had tremendous medicinal value for American Indians and herbalists, and these uses continue. The root extracts are valued as sedatives and nervines. To aid women in childbirth, the Cherokee Indians used decoctions of the yellow moccasin flower, to which they added chickweed and purslane. The Penobscot Indians used a decoction of the orchid root alone to treat nervousness, and the Tete de Boule Indians used it for stomach problems and urinary infections. Root decoctions also served the Mohawk Indians to treat respiratory problems, tuberculosis, and epilepsy, and the Chippewa (Ojibwa), Menomini, and Meskwaki used it for relieving women's disorders and easing childbirth. The dried roots were carried in medicine bundles, and some used them in love medicines along with other charms. A belief existed that the root could induce dreams of the supernatural.

Modern uses: Modern herbalists use a tincture of moccasin flower root as a sedative to treat insomnia, depression, menstrual irregularities, PMS, and nervous anxieties. Many herbalists are farming this respected wildflower in similar ways to ginseng and goldenseal to meet growing demand. As conservationists, more

Moccasin flower
Cypripedium calceolus

and more gardeners are working to establish native orchid ecosystems wherein these species can flourish.

Cautions: All moccasin flowers can cause dermatitis. Large doses are dangerous.

Growth needs and propagation: Moccasin flower grows well in moist, rich earth. In the wild, native orchids live symbiotically with specific fungi under highly specialized soil conditions. For this reason they do not grow well from seed or transplant well from the wild. It is best to purchase healthy plants from a reputable nursery with good growth starter mix including the necessary fungi. An added complication is that deer like to eat them, so many gardeners must protect them with a mesh cover. It is well worth the effort to cultivate these amazing beauties!

Companions: Moccasin flower grows well with other native orchids such as pink lady's slipper, spotted coralroot, and adam-and-eve-root. It will also accompany strawberry, yarrow, sweetgrass, and blue flag.

Take one moccasin flower for pains all over the body and skin, caused by bad blood. Boil root of one plant in three quarts of water down to half. Take one cup every hour.

—David Jack, Cayuga herbalist, Six Nations Reserve, 1912

OREGON HOLLY GRAPE

Mahonia aquifolium
Berberidaceae (barberry family)

This evergreen shrub's genus name, *Mahonia,* honors the nineteenth-century American botanist Bernard McMahon, and the species name, *aquifolium,* comes from Latin words meaning "sharp" and "leaf"—with pointy leaves. It certainly describes this native American holly, which is also called blue barberry, mountain grape, and holly mahonia. This genus embraces more than one hundred species of thornless evergreen shrubs native to North and Central America and Asia.

The distinctive leaves of Oregon holly grape, alternate and spiny-toothed, grow almost three inches long. Lustrous dark green above and green below, they turn bright red in the fall, earning the Spanish name *yerba de sangre,* "herb of blood." The creamy yellow flower clusters appear in spring, ripening into fall clusters of juicy red berries. This shrub can grow to three feet tall or more in favorable locations. *M. repens,* another species of Oregon holly grape that grows in the Southwest, is a creeping ground cover, while the related *M. trifoliata,* also called algerita in the Southwest, can grow into a sizable shrub or a small bushy tree. Each of these species has yellow inner bark and roots high in the alkaloid berberine.

Oregon holly grape
Mahonia repens

Traditional uses: Indian herbalists gathered the mature roots and stem bark from midsummer into winter. They used these botanicals for medicinal treatments for liver and digestive problems, and they made a fine yellow dye from these plant parts to color their baskets, bags, mats, and clothing.

Modern uses: Contemporary herbalists continue to seek and grow these species to make a bitter tonic of the roots in alcohol. This tonic is used as a fine digestive aid and a stimulant to liver metabolism, as well as an antimicrobial for the skin and intestinal tract.

Cautions: Do not take in large doses.

Growth needs and propagation: Mahonias are hardy in northern regions if carefully protected from the wind and hot sun. Seeds, suckers, layers, and cuttings of the half-ripe woody growth easily propagate new plants. The last three should be kept under glass in a greenhouse arrangement until secondary roots form. Healthy plants should be ordered from nurseries for best results.

Companions: Oregon holly grape grows happily with yarrow, sweetgrass, sage, and bayberry in the medicine wheel garden. It will also be a pleasing companion for strawberry and bearberry.

PIPSISSEWA

Chimaphila umbellata
Pyrolaceae (wintergreen family)

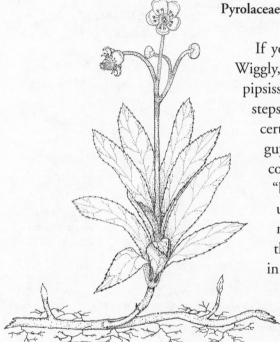

Pipsissewa
Chimaphila umbellata

If you ever played the old board game of Uncle Wiggly, maybe you remember the phrase "The bad pipsissewa shivered and shook as Uncle Wiggly three steps took." This pretty, creeping evergreen herb certainly does not deserve the reputation of bad guy! Its Algonquian Indian name, *pipsissewa*, comes from a Canadian Cree word meaning "breaks it into small pieces," such as breaking up a stone in the bladder. Its official genus name, *Chimaphila*, means "winter-loving," as these tiny shrublike plants are often prominent in winter snow. The species name, *umbellata*, points to their little umbrellalike flowers.

Also called wintergreen, ground-holly, wax-flower, and prince's pine, pipsissewa is native to the eastern woodlands and thrives in a mixed hardwood forest. The stems can stand ten inches tall, topped in midsummer by one to three small, fragrant, drooping, white-to-pink blossoms. These small, waxy flowers eventually stand straight up in climax form and become woody and fibrous as each plant projects its ripe seedpod aloft. Striped or spotted pipsissewa, *Chimaphila maculata,* also called ratsbane or rheumatism root, is a close relative.

Traditional uses: Native peoples chewed and sometimes smoked the leathery leaves of pipsissewa to treat numerous conditions. Leaves and roots were steeped in strong teas (decoctions), sometimes formulated with other native herbs, to relieve coughs, colds, bladder complaints, and kidney problems. Eastern Algonquians used the tea to season other medicines, to relieve PMS problems, and as a diuretic, astringent, and sudorific (to induce sweating) for the sweat bath. Iroquois herbalists used this to treat stomach cancer and rheumatism. Some tribes used leaf decoctions to treat eye problems, and drank them as spring tonics. Along the West Coast, from British Columbia to southern California and into Idaho, is found the western *C. menziesii,* a whorled, often variegated species that stands six inches tall. The Thompson Indians of British Columbia poulticed the whole pulverized plant to reduce swelling in joints, legs, and feet. Native peoples also poulticed the leaves on skin tumors, ulcers, and sore muscles, especially as a backache remedy.

Modern uses: A decoction made from pipsissewa leaves was an original ingredient in traditional root beers, and pipsissewa extract continues to be used as a flavoring agent in some candies and soft drinks as well as in various health care products. It provides an earthy, musky taste.

Cautions: The biologically active compounds arbutin, sitosterol, and ursolic acid can produce various healing benefits but also irritate sensitive skin.

Growth needs and propagation: Pipsissewa favors dry woodlands and sandy soils. Across most of our northern temperate regions, their shiny green toothed leaves are signs of healing through winter snows. However, pipsissewa is now endangered throughout much of its natural range, making it especially important to cultivate in our medicine wheel gardens. It is difficult to propagate from seed. Propagate from one-inch pieces of underground rootstock left under leaf mulch.

Companions: Pipsissewa grows well with most of the shade-loving plants in the medicine wheel garden, especially mayapple and maidenhair fern.

When a pregnant woman feels feverish and drowsy, she is not sick, her baby is. Make a small bundle of pipsissewa about one inch thick using the whole plant. Put this in one-half quart of water to steep. Take a cupful four times a day until it is used up.

—Sam Hill, Onondaga herbalist, Six Nations Reserve, 1912

Phytolacca americana
Phytolaccaceae (pokeberry family)

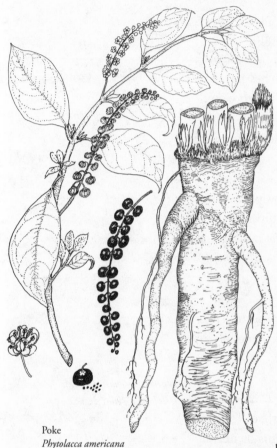

Poke
Phytolacca americana

This powerful medicinal plant has a battery of regional names: pokeweed, scoke, poocan, garget, pigeon berry, pigeon-blood, poke-salat, cancer root, and cancer jalap. Its Latin name, *Phytolacca,* refers to the family it belongs to: *phyto,* meaning plant, and *lac,* meaning a crimson dye; *americana* speaks for itself, identifying the species as a native. This widely spread perennial grows from Maine to Florida and Mexico, and across the West, except in the Dakotas.

Mature poke plants, multibranched with ruby-red stalks and stems in late summer, can grow up to ten feet tall. Earlier, small flowers appear in long, often curving or drooping spires. Each tiny greenish-white, petal-like sepal ripens into a purple-black, fleshy berry. Songbirds favor the ripe, dark purple berries and excrete the fertile black seeds indiscriminately, thus assuring a wide distribution for this amazing herb. After killing frosts arrive, it dies back to the ground.

Poke's genus embraces about twenty-five species of coarse herbs, shrubs, and treelike perennials native to the tropics and warm regions. The Brazilian species, *Phytolacca dioica,* is an evergreen tree that can grow to sixty feet tall and develop a thick trunk. Two East Asian species, *P. acinosa* and *P. esculenta,* are grown as ornamentals and potherbs. American poke is one of our most rugged, enduring herbs, with many historical and contemporary uses.

Traditional uses: American Indians made use of all plant parts in their specific seasons of optimum strength. Throughout the winter, even year-round, the often-huge taproots, fresh or dried, were pounded and poulticed on wounds, tumors, bruises, rheumatic swellings, and sore breasts. Poke root was vital in many cancer and diabetes remedies.

Pokeberry tea served to treat rheumatism, arthritis, and other joint infirmities; the warm tea was helpful as a skin wash to treat bruises, swellings, and sprains. Many believed this spring tonic was also a powerful preventive medicine.

Young spring shoots of American poke provided delicious, asparaguslike greens for our ancestors, and still do for us. When only six inches high, they are easily collected and stewed as a potherb. I remember my grandmother and mother enjoying this spring ritual and teaching us to pick the youngest green spears before the leaves fully form. The cooking water should be brought to a boil and poured off at least once to discard the dark, bitter elements.

The plant's simple, ovate, alternate leaves exude bright green ink when crushed or rubbed. Crushed pokeberries yield one of nature's most brilliant magenta colors. Exciting ranges of inks and dyes come from some of the poke species, but unfortunately they are not sun-fast. Unless overdyed, the colors will fade.

Modern uses: Contemporary herbalists view poke with both respect and caution. A tincture of poke root is used as a blood cleanser in very small amounts and also taken to relieve lymph congestion and swollen lymph nodes. American pokeweed contains numerous alkaloids and complex chemicals, some of which are quite harmful to human systems. A pokeweed mitogen is being studied in antitumor immunity research, as it seems to stimulate cell transformation. Poke root is used in several herbal cancer remedies, including essiac and floressence.

Cautions: The whole plant is toxic. Never use during pregnancy. Plant juice of pokeweed can cause dermatitis in very sensitive individuals.

Growth needs and propagation: Poke grows readily from seeds and root cuttings. The main effort needed is to keep this

Take the berries of pokeweed, or cokum, squeeze out their juice, add it to the same quantity of cream and simmer it down to the consistency of an ointment. If this is used in the early stages of the disease [cancer], it is a certain safe and easy cure. It should be rubbed on every six or eight hours until it has some effect.
—John Williams, a "celebrated Indian doctor," in his 1828 book *New and Valuable Recipes for the Cure of Many Diseases*

For sprains and bruises, a
poke root was boiled and
applied, mashed, as a poultice.
—David Williams, Oneida
herbalist, Oneidatown, 1912

plant under control in the garden, where it will grow up like a
shrub, towering six to ten feet tall from mature roots.

Companions: Poke grows well with almost everything, especially yarrow and strawberry. It seems to enhance the growth of
gourds.

PRICKLY PEAR CACTUS

Opuntia polycantha
Cactaceae (cactus family)

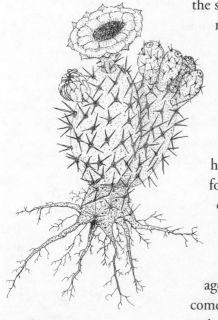

Prickly pear
Opuntia polycantha

The genus name of this spiky plant, *Opuntia*, was given in respect for the ancient city of Opus or Locris, Greece. *Polycanthos,*
the species name, in effect means "many corners," perhaps referring to the structure of this cactus, whose jointed series of flat
pads grow at angles to one another. The common name
prickly pear refers to the pearlike fruits, often sold in fruit
stalls and vegetable markets across the country. To add further confusion, the tasty fruits are commonly called "tunas"
in the Southwest, or "tuna pears" . . . so much for names!

The large, bristly *Opuntia* genus embraces perhaps three
hundred species of prostrate to treelike, mostly jointed cacti,
found from Massachusetts and British Columbia to the Straits
of Magellan. These mostly awkward and coarse plants, also
called cholla cacti, have formidable spines and showy flowers and fruits. I have encountered great colonies of opuntia
in full, glorious bloom on islands of the Norwalk Archipel-
ago in Long Island Sound, where they overwinter well and welcome the seabirds back to their rookeries with their large yellow
spring blossoms. Their ability to withstand unfavorable growing
conditions make them useful ornamentals, especially in rock gardens, sandy banks, and the medicine wheel garden.

O. ficus-indica, the Indian fig or tuna, is widely grown for its
abundant edible pads and fruits. Centuries ago, the Spanish

adopted the Taino Indian word *tuna* for this plant's small red fruits, long a favored food in tropical America. The teddy bear cactus, *O. bigelovii,* grows three to eight feet tall in the West and produces pale yellow flowers in spring. The flapjack cactus, *O. chlorotica,* grows up to six feet tall with long spines and yellow flowers. The beavertail or rose tuna, *O. basilaris,* has yellow- to rose-colored blossoms. There are so many fascinating species of cholla, hedgehog, and prickly pear to consider for the xeriscape garden.

Traditional uses: Throughout the Indian pueblos, both the pads and the sweet, delicious fruits of the prickly pear and many other native cacti were and continue to be eaten. The Zuni made a fine red dye from the prickly pear fruits and the bee plant, dried and ground together. The pads and fruits are best gathered with sharp shovels and gloved hands; then the spines may be roasted or burned off. The peeled pads are used in the mouth to ease inflamed gums and mouth sores, and can be applied as poultices to tumors and skin injuries. The dried flowers are also used in poultices, and are applied to skin as anti-inflammatory treatments. These dried-flower poultices can improve hair and scalp conditions as well. The mucilaginous juice is an anti-inflammatory diuretic, and the fruits are often mixed with corn-meal in various dishes. Native people also use the juice, pads, and fruits of the prickly pear to treat diabetes.

Modern uses: Today there is a cultivated spineless prickly pear cactus grown and sold for the gourmet markets, especially in the Southwest, where these pads and fruits are frequent ingredients in regional foods. Pickled opuntia pads provide the *nopales* enjoyed in Mexican cuisine. Often available in supermarkets, the rosy red tuna pears are delicious raw or cooked into various sweet dishes and jellies. The mucilaginous exudations from the cactus pads are used directly on the skin to ease rashes and many skin problems.

Cautions: Be careful to avoid cactus spines. Handle these cacti with great care, wearing thick garden gloves; you can make a

The Aztec City of Tenochtitlan, "place of the prickly pear cactus," was founded in A.D. 1345, later becoming Mexico City. Its symbol of the prickly pear is on the heart of the Mexican coat of arms, and most Mexican coins. This cactus is ubiquitous in the desert Southwest and across the Mexican countryside.

The Aztec dye *cochineal* is made from the female insects found on the prickly pear cactus, and results in beautiful shades of purple, red, and magenta.

Prickly pear grew so thick that in summer, when you picked the fruit, it was only four steps from one bush to the next.
—Maria Chona, Papago medicine woman, 1930

corset of rolled newspaper to wrap around the plants when handling them.

Growth needs and propagation: Prickly pears will grow well in sandy, loamy soil in full sun. They may be easily propagated from the joints (from which they readily grow roots in good soil), and grow just as readily from seeds. They grow as far north as Connecticut and Massachusetts. Prickly pear colonies are relatively slow-growing and don't usually take over a large area. Many gardeners want them, so you may often be cutting and giving away pads to root new plants. That is how I got mine—from "friendship" gardens. Perhaps your medicine wheel garden will become a friendship garden as you share your plants with others.

Companions: Prickly pears grow well with yucca, yarrow, Oregon grape holly, and poke. They will also make good companions for many other plants in the garden, but they do not like to be crowded and overshadowed. Hummingbirds love the opuntia blossoms.

SAGE

Artemisia tridentata
Compositae (daisy family)
Salvia spp.
Labiatae (mint family)

The ancient Romans associated sage with immortality, longevity, and strong mental capacities. The Latin verb *sapere*, from which the common name derives, means both "to have a good taste" and "to have good sense," thus linking the plant with wisdom. Artemis, the Greek goddess of forests and hills, inspired the genus name *Artemisia,* which is also the Latin word for "mugwort."

Most of the herbal and ornamental sages fall into two great camps: the genus *Salvia,* which lies within the great Labiatae (Lamiaceae), the mint family, and the genus *Artemisia,* which belongs to the compositae, or asters. The dominant sage across Europe, a *Salvia,* differs markedly from the American prairie sage, or sagebrush, an *Artemisia.*

Artemisia includes about two hundred species of aromatic annual, biennial, and perennial herbs and shrubs native mostly in dry, stony areas of the Northern Hemisphere. Many species create their own colonies, or econiches, quickly taking over disturbed ground in the wild. They are grown as ornamentals and for their medicinal, insecticidal, and aromatic qualities, and we know them mostly as the sagebrush, mugworts, wormwoods, and fragrant annies. Southernwood, absinthe, dusty miller (beach wormwood), and garden tarragon are striking Eurasian species of *Artemisia* familiar in many of our perennial gardens. Their small flower heads are generally in spikes or racemes of tiny disklike flowers that can range from white to yellow-green, and even brownish to purplish. The alternate leaves can be lobed or dissected, and most have unusual fragrance.

Sagebrush
Artemisia tridentata

The most common species west of the Mississippi River—and the most sacred smudging herb—of the rugged, attractive native sages growing in dry areas of North America is the classic sagebrush, *A. tridentata.* This rounded evergreen shrub can grow up to ten feet tall, and its silvery-gray foliage and branches are highly aromatic. Nineteen species of sage are native to the greater California–West Coast regions. Sand sage, *A. filifolia,* can grow to five feet tall in the desert Southwest regions, while Alaskan sage, *A. frigida,* is a more prostrate, mat-forming species, which grows south into Kansas and Arizona. The highly aromatic white sage, *A. ludoviciana,* found across the West, has been hybridized into garden varieties called Silver King and Silver Queen. This native herb was first collected in the Louisiana Purchase regions in the eighteenth century—a bit of history reflected in its Latin species name.

The genus *Salvia* embraces more than 750 species of herbs, some growing as shrubs, widely distributed throughout the world's dry, stony regions. *Salvia* comes from the Latin *salvare,* meaning "to cure," and these are certainly healing plants. Some *Salvias* are cultivated as ornamentals and for culinary, perfumery, and medicinal uses. Our native scarlet or Texas sage, *Salvia coccinea,* is one of the most widely cultivated ornamental sages, along with the aromatic native pineapple-scented sage, *S. elegans,* which can grow to more than three feet tall.

Common (culinary) or garden sage, *S. officinalis,* is the familiar Mediterranean herb we use in cooking and some teas. This species was a favorite ancient potherb, cultivated for many centuries. Attractive cultivars grown today in varieties of purplish-red variegated leaves are *purpurascens* and *purpurea* along with the gold/white/green *tricolor* and the *albiflora,* which are favored in many of our kitchen gardens and are welcome additions to the medicine wheel garden. A California native, the aromatic blue sage, *S. clevelandii,* is often recommended as a substitute for culinary sage.

Many more native *Salvia* species are used ceremonially and medicinally, especially the southern California greasewood or white sage, *Salvia apiana,* which can grow three to eight feet tall, with oblong leaves covered in white hairs and white to pale lavender blooms. The Great Plains blue sage, *S. azurea,* has been naturalized in the East and hybridized into several showy varieties. The white woolly Mexican bush sage, *S. leucantha,* and the tall rosy-leaf sage, *S. involucrata,* are stunning southern perennial shrubs. In the Northeast, our native cancerweed, *S. lyrata,* is a diminutive perennial with noted medicinal uses. Wide-ranging historical uses for these herbs span the broad spectrum of human needs.

Traditional uses: Indians throughout the Americas extensively use numerous species of native sage. For example, in the

Artemisia genus, many western tribes use Alaskan sage, *A. frigida,* and sand sage, *A. filifolia,* medicinally and ceremonially. Rocky Mountain sage, *A. arbuscula,* and California sage, *A. Californica,* are collected and dried for ceremonial smudging, and their leaves are chewed for relief of congestion and sore throat. Native peoples have long exploited *Salvia carducea* for its aromatic qualities and cooling, fever-reducing principles, along with gray or purple sage, *S. leucophylla,* the West Coast gray ball sage, *S. dorrii,* and the stout thistle sage. Some sage species are now commercially grown to meet the growing demand for their use in sacred and ceremonial rites.

Dried sage leaves, stems, blossoms, and seeds have long been used as sacred smudging herbs, and many tribes traded for favorite species to use for medicinal teas, sedatives, insecticides, and fumigants. Special clothing, especially ceremonial apparel and masks, was often packed away between layers of dried sage to protect it and keep it fresh. The spirits associated with ceremonial items were and are blessed with sage, and these items were often tied with a sprig of sage for strength and respect. Sage was and is one of the foremost sweat lodge herbs, used by American Indians to banish all negative spirits and emotions and to smudge over the fire. This beneficial herb has long been important on tribal and personal altars and carried in the medicine bag and the car.

Modern uses: Today herbalists around the world use the sages to relieve many problems. Chinese red sage, *Salvia miltiorrhiza* (dan shen), is traditionally used for heart and circulatory problems. Many of the European and native American species serve similar needs and also as digestive tonics, gargles, and a valuable hormonal stimulant for women throughout their childbearing years and menopause. Culinary sage, *S. officinalis,* is also a traditional treatment for asthma, and is drunk as a tea to clear the mind and stimulate thought. Many of us wear a sprig of sage in the garden as an insect repellent.

Cautions: Some individuals can suffer respiratory problems, such as hay fever, and some may even experience slight dermatitis from handling certain species in these two large families. Yet many people rub sage leaves on their bodies to ward off insects and never have any skin problems.

Growth needs and propagation: Most species of sage tolerate sandy, alkaline soil that is well drained. They flourish in rich soil and full sun. Plants do not seem to come as well from seed as they do from root and stem cuttings; they take a good two years to come to maturity from seeds. Once mature, the blossoms and leaves can be clipped repeatedly for ritual or medicinal use. Check them carefully for plant pests, and spray with an organic soap mixture if you detect spittle bugs or spider mites. Sage has many antibacterial properties and usually remains pest-free.

Companions: Sage grows well with other gray-leaved herbs that like slightly alkaline soil, such as coneflower, evening primrose, yarrow, rosemary, and lavender.

The Great Spirit is our Father, but Earth is our Mother. She nourishes us; that which we put into the ground she returns to us.
—Big Thunder, Wabanakis, Maine

SKULLCAP

Scutellaria lateriflora
Labiatae (mint family)

Mad-dog skullcap was the historical name for this native perennial herb, an early folk remedy for rabies. The name skullcap comes from the blossoms, which resemble a type of military helmet worn during the colonial period, when Europeans were learning of and naming most native herbs. The genus name, *Scutellaria,* comes from the Latin meaning "drinking bowl," a shape similar to a skullcap; and *lateriflora,* the species name, means "flowering on the side."

Found growing throughout the East in rich woodland openings and moist hedgerows, skullcap is a favorite in my American Indian medicine wheel garden and is cultivated in many herb gardens. It will grow up to three feet tall with opposite leaves (oval to lance-shaped) and branching racemes of violet-blue flowers blooming from May through September. It can often create large colonies in favorable locations.

Of some three hundred species of skullcap all told, there are nine noteworthy wild species in the eastern states, and each holds some native medicinal values. All flower in late spring and summer in shades of violet to blue, with occasional varieties of pink or white flowers. Hyssop skullcap, *S. integrifolia,* has slender, untoothed leaves and grows from six to thirty inches tall in clearings and woodland edges from Connecticut to Ohio and Missouri and south. Heart-leaved skullcap, *S. ovata,* is a robust, softly downy species favoring limestone soil and wooded riverbanks from Connecticut to Minnesota and Wisconsin to West Virginia, and south. It can grow from one to three feet tall. Downy skullcap, *S. incana,* is minutely fuzzy and can develop many branches. This species favors dry woods and clearings from New Jersey to Iowa and south, standing up to three or more feet tall. Hairy skullcap, *S. elliptica,* is much more hairy, branched, and favors similar soils and the same general range as the downy skullcap.

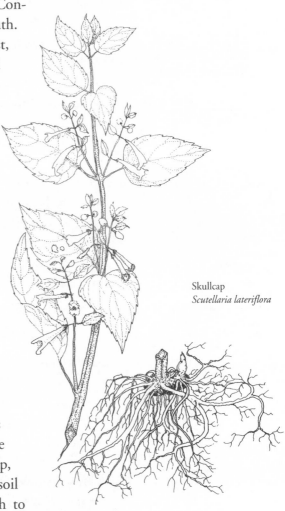

Skullcap
Scutellaria lateriflora

Showy skullcap, *S. serrata,* is a smooth, slender herb that grows up to two feet tall in woods and along streambanks from New York south along the Appalachians, while the tiny smaller skullcap, *S. parvula,* barely twelve inches tall, favors limestone soils from Quebec and Maine south and west to Minnesota. Veined skullcap, *S. nervosa,* can reach two feet tall in damp soil of thickets and woods from Ontario south to

Pennsylvania, and west to Indiana and Illinois. Widespread throughout eastern wet areas from Canada to Delaware to Missouri, common or marsh skullcap, *S. epilobiifolia,* can grow from one to three feet tall.

Traditional uses: Strong teas of skullcap were used by the Indians to treat headaches, epilepsy, and insomnia, and for general pain relief. The leaves and blossoms also went into tonics, tinctures, and salves. The Cherokee used skullcap to relieve cramps and promote menstruation, as well as to relieve certain taboos.

Modern uses: Modern herbalists continue to take advantage of the healing powers of these native perennial herbs. Our native skullcap, *S. lateriflora,* and Baical skullcap, *S. baicalensis* (huang quin), are the principal medicinal herbs of commerce. Their tinctures, infusions, and capsules, with a bitter, astringent taste, serve to treat ailments from migraines and headaches to panic attacks, tension, and depression. It is mainly used as a nerve tonic and sedative. Skullcap medicines have restorative properties that help to nourish and support the nervous system. Often prescribed alone or in formula with other herbs, they also help relieve insomnia and menstrual pain. Teas, capsules, and tinctures made from *S. lateriflora* act as an antispasmodic for all types of nervous conditions, especially asthma.

As a smallpox preventative, mad-dog skullcap keeps the throat clean. Dry the root and take one tablespoon of powdered root and steep it in one quart of water. Drink a wineglassful three times a day.
—Sam Hill, Onondaga herbalist, Six Nations Reserve, 1912

Cautions: Large doses of this herb are harmful.

Growth needs and propagation: Skullcap favors rich, moist earth and semishaded areas in the medicine wheel garden. This herb will grow well in most kinds of soil and is easily propagated from root divisions. Also consider purchasing healthy young plants from good garden centers and plant nurseries.

Companions: Skullcap grows well with strawberry, mayapple, maidenhair fern, blue flag, and ginger.

Fragaria virginiana
Rosaceae (rose family)

These rugged little members of the rose family are some of our most common healing herbs. The name strawberry derives from an Old English word meaning "strew over the ground," and ripe strawberries can appear to be strewn across the ground. *Fragaria* comes from the Latin word for "fragrance," and *virginiana* means "from Virginia." The first specimen identified was probably from the Virginia regions. Most of our native plants were identified and named by European naturalists in the 1600s and 1700s. Enthusiasm for the plants and wildlife in the New World, as America was called during the historic period, brought countless explorers to these shores.

There are perhaps twelve species of these low-growing perennial herbs, with rooting runners that can carpet a whole area. The classic compound leaves divide into three leaflets with serrated (toothed) edges. The wood strawberry has pointed leaflet tips, whereas the common or Virginia strawberry has rounded leaflet tips. The classic white flowers have five petals surrounding the center, which expands and ripens into the fleshy red fruits, which are not true berries, bearing seedlike achenes on the fruit surface. Native to northern temperate regions, strawberries will grow in

Strawberry
Fragaria virginiana

almost any soil and are widely distributed across North America. Field biologists noted that the wild strawberry was the first plant to colonize the rim of Mount St. Helens, growing in volcanic ash, after the volcano subsided following its eruption in 1980.

A native Indian symbol of fertility and sacred renewal, the wild woodland strawberries are reproduced and honored in baskets, wood carvings, quillwork, moosehair embroidery, and beadwork designs. We see our wild strawberry plants, blossoms, and fruits pictured everywhere from cradleboards to traditional clothing, as it is believed that they carry special blessings.

Traditional uses: The medicinal virtues of these plants were well explored by the Indians. In the early 1600s, Jesuit missionaries working among the Huron in southern Canada described one of the Huron curing ceremonies with obvious amazement. Tscondacouane, a blind Huron man, dreamed that it was important for him to fast in order to end a raging epidemic among his people. He fasted for seven days, whereupon the spirits said to him, "We can do nothing more to you, you are associated with us, you must live hereafter as we do; and we must reveal to you our food, which is nothing more than clear soup with strawberries." After this the Huron ate dried strawberries during the winter months in order not to get sick. This was also the practice among other tribes, as wild strawberries were incredibly numerous centuries ago and easily collected and dried for future use, as were cranberries, blueberries, blackberries, and many types of raspberries.

Roger Williams, living among the Narragansetts in 1643, wrote about the ubiquitous wild strawberries, extolling their many virtues. He noted that they were so prolific in some areas, where the Indians had planted them, that there was fruit "enough to fill a good ship." The French traders noted the importance of trading for fresh and dried strawberries with various northern tribes.

The soothing, astringent leaves were used by most tribes in

teas or decoctions to relieve stomach ailments, cramps, menstrual difficulties, and as a therapeutic body wash to relieve sunburn, rashes, and other skin irritations. Root teas were taken as blood purifiers, diuretics, and digestive aids, and the roots were chewed to relieve toothaches and sore throats, coughs, and upper respiratory distress. Some tribes used strong leaf decoctions as nerve tonics, to treat kidney and bladder problems, and to cure diarrhea.

Modern uses: Today strawberries are cultivated as ornamentals, ground covers, for herbal needs, and especially for their edible fruits. Both fresh fruits and leaves are high in vitamin C. Strawberry flavorings, essential oils, and essence have great commercial value in everything from ice cream and yogurt to shampoos, aromatherapy, herbal skin care, and soothing herbal healing formulas.

Modern herbalists honor the many therapeutic qualities of these wild plants. The ripe fruits can prove to be laxatives for some people, and some folks are sensitive to strawberry seeds. Strawberry leaf tea is a trusted, mild aid to digestion and can also stimulate the appetite.

Cautions: Some people have sensitivity to the minute strawberry seeds and find that the fruits can be diuretics. A few individuals are allergic to strawberries.

Growth needs and propagation: Strawberry grows best in rich, sandy, humusy soil, yet will do well in most soil types. It is easiest to propagate from runners cut from healthy plants. These root readily and are useful in forming great strawberry colonies. They make fine ground covers in the medicine wheel garden.

Companions: Strawberry grows well with most plants in the medicine wheel garden, especially skullcap, moccasin flower, yarrow, and yellow dock.

Use wild strawberries to cure canker sores and sties; boil roots for five minutes, and wash eyes and mouth with this cool solution.
—Delia Carpenter, Onondaga herbalist, 1974

Rhus typhina and other species,
Anacardiaceae (sumac or cashew family)

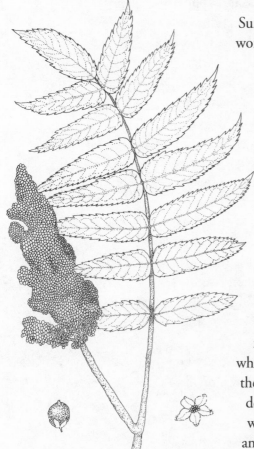

Smooth sumac
Rhus glabra

Sumac, spelled also *sumach,* comes from the Arabic word *summaaq.* The genus name, *Rhus,* comes from the Greek *rhous,* meaning "bushy," which certainly describes these native herbs. The species name, *typhina,* means "pertaining to fever," as these plants were used to treat fevers and colds.

There are perhaps 150 species of *Rhus,* erect shrubs, trees, or vines supported by clinging roots, native to temperate and subtropical regions. They have milky or resinous sap. Some, like the six species of poison ivy and poison oak, have simple leaves with three leaflets; other species have compound leaves with stunning foliage, which ranges from bright orange or yellow in autumn to scarlet red, along with colorful autumn/winter fruits. The small flowers are usually unisexual. The small terminal clusters of fruits are dry, one-seeded drupes, which ripen into attractive pyramid-like clusters atop the naked branches through late fall and winter. These deep red pyramids of fruit are important food for wildlife and were extensively used as food, beverages, and medicines by our early ancestors. All plant parts were used in many ways, in all seasons, by native peoples.

Traditional uses: The red berries and dried leaves and scraped bark of sumac were first exported to Europe in the seventeenth century as fragrant smoking ingredients. For more than twenty-five years they brought a much higher price (from European tobacconists and their patrons) than New World tobacco, *Nicotiana,* which would dominate this market for the next three centuries.

The sumacs are close cousins of poison ivy. Staghorn or velvet sumac, *R. typhina,* also called Virginian sumac, can grow to thirty feet tall, with densely pubescent twigs and fruits. This was an important source of tannin, used for tanning leather. Smooth or scarlet sumac, *R. glabra,* is also called vinegar tree, squawberry, and squawbush, and can grow to twenty feet tall, often forming dense thickets in favorable econiches. The Kiowa call this *maw-kho-la* (tobacco mixture), and many native tribes esteem these botanicals for their kinnikinniks (smoking mixtures). Fragrant or sweet or lemon sumac, *R. aromatica* (*R. canadensis*), is also called polecat bush and can grow to eight feet tall, with several distinctive cultivars and varieties.

Dwarf or shining sumac, *R. copallina,* is also known as mountain sumac, and can grow up to twenty feet tall, often in dense thickets. This species was also an important source of tannin.

There are numerous other regional species that were extensively used by native peoples in their regions. Less common is our poison or swamp sumac, *R. vernix,* also called poison dogwood or poison elder, and often growing to twenty feet tall in wet areas. It can be poisonous to touch, yet is easily distinguished from its nontoxic relatives by its swampy habitats, rank odor, and greenish-white fruits, although its brilliant fall foliage is beautiful.

California, Mexico, and Central America have their own unique species of sumac. Lemonade or sourberry sumac, *R. integrifolia,* is an evergreen shrub or tree that can reach heights of thirty feet. The evergreen or tobacco sumac, *R. virens,* and skunkbush, *R. trilobata,* and its variety *malacophylla,* known as squawbush, have extensive ethnobotanical interest. Sugarbush sumac, *R. ovata,* desert sumac, *R. microphylla,* and laurel sumac, *R. laurina,* are shorter, more diminutive shrubs, as is temazcal, *R. terebinthifolia,* the evergreen shrub native to Mexico and Guatemala.

A Sumac Tea

A simple preparation calls for one cup of the ripe red berries of *Rhus integrifolia* (lemonade sumac), soaked for fifteen minutes or more in one quart of hot (not boiling) water; cool and strain. This pleasing, refreshing beverage is good hot or cold and is high in vitamin C, trace minerals, and malic acid, which gives it the light, citrusy taste so distinctive of these sumacs. In Middle Eastern cuisines ground sumac berries (*zahtar*) often replace lemons in fine dishes and breads.

Wilderness beverages made from plants often acted as preventive medicines and were enjoyed routinely to maintain good health or treat particular problems. "Indian lemonade" or "sumacade" was made from ripe red berries (actually dry drupes) of *R. glabra, R. typhina, R. aromatica, R. copallina,* and/or *R. integrifolia.*

Widely distributed across North America, the sumacs have been used in almost every conceivable way by native peoples for longer than we can know. Prehistoric evidence from almost thirty centuries ago found in the Ozarks suggests that sumac fruits were a primary food.

All plant parts have usefulness. The dense, creamy wood with its pithy center was used for maple syrup spiles, blowguns, arrow shafts, hunting and courting flutes, and hunting whistles, as well as for rhythm and percussion instruments. Sumac's fragrant bark was used for scrolls, rolled for decorations, twisted into cordage, twisted and plaited into baskets, and pulverized into paper. It was also used to make a soft brown dye. The leaves, like the bark, are high in tannin, which added to their effectiveness in medicines, especially for external skin treatments, and made them equally valuable in tanning leather. Thick milky latex exudes from most broken plant parts, and this can be worked into fragrant, sticky pastes, natural glues, and fixatives for paints. Select twigs were used as dentifrices and chew sticks by many different tribes and settlers, as the sumacs also provided dependable toothache remedies. Sumac has long been a vital ingredient in native ceremonial and medicinal formulas, with wide applications.

Modern uses: The astringent and tonic qualities of various sumacs have made them widely respected in medicines, and according to Lewis and Lewis (*Medical Botany,* 1977) some specimens contain antibiotic properties and are effective in preventing tooth decay. Today the native sumacs are grown as ornamentals and extensively used as plantings along roads and highways because of their trim, graceful beauty and resistance to pollution.

Cautions: Some people experience temporary dermatitis from handling these plants, which are closely related to poison sumac and poison ivy, and both have gray-white berries.

Growth needs and propagation: Sumacs are easily cultivated from root divisions, and healthy new plant varieties can be readily gained from garden suppliers and nurseries.

Companions: Sumac grows well with many plants in the medicine wheel garden, especially wintergreen, pipsissewa, skullcap, tobacco, and yarrow.

SWEET FLAG

Acorus calamus
Araceae (arum family)

Acorus is Latin for "aromatic plant," and *calamus* means "reed." Flag comes from the Middle English word *flagge,* meaning "reed." Indeed, these highly aromatic reeds were quite sought after in weaving chair seats, ropes, mats, and baskets. This is also the famous "calamus root," used for pain relief in the folktale classic from the Deep South, *Uncle Remus.*

Calamus, muskrat root, beewort, sweetgrass, sweet root, sweet cane, flagroot, and sweetrush are some of the many regional names. Our native sweet flag, *A. calamus,* is a distinctive member of the arum family, Araceae, which has about two thousand species worldwide that primarily live in wet regions. Its close relatives are jack-in-the-pulpit, green dragon, arrow arum, golden club, and skunk cabbage in the Northeast. When sweet flag is not in bloom it resembles blue flag, and like the latter it has been a highly valued root medicine among Eastern Woodland Indians and other tribes throughout its broad range for a long time.

The arum family, Araceae, includes more than 115 genera, and many of its species are cultivated ornamentals from the trop-

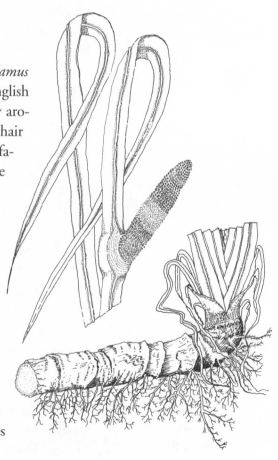

Sweet flag
Acorus calamus

ics. The native perennial sweet flag is found in wetlands, often standing in water along streams and riverbanks across southern Canada from James Bay to Nova Scotia, south to North Carolina, and west to Texas and the Oregon coast. Its long, swordlike leaves are pale glossy green, with a stiff midrib running the entire length. The plants may grow up to five feet tall.

Mature stalks may produce halfway up an outward-jutting clublike spadix (a fleshy cylindrical bloom structure) between May and August that bears tiny clusters of yellowish-green flowers. These ripen into small gelatinous berries that quickly dry up and disappear. All plant parts are fragrant when brushed or bruised, especially the highly aromatic underground rootstalks so prized in Native American medicines.

The long, creeping rootstocks, with many tiny rootlets along their lower half, are usually dug from sand or wet mud, where these plants grow in dense colonies. Old colonies of sweet flag can take over an entire econiche in low, wet pasture or marsh areas, crowding out almost all other plants. Transplanted into the garden, it becomes a delightful, slow-growing ornamental.

Traditional uses: Some observers speculate that native peoples carried these valuable roots with them, establishing new stands of sweet flag near their settlements as they moved and traded. The plant was so valuable to American Indians, possessing countless medicinal and spiritual qualities, that it was a primary trade commodity.

The roots are warm, aromatic, pungent, and bitter, and much better infused in water than in wine or spirits, as they resist the latter. Indian children were especially fond of calamus root, and would chew on a small piece, which was excellent to relieve colic, upset stomach, even toothaches. Calamus root was an early export from the colonies, being much sought after in England and China.

The Cheyenne called calamus *wi'ukh is e'evo* (bitter medicine), and they traded with the Sioux to obtain the plant. They tied a small piece of calamus root on their children's necklaces, dresses, or blankets to keep away the night spirits and bless their dreams. Men and women in many different tribes wore the long leaf blades as garlands and to adorn their hair. The Great Lakes tribes used sweet flag extensively. Small pieces of the root were chewed and held in the mouth to numb toothaches and other mouth problems, and to treat stomachaches, other digestive problems, sore throats, and colds. Infusions of calamus root were also drunk to treat these same problems. Calamus water was often sprinkled on sacred items and throughout dwellings while prayers for renewal were offered.

The Hudson Bay Cree called calamus *pow-e-men-arctic*, meaning "fire or bitter pepper root." The Penobscot and Nanticoke called it muskrat root, and early in the twentieth century it was noted that calamus was perhaps the most important herb in Penobscot pharmacology. A Penobscot legend told that a plague of sickness was sweeping the Indians away and no one knew how to cure the people. Then one night a man was visited by a muskrat in a dream. The muskrat told him that he was a root and where to find him. The man awoke, sought the muskrat root, made a medicine of it, and cured the people of the plague. Sections of the dried root were cut up, strung together, and hung up for the preservation of nearly every house. Stan Neptune, a contemporary Penobscot artist, wood carver, and historian, recalls the importance of eating muskrat in winter, after the animals have been feeding on sweet flag root and their meat tastes "like sweet medicine."

Gladys Tantaquidgeon, a Mohegan medicine woman, noted that the Delaware and other Eastern Algonquians made a sweet flag tea that was used to treat coughs, colds, and suppressed menses. Sweet flag was combined with sassafras root for intestinal pains among the Delaware and other Eastern Algonquians. She described the practice of Eastern Algonquian people carrying a piece of muskrat root as a disease preventive, to chew in case of sudden illness, and just to ensure good health. Gladys also recorded the muskrat root as one of eleven botanicals steeped together for a spring tonic. The Connecticut Mohegan also used small pieces of calamus root to treat rheumatism and colds. From talisman to sophisticated compounds, sweet flag continues to be a most valued health aid.

The Pawnee name is *kahtsha itu* (medicine lying in water), and they have songs about the calamus in their mystery ceremonies, as these plants were considered to have mystic powers. The long blades were used ceremonially for garlands and attached to important objects to bring good luck and power. The Osage called this *pexe boao'ka* (flat herb), and the Omaha and Ponca called it *makan-ninida;* the roots were chewed to treat diabetes, especially among the Dakotas. Potawatomi powdered the root as a styptic.

Calamus is found worldwide, mainly in the northern latitudes, and has an ancient history of uses. The unpeeled, dried rhizome was officially listed in the *U.S. Pharmacopoeia* from 1820 to 1916 and in the *National Formulary* from 1936 to 1950. Doctors prescribed it for indigestion, stomach ailments, and gas, and as a general tonic.

Modern uses: Extracts and bitters made from calamus root continue to be taken to relieve stomach cramps and indigestion. Calamus has long been valued as a flavoring agent and tonic, especially in aromatic bitters, and as a stimulant and carminative. Calamus continues to be a very valuable addition to many American Indian healing formulas, ceremonies, and health care practices, and is still used, alone, in essential ways of healing from tribe to tribe. Many American Indian traditional singers carry the dried root to chew on in order to improve their singing.

Sweet flag is an important component in Chinese, Ayurvedic, and Western herbalism. The rhizome is a valued remedy for indigestion and a tonic for the nervous system. It stimulates the appetite, relieves gas and colic, and is formulated in tinctures and decoctions as well as powders. The aromatic qualities make the leaves a valuable insect repellent.

Cautions: Some Asian varieties have been labeled as unsafe because they have been associated with tumors found in some laboratory rats. The carcinogenic agent is considered to be asarone, a constituent in the volatile oil. Apparently this is not present in the American species.

Growth needs and propagation: In the wild, sweet flag can form dense, intertwining mats in shallow water. Spring or fall is a good time to dig and gather the outer rhizome tips, three to six inches long. Place them about two inches deep in garden soil. The young sprouts can grow rapidly, sending out many white hairy roots. These plants are handsome garden additions, especially in the medicine wheel garden, where their foliage is striking.

Companions: Sweet flag grows well in the company of blue flag, cardinal flower, goldthread, and jack-in-the-pulpit. It will also grow fairly well with other moist-ground-loving herbs.

SWEETGRASS

Hiërochloe odorata
Poaceae (grass family)

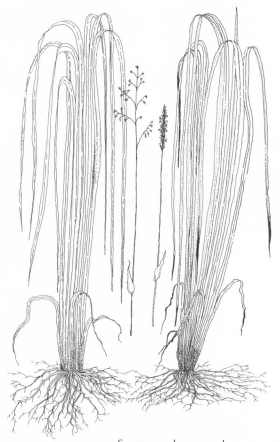

Sweetgrass is one of North America's most sacred plants. It is also called holy grass, vanilla grass, and Seneca grass, and is most desirable because of its vanilla-like fragrance. The genus name comes from the Greek *hieros,* meaning "holy, sacred, or supernatural," and the Greek word *khloros,* meaning "greenish yellow." The species name comes from the Latin word *odor,* meaning "having or giving off odor." The name of the related sweet vernal grass, *Anthoxanthus odoratum,* comes from the Greek for "flower" and *xanthos*, meaning "yellow." These words come to life in the minute yellowish flowers of these grasses, which are filled with yellow pollen in the spring.

These two fragrant grasses are strong perennials that grow in moist, rich earth. Sweet vernal grass will grow in dry sandy pastures and is more widespread than sweetgrass. Both have flat, smooth, shiny green blades that grow to a yard long by late summer. If you run your fingers down the leaf blades toward the roots you will feel the minute barbs (teeth that catch). Sweetgrass, *Hiërochloe odor-*

Sweetgrass and sweet vernal grass
Hiërochloe odorata and
Anthoxanthus odoratum

ata, grows naturally from Nova Scotia to Pennsylvania and west to Ohio, Iowa, and South Dakota.

Traditional uses: As you travel across the country you will find that many Indians use an herb they call sweetgrass, but it is not always the same botanical. Out west there are many more rushes and sedges that also have fragrance, and these are called sweetgrass. Native Americans perceive these grasses to be the "hair of Mother Earth," and so they are considered holy. Both species produce three-foot-long green blades in late summer, when they are ripe for harvesting. The long, slim blades were grouped together and braided to use on altars, to carry with medicines, and to pack with clothing. Indian men and women often braided sweetgrass into their hair during courting and ceremonial times.

Sweetgrass is used in fine basketry, mats, and ceremonial items. It is widely used as smudge (incense) for purification, and blessing ceremonies. Medicinally, sweetgrass is used in teas to treat colds, coughs, and sore throats, and also to help stop bleeding after childbirth.

The Cheyenne used sweetgrass in many of their ceremonies, especially the Sun Dance. Burning smudge of sweetgrass symbolized life's growth and changes. They renewed their arrows during the Sacred Arrow ceremony by passing them through sweetgrass smoke. Ceremonial rattles and other accoutrements were passed through the smoke of sweetgrass.

Centuries ago sweetgrass was the most popular perfume of the Blackfeet and Flathead Indians. They braided it and kept it with them in small leather bags. A mild sweetgrass tea was used as eyewash and on the skin to treat sunburn.

Modern uses: The roots and blades contain coumarin, a fragrant compound that is sought for flavorings and perfumes. Some modern research shows that coumarin and related compounds are effective in reducing high-protein edemas, especially lymphodema. Sweetgrass is sacred to Native Americans and used in many of their ceremonies. It is carried for protection and woven into many baskets.

Cautions: Roots and blades contain coumarin, a blood thinner, which is given to heart patients today.

Growth needs and propagation: These two sweetgrasses are easy to grow, as they usually prosper in sunny meadows. It is best to grow them from healthy rhizomes, which you can buy from a native plant nursery.

Companions: Sweetgrass tolerates competition and will grow well with yarrow, yellow dock, yucca, blue flag, and tobacco.

TOBACCO

Nicotiana rustica and other species,
Solanaceae (nightshade family)

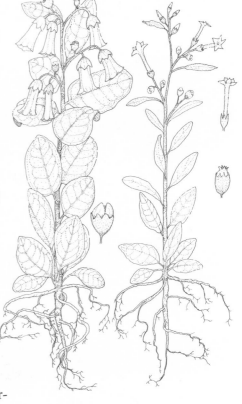

Wild tobacco and coyote tobacco
Nicotiana rustica and *Nicotiana attenuata*

The genus *Nicotiana* was named after Nicot, a Frenchman who first brought the seeds to Europe from the West Indies, thus dispersing the commercial opportunities for growing tobacco—a crop on which numerous fortunes have been made and to which even more deaths have been attributed. Pocahontas's second husband, John Rolfe, and their only son, Thomas Rolfe, established a lucrative tobacco farming/exporting business in colonial Virginia. The species name, *rustica,* means "rustic" or "of the country."

The genus *Nicotiana* yields numerous tobacco species, including the highly fragrant ornamental species cultivated for our annual gardens. Connecticut, for example, was once famous for growing the large-leaved "shade tobacco," used for cigar wrappers, and the broad Connecticut River Valley was historically called "Tobacco Valley." Indeed, tobacco has shaped the character of many states' economies during the past three centuries.

More on Tobacco

Tobacco is one of many Taino Indian words adopted into English and carried forward through time. Tubular stone pipes have been dated as early as 1000 B.C. from archaeological sites in eastern North America. Jacques Cartier, while exploring the St. Lawrence River in 1535–36, noted that the Iroquois Indians in that region called their tobacco *quyecta*. The Virginia Indians called it *uppowoc*. Explorer Henry Hudson noted in 1609 that the native people had copper tobacco pipes and "green tobacco, which is strong and good." The Huron called it *anondahoin*.

Traditional uses: Both sacred and holy to American Indians, tobacco has always been a plant whose leaves were prayed with and seeds carefully saved for spring planting. The dried leaves were crumbled and given as offerings before wild herbs, especially medicine plants, were harvested or game animals killed. Dried, cured leaves were also used in tribal council meetings and in traditional religious ceremonies. When smoked (or burned) the upward-drifting smoke carried prayers to the Creator in the Sky World above, thus enabling one to communicate directly with the Creator and the ancestral spirits. Tobacco smoking calmed the spirit and relaxed the body. The leaves, when chewed and applied to the skin, were a favorite Indian bee sting remedy and an insect repellent. The dried, powdered leaves are still an effective insect repellent.

American Indians introduced the early settlers to smoking, which they used both medicinally and ceremonially. Pipes were most often used, although some tribes prepared and smoked corn-husk cigarettes. Pipes and tobacco were items of status and trade in colonial times. They were often used in treaty-signing ceremonies.

The Indians smoked a variety of dried wild herbs, including wild mints, colt's foot, and goldenrod, blended with a very small amount of tobacco. Consequently, the nicotine content of their smoking materials was minor. By contrast, modern smoking materials use flavorful tobacco, rolled in chemically treated papers to assist burning and prevent flavor loss, and the nicotine content is considerable.

Prehistoric tribes in the regions now called Mesoamerica, where more species of tobacco flourish, honored "tobacco gods." Many were aware of tobacco's mind-altering capacities, and some of the southern tribes considered these herbs to be "flesh of the gods," with the leaves ritually smoked in ceremonies. *N. tabacum* is a stout, viscid annual (in northern zones) or perennial (in southern zones). This species can grow from three to ten feet tall, with large ovate leaves and greenish-cream to pink or red tubular flowers that grow to one inch long and open to one inch across.

Western Indians used their potent native *N. attenuata* and *N. bigelovii* for tobacco. There is a striking tree tobacco, *N. glauca,* also called mustard tree, of southern Bolivia and northern Argentina, which is sometimes grown as an ornamental in North America. Also from South America is the long-flowered tobacco, *N. longiflora,* sometimes grown in the eastern United States, along with hybrids of South America's *N. acuminata.*

Modern uses: Certainly more has been written about tobacco than about any other native plant. As a sacred, ceremonial, and medicinal herb for perhaps thousands of years, it has certainly been exploited and abused as a recreational drug for the past three hundred to four hundred years.

Nicotine, when inhaled, inhibits hunger-related contractions of the stomach and slightly increases blood sugar levels; it also deadens the taste buds.

Cautions: Smoking is hazardous to the health. Tobacco is a noted toxic herb. Nicotine is more addictive than alcohol, causes lung cancer, makes heart disease worse, increases the risk of dying of other diseases, hurts the child in the womb of the mother who smokes, and lowers the skills of those who smoke, according to Walter Lewis and Memory Elvin-Lewis in their book *Medical Botany.*

Growth needs and propagation: Tobacco is very difficult and time-consuming to start from seed. The very fine seeds must be spread in soft, sifted soil, barely covered, and misted to enable germination. Growing tobacco requires a good deal of work, and tobacco is a "heavy feeder" requiring rich soil, shade, and fertilizers during the growing season. In the case of the delicate garden nicotianas, with their beautiful, tubular, fragrant flowers, tobacco

Moshup [a mythical giant credited with forming much of the region's unique landscapes] loved his great stone doorstep. Frequently he would stand thereon and smoke his peudelah [pipe]. Once an offering had been made to him of all the tobacco grown on Martha's Vineyard, which was then called Nope by the Indians. With his peudelah filled with the last of this great gift he one day stood in the sunshine and smoked while he mused of his past . . . his big peudelah suddenly tilted sidewise, and, as the tide was high, the falling ashes therefrom were carried out and down to the east by the swift-running tide, until at last, caught by some drift on a shoal, they became fixed, and in time Nantucket—or the Devil's Ash-Heap, as it is called by the older natives—grew little by little.

—Mary A. Cleggett Vanderhoop, Gay Head Wampanoag, from her Gay Head legend and folklore collections, 1904

is worth the effort. When the old, wild species become established in the garden they will self-sow.

Companions: Tobacco grows well among yarrow, sweetgrass, sage, and mayapple.

WILD GARLIC AND OTHER ALLIUMS

Allium canadense
Liliaceae (lily family)

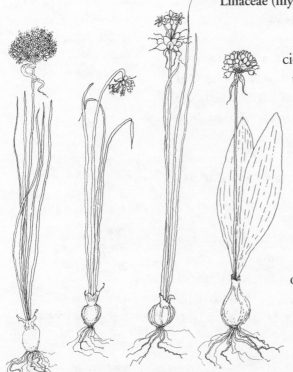

Wild onion, nodding wild onion, wild garlic, and wild leek
Allium stellatum, A. cernuum, A. canadense, and *A. tricoccum*

Species of *Allium* are among the most ancient cultivated plants. Thousands of years ago the early Babylonians, Chinese, and Egyptians noted their use for foods and medicines. *Allium* possibly comes from early Celtic origins; the word *all* meant "pungent." *Canadense* denotes that the plant is native to Canada or the northeastern United States. The great lily family holds many healing and ornamental plants like aloe, asparagus, daylily, and trillium.

Perhaps four hundred species of strongly odorous (when bruised) perennial bulbs in the genus *Allium* are native in the Northern Hemisphere. It is often hard to tell some species apart because their differences are so subtle. *A. canadense* is perhaps the most common and widespread species, found growing wild from southern Canada to the Gulf of Mexico and from the eastern shores to the Rocky Mountains.

Traditional uses: Wild garlic, *A. canadense,* is also called wild onion, wild meadow leek, prairie onion, crow onion, or Canada onion. Early explorers noted many American Indian food and medicine uses for wild onions and garlic. Archaeological evidence in North America shows that native people were eating alliums more than six thousand years ago. The Menomini and Meskwaki favored wild garlic as a choice food, especially during winter, as did many Great Lakes Indians. The Winnebago called it "shin-hop," the Pawnee called it "osidiwa," and the Tewa Puebloans called it "akonsi." Indeed, there are countless Indian names for this native staple food, flavoring, and medicine. The city of Chicago is said to get its name from the Winnebago Indian word for wild leeks, *shika'ko.*

Wild garlic, *Allium canadense,* prospers in most soils, especially sandy bottomlands. It will grow up to two feet tall, bearing tiny pink starlike blossoms in top clusters during spring. Unlike many alliums, the leaves are not hollow, long, and bladelike; they grow from the base at earth level from the small, oval underground bulb. After the bloom, the top grows into numerous tiny bulblets with long, threadlike tails. These spicy hot additions to summer foods both flavor and heal.

Field garlic, *A. vineale,* is an introduced species that has become widespread in the American wild. This one can grow up to three feet tall and blooms pink or white in clusters mixed with tiny bulblets.

Wild onion, *A. stellatum,* is also widespread across North America. Showy umbels of six-point lavender flowers top each small bulb in the spring and can stand two feet tall above grasslike green leaves.

Nodding wild onion, *A. cernuum,* grows across the northern regions, often in distinct colonies. Blooms top the two-foot slender stems during summer. Their classic "nodding" characteristic and delicate pink or white blossom clusters help distinguish this species.

Wild leeks, *A. tricoccum,* also called ramps, usually produce two or three leaves in early spring. The whitish to creamy yellow blossom clusters follow in June and July. Wild leeks are often found in little clusters or colonies in cool woodlands. The leaves are noted spring vegetables, as are the more odorous bulbs.

Modern uses: Cultivated onions, *A. cepa,* and garlic, *A. sativum,* have been garden and gourmet favorites for many centuries as well as being long acknowledged for their medicinal virtues. Modern research has confirmed their antibacterial qualities plus their ability to help lower blood pressure and cholesterol. Wild onion and wild garlic are antibiotic and anti-inflammatory as well as stimulating to the circulation. Eaten as foods, they help prevent colds and even tooth decay. Warmed onion or garlic oil, when dropped into the ear canal, will relieve an earache. This oil has even been used cosmetically to stimulate hair growth. The alliums are valuable systemic insecticides, as eating them makes an individual less appealing to stinging and biting insects.

Cautions: The essential oils from the bulbs can be irritating.

Growth needs and propagation: The alliums favor rich, moist earth but will grow almost anywhere, especially under cultivation. They can be propagated from both seeds and bulbs, but quicker, more robust results come from planting the bulbs, which are available from many native plant suppliers. Alliums do well in groupings of related species, such as a cluster of wild garlic and a colony of wild leeks.

Companions: Wild onion, garlic, leeks, and nodding wild onion grow well with moccasin flower, maidenhair fern, yarrow, and many other plants in the medicine wheel garden.

WINTERGREEN

Gaultheria procumbens
Ericaceae (heath family)

The genus name *Gaultheria* comes from the Celtic language of ancient Gaul; the meaning is obscure. The species name *procumbens* is Latin for "prostrate or flat on the ground," which describes the low growth habits of this diminutive evergreen.

Wintergreen is related to bearberry, *Arctostaphylos uva-ursi,* trailing arbutus, *Epigaea repens,* and several other native Indian wildflowers in the heath family. The genus *Gaultheria* has as many as a hundred species of evergreen, erect or prostrate shrubs native chiefly to the Andes of South America, to North America, and from Asia to Australia. Creeping snowberry, *G. hispidula* (*Chiogenes hispidula*), is also native to our regions. Alpine wintergreen, *G. humifusa,* and salal, *G. shallon,* are native to the mountainous northwestern regions.

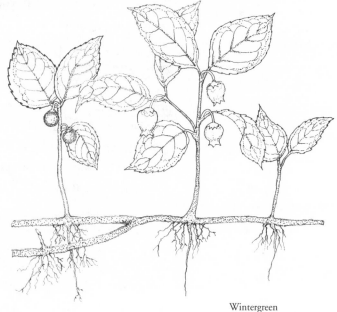

Wintergreen
Gaultheria procumbens

Wintergreen is a low-growing evergreen about six inches tall, with leathery dark green leaves. Solitary white, bell-like flowers emerge in summer, about one-quarter inch long, and hang nodding below the glossy leaves. Scarlet red berries follow in fall and are a tasty treat for humans and birds, especially when found in winter snow. These plants favor sandy or peaty soils and partial to full shade. Wintergreen is an occasional trailside plant found in the woods.

The oval, glossy leaves of wintergreen possess the characteristic flavorful oil. This was the original source of oil of wintergreen, which is now obtained from the gray birch, *Betula lenta,* or made synthetically. Cool, clean, and slightly antiseptic, the flavor of wintergreen is familiar to us in toothpastes, lozenges, candy, and gum. It is also used in some medicines.

Traditional uses: Wintergreen, teaberry, checkerberry, or Green Mountain tea was called *pockqueesegan* by Lake Superior Chippewa, *pahgezegun* by the Saultaux Indians in Minnesota, and *pollom* (for the berries) by the eastern Delaware Indians. This tiny native herb was widely used by many different tribal groups as a cooling, antiseptic pain reliever, and for much more. Several different woodland plants are sometimes referred to as wintergreen, including pipsissewa, *Chimaphila maculata,* because they are green in winter and often used in similar ways medicinally. Yet true wintergreen is *Gaultheria procumbens,* found growing wild from Newfoundland to Manitoba and Minnesota, and southward to Georgia and Alabama.

American Indians traditionally used wintergreen leaf teas to treat headaches and stomachaches, kidney ailments, colds, sore throats, and fevers. The early spring roots were chewed to strengthen teeth and gums and prevent tooth decay. A strong tea (decoction) was used for external skin and sore muscle treatments and especially for relief of rheumatism.

Modern uses: Experiments prove that the essential oil of wintergreen is anti-inflammatory, antiseptic, and analgesic, and small amounts have delayed the onset of tumors. The essential oil in liniments and ointments provides relief from swollen muscles and joints and especially from sciatica (pain in the lower spine resulting from nerve pressure) and trigeminal neuralgia (pain affecting facial nerves). This is an effective remedy for rheumatic and arthritic problems. Wintergreen teas are also valuable to relieve colic and flatulence.

Cautions: The essential oil of wintergreen is highly toxic; absorbed through skin, it harms the liver and kidneys, except in the small amounts used in flavorings or liniments. People sensitive to aspirin should not take wintergreen internally. Do not use on the skin of young children.

Growth needs and propagation: Wintergreen favors a rich, acid woodland soil. It can thrive in shaded locations in the medicine wheel garden. Propagation is generally by seed and root division, following the traditional methods for both.

Companions: Wintergreen grows well with yarrow, yellow dock, pipsissewa, and Oregon holly grape.

Achillea millefolium
Asteraceae (sunflower or aster family)

The genus name of this rugged, lacy herb remembers the Greek hero Achilles, noted for his strength, who used this plant to heal wounds more than three thousand years ago during the Trojan War. The species name *millefolium* means "thousand leaves," and the many fine dissections of these leaves do seem that numerous. The name *yarrow* comes from West Germanic and Old English origins; its meaning is obscure. Yarrow is a member of the huge Asteraceae (sunflower or aster family), which comes from the Latin word *aster*, meaning "star." These family members are very different yet all have radiating ray flowers that seem to symbolize expanding stars.

Achillea embraces about a hundred species of aromatic perennial herbs native to northern temperate zones. The finely cut leaves are alternate and in basal rosettes. *A. millefolium* is a soft, fragrant perennial that will grow from one to three feet tall. This fine fernlike foliage is covered with silky or woolly hairs. The white blossoms appear in flat, tightly packed clusters atop the sturdy stems.

Yarrow
Achillea millefolium

These plants will bloom from May through October in most gardens, making them cheerful additions. Each tiny individual flower has five petal-like rays, and each ray has three teeth at its tip. Yarrow has been hybridized into various blossom colors from pale to vivid pink, red, yellow, gold, and orange. Many gardeners have special cultivars that blossom in a bright range of colors. Variations in yarrow foliage are also interesting in garden hybrids. Yarrow has a broad geographical range. It grows all across Canada and the United States, and from Alaska, the Yukon, and the Aleutian Islands to Mexico.

Fern-leaf yarrow, *A. filipendulina,* is a stiff perennial herb that will grow from four to five feet tall. This is a favorite species in many gardens, as is woolly yarrow, *A. tomentosa.* There are many attractive species and varieties to choose from.

Traditional uses: Archaeological evidence suggests that yarrow has been associated with humans, and has grown for some sixty thousand years on every continent. The Chinese used yarrow sticks to cast the I Ching, an ancient method of divination. African cultures also used yarrow sticks for divination and fortune-telling. American Indian tribes in the Southwest used yarrow stems for divination and to create prayer feathers and prayer sticks.

The Illinois and Miami Indians used yarrow for wound dressings and to treat diarrhea and stomach problems. The Montagnais used this herb for colds and fevers, as did the Mohegan and Delaware Indians. The Iroquois and Micmac used yarrow for colds and fevers and in the sweat lodge. The Winnebago and Chippewa used the dried powdered yarrow to treat headaches, to clean cuts and wounds, and to treat toothaches.

The Navajo and Pueblo people used yarrow to treat stomach disorders and toothaches, as well as to treat burns, hemorrhoids, and for hair and scalp care. In some native communities yarrow was used to flavor foods and for its medicinal benefits. In many respects these herbal ways continue because they provide relief and actually work. Many tribes used yarrow as a birth control treatment in formula with selected other herbs, and exploration of these techniques led to our first modern birth control medications.

Yarrow was also used in medicine lodge rites. The Cheyenne Indians used yarrow infusions to treat coughs, colds, and nausea.

The Menomini and Meskwaki Indians used fresh yarrow tops to treat eczema and children's rashes. Many of the Great Lakes tribes dried yarrow to add to kinnikinnicks, or smoking mixtures. Yarrow was used as a smudge by many tribes.

Modern uses: Over a hundred biologically active compounds have been identified in yarrow. Experiments show that yarrow extracts are anti-inflammatory and help stop bleeding. Yarrow tea, made from the flowering plant, helps treat indigestion, colds, fevers, and even anorexia and internal bleeding.

The fresh leaves may be used as a poultice on sprains and swellings. Yarrow (dried) is one of the valuable "herbs of dreaming" and is sewn into eye masks and dream pillows along with mugwort, sage, lavender, and flaxseed. Yarrow is a favorite dye plant yielding a range of yellow to olive hues depending upon the mordants. Yarrow dries beautifully when cut early and hung upside down. It is used in herbal flower arrangements (both fresh and dried), and is used in a variety of cosmetic preparations for skin and hair.

Cautions: Large or frequent doses taken over a long period of time can be harmful. The plant may cause dermatitis to some with sensitive skin. Do not use during pregnancy.

Growth needs and propagation: Yarrow does best in full sun. It grows in most soil types. It is easily propagated by root division, and rarely by cuttings; seeds should give you blooming plants in the second year.

Companions: Yarrow is known as an "herb of strength" that strengthens anything growing nearby. This makes yarrow a fine companion plant in any garden. It grows very well with sage, sweetgrass, blue flag, and wild garlic and onions—perhaps making them even sweeter and more aromatic.

YELLOW DOCK

Rumex crispus
Polygonaceae (buckwheat family)

The species name, *crispus*, means "crisped or curled" and accurately describes this plant's curly leaf edges, but the original meaning of *Rumex* is obscure. Curly dock, narrow dock, or common sorrel are some of the regional names for this powerful healing herb.

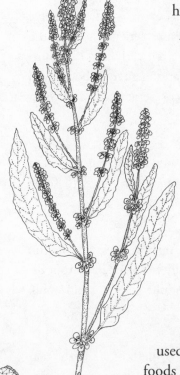

Yellow dock
Rumex crispus

Perhaps twenty species of dock are found across North America and some of them are Eurasian introduced species. All have a long history of food and medicinal uses. The juice from their crushed leaves will relieve irritations from stinging nettles as well as some insect and spider bites. Shades of bright green and yellow dyes are obtained from these roots and leaves. Bitter or broad-leaved dock, *R. obtusifolius,* is especially common along roadsides and in meadows.

Sheep-sorrel, *R. acetosella,* a diminutive relative in this same family, is one of the major herbs in the old Ojibwa cancer formula known as essiac.

Traditional uses: American Indians used all plant parts in various seasons for foods and health care needs. It is fascinating to see how readily and widely native herbalists and families adopted the uses of this plant, long considered an introduced European herb. In the mid-1880s Hoffman noted that the Ojibwa used the pounded roots poulticed on skin sores and wounds. The roots and seeds were considered laxatives, purgatives, and diuretics. The young green leaves were stewed for a spinachlike vegetable among many tribes.

The carrotlike, yellowish-brown taproots anchor these rugged perennials in almost all soils. A slender, grooved stalk rises to almost three feet tall by midsummer, supporting many branching, erect, tiny green flowers. These ripen by late summer into three-winged grains turning golden amber, then brown. These are roasted and ground fine into a delicious buckwheat-like flour for hot cereals, soups, breads, and ash cakes. Pressed into patties with herbs and raw eggs, these make memorable grilled veggie burgers. The large lance-shaped green leaves are steamed and sprinkled with vinegar. The fresh green leaves also make excellent wound dressings and can relieve skin rashes and irritations.

Modern uses: Today herbalists rely on yellow dock roots in tinctures and teas to take as blood purifiers for toxic skin conditions like acne, psoriasis, and eczema. This herb also can increase iron absorption and help our bodies with fat metabolism. The anthraquinones curb ringworm.

Cautions: Both curly dock and sheep-sorrel should be used in moderation as they can prove to be poisonous in large doses. Their high oxalic acid content can bind and eliminate calcium from our bodies, and their tannin content can cause stomach upset and constipation.

Growth needs and propagation: Yellow dock will grow in most soil, and in full sun or partial shade—nearly anywhere. It propagates readily from seed and root cuttings following standard procedures.

Companions: Yellow dock grows well with yarrow, strawberry, poke, and most other plants.

Yucca glauca
Agavaceae (agave family)

Yucca was misnamed by John Gerarde, an English physician, in the 1600s, as it was mistaken for the vegetable yucca. Like other botanical misnomers, the name has stuck. The species name, *glauca,* means "whitened with a bloom"; the leaves are covered with a whitish, waxy film.

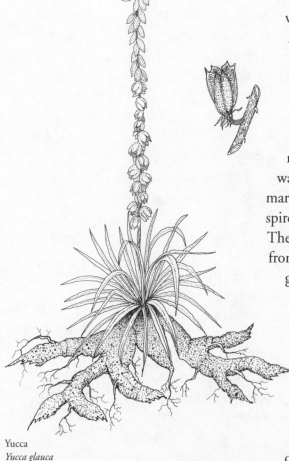

Yucca is a big family of striking plants, with about forty species native to North America. They grow primarily in the warmer regions of the South, where they are often cultivated. There are a few hardy species in the North.

These perennials grow in clumps radiating out from basal rosettes above woody rootstocks. Abundant, long, bayonet-like, waxy green leaves sometimes have whitish margins. Large flowers cluster along stout, spirelike stalks extending well above the leaves. These bell-shaped creamy-white flowers bloom from May through July, then ripen into long, green oval pods that become woody when mature and open to release numerous flat black seeds. All plant parts are valuable, but principally the large roots were used medicinally and for hair care.

Soapweed, *Yucca glauca,* is also known as beargrass, amole, Spanish bayonet, dagger plant, and Adam's needle (referring to these sharp-pointed leaves). The Lakota call it *hupe'stola* (sharp-pointed stem); the Pawnee call it *chakida-kahtsu;* the Omaha and Ponca call it

Yucca
Yucca glauca

duwaduwahi; and the Blackfeet name is *eksiso-ke.* This plant grows wild across the Great Plains regions, especially favoring the sandy areas.

Traditional uses: The Blackfeet and other Plains tribes boiled soapweed roots in water to make a tonic to prevent hair loss. This also served as an anti-inflammatory for poulticing sprains and breaks. Young emerging blossoms and new seedpods were also edible foods for many tribes. The Lakota made a strong root tea to drink for stomachache. When this was mixed with a tea of the roots of the prickly pear cactus, it made a valued childbirth remedy.

The blue yucca, or banana yucca, *Y. baccata,* is found throughout the desert Southwest, and the Joshua tree, *Y. brevifolia,* also provided medicines, foods, and soapy cleansers. Ancient fibers from these species have been found as yucca cordage, belts, rope ladders, cradle lashings, and sandals at Bandolier National Historic Park and other prehistoric sites in the Southwest.

As the name soapweed implies, fresh or dry yucca roots are pounded and thrashed in water to make a sudsy lather for scalp and hair. Zuni, Cochiti, and Jemez Pueblo men and women wash their hair with it before ceremonial dances, as do many other Indians. They take great pride in the healthy shine it gives their black hair, plus the yucca treatments are considered to strengthen the hair. Pueblo potters used yucca-fiber brushes to draw their classic designs on clay pots, especially at Acoma Pueblo.

Modern uses: Yucca tea provides valuable anti-inflammatory relief for arthritic pains according to Michael Moore, a folk medicine practitioner. He maintains that similar teas also provide relief from prostate inflammations.

Growth needs and propagation: Yucca prefers sandy, loamy soil with good drainage and open exposure to the sun and wind. Propagation is easily made from the seeds, offsets (new young plants), and cuttings of stems, rhizomes, or roots in late summer, fall, or winter. Follow standard procedures.

*May all I say and all I think
be in harmony with thee,
God within me, God beyond
me, Maker of the tree.*
　　—Chinook prayer fragment

Soapweed is an attractive, robust evergreen plant that often blooms on Memorial Day in southern regions. It is cultivated across the country. Roots of mature plants can grow to be twenty feet long. These plants have stunning cultivars, especially *rosea,* which is noted for its rose-tinted flowers.

Companions: Yucca plants are good companions for yarrow, prickly pear, Oregon holly grape, strawberry, and tobacco.

PART THREE

Gathering the Herbal Bounty

Recipes and Practical Herb Crafting

Once you start growing things, it takes you off into a whole other way of seeing the world. You have plenty of time to meditate. . . . My parents, my brothers and sisters, and me lived with my grandmother in her house. I remember my grandmother always being very happy and not wanting or desiring material things. I remember her working in her garden, living a very simple life, and eating a very simple diet. I too have discovered that contentment and happiness come from knowledge of the natural world.

—Clayton Brascoupe, Mohawk, Iroquois Six Nations, 1986

CHAPTER TEN

Harvest Times

Making Good Use of Earth Medicines

BEFORE YOU GATHER YOUR first leaves and blossoms, go into your garden and sit or kneel down with the plant(s) you wish to harvest. Quiet yourself by relaxing and taking deep, balanced breaths. Taste the air and savor the fragrances around you. Breathe in these natural fragrances and exhale all of the tension and problems out of your body. As you continue to do this balanced breathing, think about your appreciation for these plants in this medicine wheel space. You are connected with everything here. Offer a simple prayer of gratitude and renewal, so that the growing cycles will continue to flourish. Can you feel the plants' spirits? They are communicating with you.

You are never alone when you gather herbs in your medicine wheel garden. Insects, birds, and animals also frequent your garden. There are so many critters living here, many of which you might never see. Many live in and among the plants, while countless thousands live beneath the surface soil. Move slowly through your harvesting rituals, mindful of the other residents in this sacred space. You have helped to create a magical web of life. You have nourished this medicine wheel ecosystem, and it reciprocates. Come to your garden in early summer well after dark to watch the

To become a medicine person is to realize that one has the gift to share and has an inherently great capacity for carrying energy and that energy may be positive for the benefit of the people. One chooses to walk the medicine way. And it chooses you.
—Dhyani Ywahoo, priestcraft holder of the Ani Gadoah Clan, Tsalagi (Cherokee) Nation

Dancing Circles

May we live our lives
As if they were a song
For singing in the night;
Provide the music
For the stars to be
Dancing circles in the night.

fireflies dance in their emerging mating flights. Watch for monarch butterflies around your butterfly weed. Visit your garden early on September mornings to appreciate the tent spiders' webs and garden spiders' orb-shaped webs filled with dew. Plants have many companions and assistants during their own life cycles.

Harvesting and processing your herbal bounty can be almost a year-round activity. Harvesting from your garden can be combined with pruning the plants and encouraging growth. Cut or pinch growth carefully so your plants can quickly regrow and maintain their vigor. Gather only healthy, vibrant plants, and collect only the plant material that you can readily use to avoid waste and the feeling of being overwhelmed with duty.

Many plants can be pinched back several times during the summer in order to ensure fuller, stockier growth and more blooms. Actually, this is recommended for the new cultivars and hybrids of our native herbs, and it enhances the growth of old native varieties as well. Bee balm, boneset, heal-all, sage, skullcap, and tobacco will usually prosper with this treatment, unless you want tall specimens. Pinch off a half inch of top growth in June and early July to encourage stocky branching in these plants. It is especially important to pinch back certain plants during periods of drought and the withering heat of late summer when they become distressed. These pinches of herbs can be dried to make kinnikinnick.

Most garden mints and yarrows can be cut and harvested repeatedly during their growing seasons, and the plants will be healthier for it. Use these cuttings and pinchings in summer teas, lotions, and summer salads.

TIMING IS IMPORTANT

You can harvest things from your garden anytime it suits you. Yet you may notice subtle differences when you follow the folk wisdom that specifies the best times to collect certain items. When you work with these natural rhythms, you can feel much closer relationships with the plants and all that they can give you.

Plants have their peak of potency first thing in the morning, after they have regenerated all night long. My grandmother gathered most of her medicinal plants before eight o'clock in the morning, while they were still fresh with dew and before the sun could wilt them. The morning dew is a special healing attribute when caught on the blossoms and leaves you are gathering to make salves or tinctures. On the other hand, vegetables, fruits, nuts, and seeds are best gathered in late afternoon, when they have received the maximum benefits of the day's nourishing influences.

My grandfather always felt it was best to gather the above-ground plant parts during the two weeks between the new and full moons. Roots were usually collected during the following two weeks, between the full and new moons. If you are gathering produce from the garden to dry and store, you want to collect after the full moon, as the plant's water content is lowest then.

Herbs need to be processed quickly for their vitamin-rich stores and to prevent deterioration. The medicinally active plant constituents are generally the first to be affected when plant material sits and wilts while awaiting processing.

Natural products will not have a long shelf life. Herbal tinctures will last a year or two, as will some capsules and creams, but most dried herbal products should be used and enjoyed within one to six months for maximum benefits.

COLLECTING AND DRYING

Saving Leaves and Blossoms

Collect the most vibrant leaves and flowers—the ones that you feel are full of life-force energy—to make your herbal products. Move among your

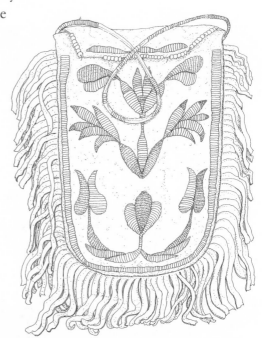

Lakota quilled and beaded medicine bag, circa 1875

The Navajo Beauty Way Chant

I walk with beauty before me.
I walk with beauty behind me.
I walk with beauty above me.
I walk with beauty below me.
I walk with beauty all
*   around me,*
As I walk the Beauty Way.
I walk with beauty all
*   around me,*
As I walk the Beauty Way.
All my thoughts are beautiful!
*   Ho!*

All my words are beautiful! Ho!
All my actions are beautiful! Ho!
As I walk the Beauty Way.
I walk with beauty all
*   around me,*
As I walk the Beauty Way.

Grandma would walk each afternoon, with a big stick, along the rims and valleys with the dogs. Sometimes she would come back with her arms full of flowers, which she boiled into a delicious tea that eased her aches and pains.

—Lori Arviso Alvord, M.D., Navajo surgeon, from her book, *The Scalpel and the Silver Bear*, 2000

plants with a feeling of happiness, and honor their healing potentials. I usually hum or sing as I work among my plants. One of my favorite chants that I repeat over and over is: *"Healer of all . . . come, Blessed One. Healer of all . . . come, Blessed One."* Another favorite song that I sing is from the traditional Navajo Beauty Way Chant. We often sing and dance this uplifting and powerful song in our circles. What better place to sing the Beauty Way than in the garden to the healing plants!

To use flower heads in teas and tisanes, collect blossoms just before or as they are beginning to bloom, as they have the highest potency then. Hang them to dry away from direct sunlight, which can rob blossoms and leaves of vital color and fragrance. Separate flower heads from stems and spread them well apart on clean muslin or paper over screens to dry, turning them often and checking for tiny insects. When thoroughly dry, pull blossoms apart, separating petals from flower centers, and store in dark containers to protect color. Leaves can be dried the same way.

I often cut fresh yarrow, sage, and boneset on long stems with leaves and young blossoms intact and tie them in small bundles. I hang them from the ceiling beams to dry for a week or two. Some of these bundles are so pretty that I leave them hanging all winter, feeling my garden's energies all around me. I can use them in teas, smudging, kinnikinnicks, tinctures, or powders whenever I need them. They are also just lovely in small, dried bouquets as gifts to friends or to patients recovering from illnesses.

Collecting Fruits and Berries

Harvest the healthiest-looking fruits and berries when just ripe. They may not dry properly and can deteriorate if too ripe. Place fruits and berries on absorbent paper on trays, and put trays in a warm oven (that's turned off). Leave the oven door ajar. Small fruits like blueberries, bearberries, and small strawberries should dry in three to four hours. Turn fruits and check carefully midway through the drying process.

Dice chili peppers and cactus fruits into one-inch pieces, or smaller, and follow the same process. These make take twice as long to dry, depending upon the humidity and weather.

Saving Seeds

If you want to save seeds, either for replanting or for consumption, look for the strongest, most robust flower heads and allow these to go to seed.

For replanting, collect fresh seeds in brown paper bags and dry them well. Store them away from strong heat and sunlight, which can rob them of their natural color and volatile oils. When thoroughly dried, sift or carefully pick out any other plant material, and pour the seeds into clean glass jars or plastic bags. Don't forget to label and date them.

I often make a circle of my finest medicine wheel garden seeds in their containers as an altar to future fertile gardens. I enjoy giving away choice selections of these seeds to friends who want some of the healing energies from my garden. Also, tiny seed packets make lovely enclosures with holiday cards.

Seeds can be saved for eating, too. Delicious tiny black seeds from ripe evening primrose pods are excellent to eat, either fresh (keep them in plastic bags in the freezer) or dried and roasted, which makes them tastier. You can use them in corn breads, biscuits, fruit dishes, and omelets. Yellow dock seeds are easily clipped and saved, too. These smell like buckwheat as they are roasting.

Roast seeds by pouring a half cup into a clean, dry iron skillet. Jiggle to evenly distribute the seeds, and then roast over medium heat on top of the stove, or in a medium oven for several minutes. The time is gauged by the size of the seeds. Tiny evening primrose seeds may only take three to five minutes in a hot skillet on top of

Seeds Art as a Record of Your Garden

You can make a seed miniature medicine wheel garden. Take a small flat plaque or white paper plate. Mark the four quarters of your garden on this, noting the pathways and other details. Using white glue, which dries clear, place a dot of glue in the appropriate space where the seed of each plant grows in your garden. Set one seed in each dot of glue and push it in with a toothpick. Allow this to dry thoroughly overnight. Write the name of each seed, if you wish, and add any colors or embellishments that suit your artistic sense. This is another fascinating way to know and honor your healing plants.

the stove. Yellow dock's fatter, winged seeds may take fifteen to twenty-five minutes in the same hot skillet on top of the stove. Jostle the skillet repeatedly while the seeds are roasting—almost like you would treat popcorn—so they roast evenly and don't burn.

Saving Roots

You can save roots for eating or for medicinal use, or to re-plant later. For consumption or medicinal uses, roots are at their peak of efficacy after hard killing frost, when the aboveground parts have died back. Indian summer—those brief fabulous days of warmth after a killing frost and before the ground freezes—is the best time to dig roots. Yet you can actually dig roots for almost six months of the year in most northern zones, from hard frost to early spring. Dig roots at any time of day, especially in late after-noon.

Remove the soil from the roots by brushing or hosing them off, then spread the roots to dry on the grass in the sun for several hours, or even overnight, if they are thick, fleshy roots like black cohosh and poke. When thoroughly dry, store for later use. Or wash the freshly gathered roots, wrap them in paper towels, and store them in the refrigerator. Use within a week or two. Evening

primrose, yellow dock, and coneflower roots may
last up to a month or more in refrigeration
if not enclosed in plastic, which will encourage spoilage.

To prepare tinctures of medicinal
roots such as coneflower, sweet flag, Oregon holly grape root, yellow dock, or
black cohosh, follow the directions for
Oregon holly grape root digestive bitters
on page 250. Tinctures use an alcohol
and water mixture to draw the maximum amount of essential constituents
out of the roots.

You can also dry and powder certain roots from your garden in order
to encapsulate them. You will need a
good industrial grinder to properly
powder dried roots. The equipment and various sizes of capsules
can be ordered from most herb
stores or herbal catalogs.

To save roots for propagation,
gently pack the freshly dug roots
in generous bushel baskets or
large pots. Surround the roots
with some soil and autumn leaves
or mulch. You may even use damp-

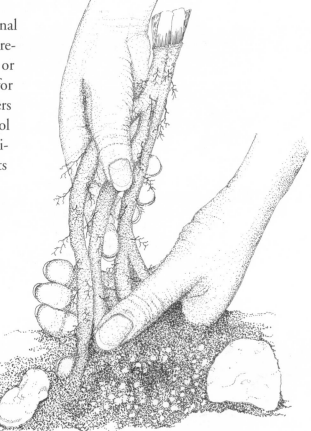

Planting black cohosh roots

ened newspapers to pack around the roots. Save in cool, dark root
cellars or sheds where they are protected from deep freezes.

Fall is a great time to trade roots with other gardeners. I am so
grateful for these offerings from gardens of friends. The subse-
quent plants seem to bring along a little bit of the friend who
shared them.

If you need to pack and ship your roots, dry them briefly and
wrap them in newspaper or pack them in peat moss or sawdust. It
is best not to use plastic, as it can cause mold and decay.

Dried Flowers

As noted earlier, if you are saving flowers for medicinal use, you should harvest them just before or as they begin to blossom. But for display, choose flowers that are at their peak.

Another way to preserve the bounty of your garden is by saving seedpods. For example, the seedpods of blue flag, coneflower, butterfly weed, and angel's trumpet develop their own unique woody, sculptural beauty. These are nicely offset by the more delicate pods of tobacco, and the fully mature flowers of fairywand, bee balm, and yarrow. The dry wintry branches of bayberry, with their small clusters of tiny white, waxy berries make nice additions to winter bouquets. To preserve these, cut the individual herbs with long stems after killing frost. This work is best done on a warm Indian summer afternoon, when all of the plant's leaves have fallen off and you can appreciate each plant's architectural beauty. Tie each small grouping together loosely with twine and hang upside down, inside, in a warm, dry, shady place where lots of air can circulate around them. These look nice tacked along ceiling beams in an old house, or suspended from cabinets. Thorough drying can take several days to a week.

Pressed flowers and leaves are also lovely. Choose examples from each plant before frost and press them between sheets of yellow paper and blotters in plant presses. (Yellow paper helps to keep specimens from fading.) You can also use old telephone books, especially the yellow pages, and place a weight of additional books on top of them. These may take a week to dry. (Check them every day to make sure they are drying without mold, mildew, or bugs—I have dried many fine specimens only to open the plant press and find that tiny bugs were eating the dried herbs! If you check your work often, you can arrest problems before they spread.) These flattened herbal samples are easily glued into notebooks or journals, or composed into beautiful pictures and cards. You are only limited by your imagination and time.

A tiny sprig of sage and yarrow can make a delicate arrangement. The Japanese call this art form *oshibana*, especially when the herbs are topped with a translucent piece of fine rice or mulberry paper. You may even feel moved to add a *haiku* to this artistry. *Haiku* is a brief Japanese nature poem expressed in seventeen or fewer syllables that captures a special moment, and conveys a seasonal touch.

> *Monarch butterfly*
> *alights to sup atop*
> *pink coneflower.*

Drying herbs from the medicine wheel garden is important for winter teas and health care preparations in other seasons. Avoid drying herbs in direct sunlight or near the heat, as these can rob herbs of vital color and fragrance. Hang small bundles to dry where air circulates, or suspend bunches of herbs tied in brown paper bags. You might dry some herbs spread thinly on cookie sheets in a warm oven overnight. I have an old gas range with a pilot light, which is perfect for drying produce. As you dry your valuable produce, bag and label each herb with the date. I love to see my shelves lined with large glass jars and plastic bags filled with dried garden herbs.

HERBAL CREATIVITY

Many of the medicine wheel herbs you have cut and gathered repeatedly throughout the growing season can be worked into yummy recipes, fabulous health and beauty items, and ceremonial items like smudge sticks and kinnikinnicks (aromatic botanical mixtures). Directions and recipes for a variety of items follow in the next few chapters. Here I provide basic information about working with plants from your medicine wheel garden.

Herbal Healing Awareness

I do not advocate self-treatment with your own herbs for any medical condition. What I offer here is information about using the bounty of your medicine wheel garden to prepare healthy

Expanding Cultivation of Native Plants

My late friend Claude Medford Jr., a Choctaw-Apache artist and historian, used to say, "When you see an increase in certain medicine plants, this is the Creator's way of showing that there will be an increased need for these plants. It is up to us to figure out how best to use them." I always think of Claude and his traditional wisdom when I see numerous wild herbs taking over new areas. We cannot safely harvest edible or medicinal plants from many places, especially not from roadside edges and public areas, where they can build up risky levels of toxins and poisons. So we must bring these therapeutic herbs into safe organic cultivation. Just associating with them can make you feel stronger.

foods, teas, tinctures, soaps, creams, and other basic homemade herbal products. Used in this way, products from your garden harvests enhance your health and provide sensory pleasure. In general, herbs tonify, support, and strengthen rather than treat specific conditions or illnesses. This is quite a different approach to healing than we are accustomed to in conventional medicine.

Herbal medicine has become more scientific in the last two decades, and it is certainly an increasingly valuable source of complementary healing to augment conventional allopathic medicine. The standardization of strengths in herbs, which is impossible in the home garden, has added another level of scientific awareness. "Standardized herbal preparations refer to products guaranteed to contain a standardized level of active compounds," according to Dr. Michael Murray, an expert on modern herbal medicine. But "standardization is only possible when research has identified the components responsible for the desired therapeutic effect," Dr. Murray points out.

In some ways this isolation of standard compounds seems to fly in the face of herbal healing, which depends upon the synergis-

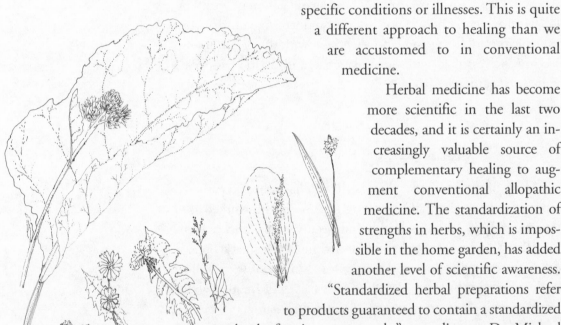

Burdock, chickweed, chicory, dandelion, sheep's sorrel, common plantain, and narrow-leaf plantain

tic qualities within herbs that work for us in many ways. Having said this, it is also responsible to note that there are valuable herbal treatments and formulas that work for countless thousands of people in treating many serious diseases and disorders. Some of these healing herbs work well along with prescription drugs under a doctor's strict guidance, and others do not.

Perhaps by including bloodroot, poke, yellow dock, and Oregon holly grape in your medicine wheel garden you will enjoy developing deeper relationships with these therapeutic herbs. I know gardeners who have confessed to me that they've worked a lifetime trying to eradicate poke, burdock, plantain, and yellow dock from their property—only to find out later that these "weeds" were medicines that could save their lives!

Cancer and Diabetes Remedies from Folk Wisdom

There are herbal healing formulas that function as lymphatic cleansers, strengthening the immune and endocrine systems and targeting cancer cells. Like all vital medicines, the proportions and dosages need to be adjusted and administered by health care professionals who understand each individual's total needs. *It is important that you do not self-medicate in this field.*

Essiac is a therapeutic herbal formula based upon an old Ojibwa anticancer and antitumor treatment that was observed by a Canadian nurse, Renée Caisse. (*Essiac* is her name spelled backward.) She worked with doctors to develop this valuable formula in Canadian hospitals. Both the dried and liquid formula products are available today, and may be found in most herbal shops in the United States and Canada. Many of my friends have experienced help with their diabetes or cancer remissions while taking this formula as a therapeutic daily tea. I take Essiac for a month each year in the spring to detoxify my system, especially my liver, after the long winter.

The Essiac formula contains key healing herbs: burdock root (*Arctium lappa*), sheep sorrel (*Rumex acetosella*), slippery elm bark (*Ulmus rubra*), Turkish rhubarb (*Rheum palmatum*), and red clover blossom (*Trifolium pratense*). Elaine Alexander, a Canadian health researcher, added three more therapeutic herbs to the original formula: watercress (*Nasturtium officinale*), kelp (*Laminaria digitata*), and blessed thistle (*Cnicus benedictus*). Her formula is now marketed as Flor*Essence.

An old formula, the Hoxsey cancer treatment that emerged in the late 1800s, is also based on three of our medicine wheel garden herbs: Oregon holly grape root, poke root, and bloodroot, along with the addition of the roots of barberry, licorice, queensroot, and prickly ash, with the bark of buckthorn. This was developed after successful veterinary work in reducing cancerous tumors in horses.

BASIC HERBAL PREPARATIONS

From teas and tisanes to tinctures and extracts, garden herbs can fit your every health need. Create your own unique medicine wheel garden wellness kit filled with delightful, useful homemade products. And remember that the more love you put into your creations, the finer the healing benefits will be.

Teas, Tisanes, and Infusions

Teas and tisanes are the simplest preparations of blossoms and leaves in hot water. These are usually made from 1 teaspoon of dried or 2 teaspoons of fresh herbs or flowers steeped in 1 cup of freshly boiled water for five minutes. Sweeten with honey, if desired.

Make solar infusions by filling an 8-ounce jar with water and a small handful of fresh herbs; cap tightly and place this on a flat rock or brick in the garden in full sun for a day or two. Then filter, serve, and enjoy, hot or cold.

You can also infuse herbs and blossoms in oils, vinegars, wines, and syrups. For herbal vinegar, place a large handful of fresh herbs and herbal blossoms in a gallon jug and cover with apple cider vinegar, and cover tightly. Warm in the sunny garden for three to six days. The plant material is then strained out and the infused herbal product is bottled in sterile jars or bottles. You might make bayberry–bee balm wine, elderberry vinegar, strawberry-fairywand syrup, and bayberry-chili oil. Tasty cooking oils, soothing body oils, and fragrant massage oils are other possibilities.

Lotions and Creams

Homemade herbal lotions may seem lighter and perhaps more watery than commercial versions because they are made without preservatives, fillers, or emulsifiers. Still, they bring the essence of your medicine wheel garden to you in a different way. Lotions combine strong herbal infusions or decoctions with water; these are excellent for facials, smoothing rough skin, or combing through hair to improve texture and luster and stimulate growth.

Homemade creams combine selected herbal infusions in an emulsion with oil or another fat and water. They are usually slowly cooked, often in the top of a double boiler, for two to three hours, then whipped until cool. Several drops of tincture of benzoin may be added to counter spoilage and extend a cream's shelf life.

Extracts and Tinctures

Tinctures are made by soaking fresh or dried herbs in a strong alcohol and water bath for several days to several weeks, in order to extract even more of the vital alkaloids and constituents from the herbs. Some tinctures are made in glycerin for children and people who are alcohol-sensitive.

Create a Medicine Wheel Garden Wellness Kit

Algonquian lip gloss to protect chapped lips and soothe rough skin (page 266)

Arnica lotion for bruises, muscle pain, joint discomfort, and sore feet (page 271)

Bayberry-yarrow deodorant powder for underarm and general body use (page 274)

Bee balm–bay berry–sage–yarrow tooth powder for sensitive teeth and gums (page 275)

Cold-care capsules to boost the immune system and target colds (page 270)

Eyebright-bearberry tea and eyewash to reduce inflammation (page 251)

Medicine wheel herbal soaks to relieve fatigue and pain (page 283)

Oregon holly grape root bitters for digestive aid and to calm the stomach (page 250)

Sage-cornmeal facial scrub to cool and soothe skin irritations (page 268)

Strawberry skin cream to soothe, cool, and clear skin (page 263)

Sweetgrass–sweet flag braid for smudging, purification, and antiseptic use (page 291)

Witch hazel lotion for cooling antiseptic skin treatments and poison ivy treatment (page 272)

Yucca root shampoo for clean, glossy hair (page 273)

Extracts are even stronger and more concentrated than tinctures. They are commercially available in liquid or solid (powdered) forms. Extracts and tinctures are much more concentrated forms of herbal medicines and must be treated with respect. These are sometimes prescribed by naturopaths or health care practitioners to treat specific problems.

HERBAL HEALTH SUPPLEMENTS FOR OUR ANIMALS

Pet lovers are always concerned to find more gentle and effective remedies for many common pet problems. Those of us who work with animals, especially domestic cats, dogs, goats, sheep, rabbits, and horses, know the importance of balancing herbs in their diets for better health, vigor, and general well-being. There are a few gentle herbal remedies and helpful treatments that you can create using products from the medicine wheel garden and other herbs to target pets' special needs. As with yourself, do not treat serious problems that require a veterinarian's care.

Most of the following herbal suggestions target small cats and dogs. Cautiously increase the herbal supplements to suit the size and weight of your pet and his appetite. Many of these suggestions may need balancing to suit your own pet's unique tastes and requirements. Please bear in mind that herbs have subtle influences; it may take a while for effects to become apparent.

Herbal Food Supplements and Digestive Aids for Pets

Herbal formulas added to your pets' food daily can enable them to avoid some debilitating skin and respiratory disorders as well as arthritis, digestive problems, and other common disorders. Many of our finest veterinarians treat animals holistically—they are often the first to advocate certain herbs and herbal products. Remember that with herbs, less is best—and be patient.

Prepare 1 cup raw brown rice for your pet, using chicken or vegetable stock. Add 1 tablespoon each of cornmeal, oatmeal, and hulled sunflower seeds. During the last ten minutes of cooking time, add a tablespoon each of dried crumbled bee balm, peppermint, Oregon holly grape root, heal-all, nettles, and coneflower (you may leave some out, based upon what you have on hand). Also add one small diced garlic clove. Stir this in thoroughly, cover, and finish cooking. Cool and store in the refrigerator for up to a week. Depending upon your pet's size and appetite, give a small dog or puppy ½ cup of this each morning. I pour 2 tablespoons of soy milk over this; you could also add ¼ teaspoon of tincture echinacea (the alcohol will evaporate in five or ten minutes).

Another delicious preparation for your pets is the addition of small pinches of garlic and choice digestive herbs to fresh scrambled eggs. This makes a nice change-of-pace breakfast for pets that need extra protein. I occasionally add tofu or soy milk to this. The garlic makes pets less susceptible to fleas and ticks.

Make a mild echinacea and bee balm tea for your pet to drink once a week to help strengthen its immune system.

Chickweed, peppermint, German chamomile, and witch hazel in lotions or creams provide gentle relief for various skin rashes and eczema. Make a mild infusion of these gentle teas to spray on your pet's coat or to bathe your pet in.

Chickweed and plantain leaves are excellent, fresh or dried, for rabbits and chickens. The plantain seeds are especially beneficial for them.

Respiratory and Skin Treatments for Pets

Surprisingly, dried nettles deliver the most relief for animals' respiratory difficulties and skin irritations. (The same is also true for humans!) For goats, sheep, and horses, a small handful of dried, crumpled nettles along with ¼ cup dried peppermint or bee balm in the morning feed can work wonders for their coats and relieve

Shoshone Bear Chant

Hey ya tua a ra

Tua a ra

Tua a ra

Hey ya

Tua a ra

Tua a ra

Hey yaaaaaaaa

many skin problems. You might also include a tablespoon of dried garlic in order to build systemic resistance to fleas, flies, ticks, and other harmful insects. These herbal supplements also add some vital nutrients and minerals that domestic animals need.

For cats or dogs, these same herbal supplements can be made into mild teas and added to the pets' drinking water. They can also be cooked into brown or white rice, oatmeal, eggs, and diced meat preparations.

Herbal Treatments for Skin Sores on Pets

Some of the gentlest skin treatments to relieve insect bites are the crushed fresh leaves of sage, basil, thyme, German chamomile, and lavender, or a daub of one of these essential oils. Simple ointments or creams made from calendula, comfrey leaves, or St. John's wort flowers also provide relief that can last up to two hours or more. Like most herbal preparations, these gentle remedies need to be reapplied every three hours or so. Do not use comfrey where the skin is broken.

Aloe vera gel provides healing relief for insect bites and most skin sores and burns. In a pinch apply a few drops of lemon or lime juice to the problem, *if it is not an open wound,* for cooling, soothing relief. Wash irritated skin with witch hazel lotion, as long as the skin is not broken.

Insect Repellents for Pets

One of pet owners' biggest headaches is fleas and ticks. As I work with my new little farm kitten to help rid her of these irritations, I am even more aware that most conventional commercial products cannot be used on kittens and puppies under twelve weeks of age. This is a valuable instance where herbal applications can provide gentle relief.

Lavender and bee balm spritzer is a fine topical spray treatment for fleas and ticks. Make this with 3 to 6 drops of each of these two essential oils in 1 or 2 ounces of water. Get your cats and dogs used to this spray relief. It is especially handy for kittens, can be applied frequently, and makes them smell nice. Spray the face, stomach, and rear end first to prevent fleas from escaping to these more sensitive regions. Then spray your pet until damp, gently rubbing the solution into its coat. Make this a special time of bonding so your pet will think this is a pleasure rather than a punishment.

Make an effective flea and tick collar for your pet by taking a small cotton scarf, like a common bandana, and laying fresh or dried stems of pennyroyal, sage, and basil inside it. Fold the herbs within, roll and twist this little bandana, then tie it comfortably around your pet's neck (make sure you can fit at least two fingers between the neck and the collar). Do not use pennyroyal if you or your pet are pregnant.

Ear and Eye Treatments for Pets

General care of eyes and ears is essential and easy. Gently wipe ears with a witch hazel gauze pad (do not use this around the eyes). You can make fine ear oil by soaking fresh mullein flowers in 4 ounces of mineral or olive oil. Place this in the warm sun on a windowsill for five or six days. Then strain through a fine filter and bottle the clear oil in a small amber eyedropper bottle. Use a drop or two in each ear (for kittens or puppies) if you suspect ear mites or need to clear out ear wax. Once you put the drops in, your pet will shake her head frequently; this helps to dislodge the wax, which you wipe away with clean cotton balls or small gauze pads. If you suspect an ear infection or pain, add several drops of garlic oil or juice to the mineral oil. This is an antiseptic and a mild antibiotic, and it helps relieve pain.

Weeping or irritated eyes can be helped with a mild solution of eyebright and bee balm. Place a small handful of each herb (fresh or dried) in a glass bowl and cover with ½ cup of boiling water. (Or you can open 1 capsule of dried, powdered eyebright.) Add ¼ teaspoon of sea salt. Stir this thoroughly and allow it to sit

Teach your children what we have taught our children, that the earth is our mother. . . . The air is precious to us, for all things share the same breathing—the beast, the tree, the people, they all share the same breath.

—Chief Seattle, 1854, addressing the tribal assembly prior to signing the Indian treaty

fifteen minutes until cool. Strain this through a fine coffee filter and pour into an amber dropper bottle. Label, date, and store in the refrigerator. Place one drop in each eye three times a day if your pet has eye problems.

Herbal Pain Relief for Pets

It is best to try to determine the cause of the pain and have your pet seen by a veterinarian as soon as possible. In the meantime, powdered willow bark, slippery elm bark, or feverfew can provide pain relief and readily lower a fever. Use it in capsules if your pet is not eating. Otherwise sprinkle ½ teaspoon of one of these dried herbs over the pet's food. Encourage your pet to drink more water.

If the skin is not broken, topical pain treatment calls for washing the painful area with witch hazel lotion or willow bark tea. Try arnica oil, lotion, or ointment as well.

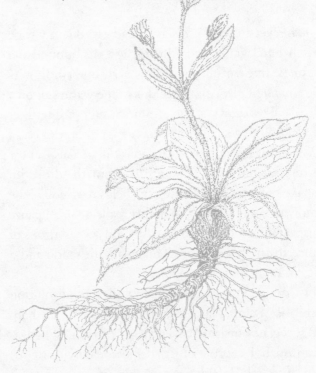

CHAPTER ELEVEN

Nutriceuticals

Foods, Beverages, Bitters, and Seasonings

NUTRICEUTICALS ARE HEALING FOODS and food supplements that have nourishing effects on the body, mind, spirit, and even one's rhythms and balance. Nutriceuticals can range from energy-enhancing supplements or foods such as American ginseng to digestive aids such as Oregon holly grape bitters.

Many everyday foods can be spiced up with a light touch of dried (or fresh) herbs from the medicine wheel garden. Try dried crumbled bee balm, bayberry leaves, fresh or dried chili peppers, and wild onions and garlic. Evening primrose seed, American ginger root, angelica stems, strawberries, and blueberries can also add great taste and wholesomeness to everyday foods and therapeutic preparations. It is a pleasure to explore these seasonal tastes and fragrances.

Kitchen medicinals have the virtue of nourishing the body, mind, and spirit, as well as one's rhythms and balance. This is enhanced when you prepare each recipe and its ingredients in a loving, thoughtful manner. All of your gardening, gathering, preparing, and serving time comes full circle in a magical embrace of profound nourishment.

I remember my grandpa was probably the happiest and funniest person I ever knew. We lived with him for a while at Akwesasne and he taught me so much about gardening, basketmaking, building, and just living with the land. I think he was happiest when he was working in his cornfield or pounding black ash logs for their splints. He kept my mother busy making baskets. He lived to be more than ninety-nine years old and was the oldest basketmaker on the reservation.
—David Richmond, Snipe Clan, Akwesasne Mohawk from Hogansburg, New York, 1983

Awendaw

2 cups water

7 tablespoons dry grits

1/2 teaspoon salt, or to taste

4 tablespoons butter

1 1/2 cups milk

1 cup fine yellow cornmeal

butter (or oil) and cornmeal
for a loaf pan

3 eggs

1/2 teaspoon dried,
powdered bee balm leaves

1/2 teaspoon fresh or dried
bee balm blossoms

1 cup ripe blueberries or
strawberries, or 1/2 cup chili
peppers

This southern herbal corn bread takes its Algonquian name from an ancient Indian settlement outside of Charleston, South Carolina. The late, legendary food historian Bill Neal, author of *Southern Cooking,* inspired this recipe.

Preheat oven to 350 degrees. Bring water to a boil in a medium saucepan. Stir in the grits and salt. Cook over medium heat for 20 minutes, stirring frequently. Remove from heat and stir in the butter. Combine the milk and cornmeal in a small mixing bowl and let this stand for 15 minutes. Also, line the bottom of a medium loaf pan with brown paper. Grease it and the pan's sides with oil or butter, and lightly dust with fine cornmeal.

As the saucepan of grits cools, slightly, stir this mixture into the cornmeal-milk mixture, then beat in the eggs, one by one. Add the remaining herbs and fruits or chili, depending upon whether you want sweet or spicy bread. Blend well and pour the batter into the loaf pan, distributing it evenly. Bake in the middle of the oven for about 50 to 60 minutes, until a table knife inserted in the middle comes out clean. Allow to cool for 5 minutes on a rack, then turn out carefully onto a prepared board or platter. Garnish with additional fruits, if desired, and serve hot with spicy or herbal butter and herbal cream cheese.

YIELD: 6 SERVINGS

In some regions this early Algonquian corn bread would contain hominy corn, too, and was served as a spoonbread. Perhaps you will enjoy developing and personalizing this old recipe to incorporate other herbal influences from your medicine wheel garden.

It is our desire that we and you should be of one heart, one mind, and body, thus becoming one people.
—Kanickhungo, Cherokee

Evening Primrose Seed Scones

Evening primrose seeds are tiny powerhouses! The oil supplies the omega-6 fatty acid and gamma-linolenic acid (GLA), which is not found in many other foods. It can lower blood pressure and may provide benefits to people suffering from multiple sclerosis and rheumatoid arthritis. The seed oil serves as a digestive aid, promotes healthy skin, and helps hormonal balance, especially for PMS sufferers. These easy scones are richer than ordinary biscuits, yet still light and tasty. What a delicious way to feel healing delights!

Preheat oven to 450 degrees. Sift flour, baking powder, maple sugar (if using), and salt together in a medium bowl. Cut in butter until mixture is the size of small peas. Make a well in the middle and add eggs, cream, honey (if using), blueberries, and seeds. Combine all ingredients with a few fast strokes, blending all together thoroughly. Drop by tablespoonfuls onto a lightly oiled cookie sheet. Sprinkle the top of each scone with a spot of honey or maple syrup and a pinch of evening primrose seeds. Bake for about 15 minutes, until just golden.

Yields 12 scones

2 cups sifted all-purpose flour

2 teaspoons double-acting baking powder

1 tablespoon honey or maple sugar

pinch of salt

1/4 cup butter

2 well-beaten eggs

1/3 cup cream

1/3 cup fresh or dried blueberries

2 tablespoons evening primrose seeds

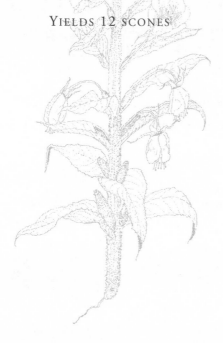

Herbal Cranberry–Bee Balm Polenta

2 cups water

2 cups cranberry juice, unsweetened

1 cup cornmeal

1 cup cold water

1/2 cup chopped cranberries

1/2 cup chopped fresh parsley or cilantro stems

1/4 cup chopped fresh bee balm leaves

1/4 cup orange zest

1 tablespoon corn or sunflower seed oil to coat the pan

herbal seasonings or salt and pepper to taste

toppings (optional), grated cheese, sunflower seeds, chopped garlic, chopped green onions

This recipe is actually a classic American Indian cornmeal mush developed in an herbal medicine wheel garden variation. The herbs can help strengthen the bladder and kidneys and improve digestion. Polenta is comfort food, and this version is especially soothing for children when they are feeling under the weather or just cranky. This can be a hot winter treat or a chilled summer surprise, and is interestingly reconfigured as an appetizer for the following day, if there is enough left over. If you do not have fresh herbs and cranberries, substitute half the amount of dried herbs and cranberries.

Preheat the oven to 350 degrees. Place the water and cranberry juice in a medium saucepan and bring them to a boil. Blend the cornmeal and cold water together in a small bowl. Carefully pour the cornmeal and water into the boiling liquid. Reduce heat to medium low. Simmer, stirring constantly, until the polenta thickens, about 5 minutes.

Add the remaining ingredients, except for the oil and toppings. Blend all together thoroughly and balance the taste to your liking.

Spread the oil evenly around the bottom and sides of an 8-inch-square baking dish. Sprinkle the top with grated cheese or your favorite toppings.

Bake for 30 to 40 minutes. Serve piping hot. (Or cool and cover with plastic wrap and refrigerate until firm, at least an hour or two.)

YIELD: 6–8 SERVINGS

If there are any leftovers, spoon them into a tall glass or can and refrigerate overnight. The next day make Herbal Berry Oven Cakes.

Herbal Berry Oven Cakes

My grandmother's favorite dish was fried or baked cornmeal mush. Leftover mush or polenta makes delicious little fat fingers or wedges as hotcakes for breakfast, lunch, or dinner. This would also provide a wholesome snack or appetizer.

Run a clean dinner knife around the inside of the cylinder of leftover polenta to loosen it. Turn this out on a lightly oiled cookie sheet and slice into 1-inch-thick circles, laying them out flat, side by side, yet not touching. Sprinkle the tops of each round cake with grated cheese or favorite herbs. Then, using the same dinner knife, cut each cake into quarters or eighths, gently separating these little sections just a bit. Place the cookie sheet in a preheated 350 degree oven for 30 minutes. Remove and cool briefly. Loosen each small cake with a knife or spatula and remove it to a warm plate for serving. These are great just hot from the oven, or cooled and topped with a small dab of cranberry relish or maple syrup.

Yield: 12–14 cakes

Oregon Holly Grape Root Digestive Bitters

2 ounces dried Oregon holly grape root, chopped

1 ounce dried sweet flag root, chopped

2 ounces vodka or brandy (or enough to cover)

Ellen Carr, a traditional herbalist in Jackson, Wyoming, who is noted for her special formulations, inspires this marvelous digestive aid. A half teaspoon of this tincture following a big meal (or any meal) will aid digestion and help relieve a "full feeling." You may not want to dig the valuable roots from your medicine wheel garden to make this; the roots can be purchased at many health food stores.

Place the dried roots in an 8-ounce glass jar and cover them with 3 parts vodka or brandy plus 2 parts spring water. Cover the jar with a tight lid and shake it vigorously. Place it on a cool shelf to infuse for 6 weeks. Remember to shake it once or twice daily.

At the end of 6 weeks, strain off the liquid and bottle it in 2-ounce amber bottles with eyedroppers (standard tincture bottles). Label and date your medicine wheel digestive bitters. You may want to carry a bottle with you wherever you go.

YIELD: ABOUT 4 OUNCES

Always lay out your tools and equipment before you begin, and sterilize the tools and jars for best results.

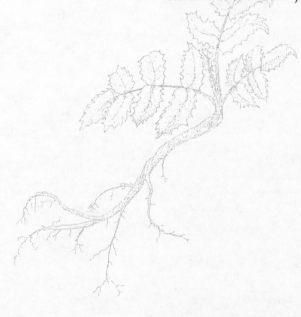

Eyebright-Bearberry Tea and Eyewash

Relieve tired eyes and soothe eye problems or infections with this valuable treatment, which requires just two essential ingredients from your medicine wheel garden. For the eyebright, I find it most effective to empty the contents of an herbal supplement capsule from my local natural foods store.

10 healthy bearberry leaves

5 shiny bayberry leaves

2 cups water

1 380 mg capsule powdered eyebright

Wash the leaves and place them in a small saucepan with the water. Add the powdered contents of 1 opened eyebright capsule. Place the pan over medium heat and bring it almost to a boil. Remove it immediately from the heat and cover. Let the mixture steep for 5 minutes. Strain out the herbs and pour yourself a soothing cup of garden tea. Cool the remaining liquid and keep in a clean glass jar, chilled. Use within 2 weeks.

For a soothing eyewash, pour a small amount into a sterile eyecup. These three antiseptic herbs also make a fine face wash and body lotion.

YIELD: 2 CUPS

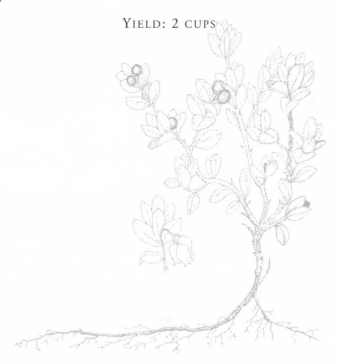

1-inch section fresh ginger
root, sliced very thin

1 pint brandy

Ward off the blahs, a head cold, or sore throat with this bracing drink. Master gardener and dear friend Peter Dubos shared this recipe.

Add slices of ginger to brandy in a clean jar. Cover and shake vigorously. Allow this to infuse for two weeks.

Use 1 teaspoonful in a cup of hot water, as a sipping tea, whenever you feel a cold, headache, or sore throat pressing in on you. Fish out a slice of ginger and chew it slowly to treat a sore throat or sinus problems.

YIELD: 1 PINT

To make an energy tonic to use when you must have maximum concentration and alertness, substitute sliced ginseng root for the ginger.

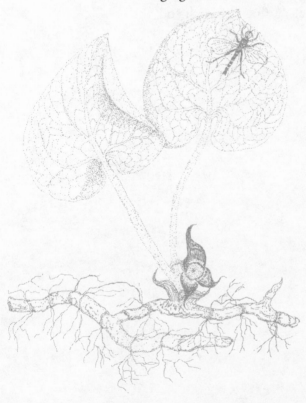

Boneset-Coneflower Immune-i-Tea

Ward off colds and flu and ease coughs and sore throats with this delicious tea. It is filled with natural strength and goodness, with or without honey. Make extra amounts to store in the refrigerator in a small spray bottle (unsweetened) to use as a throat spray and to occasionally mist your face and hair.

3 large boneset leaves

3 medium coneflower leaves

1 quart water

1 teaspoon honey or maple syrup (optional)

Wash the leaves well and place them in a 2-quart saucepan or large teapot. Pour 1 quart of boiling water over them and cover. Infuse for 5 to 10 minutes.

Strain some into a large teacup and enjoy warm. Put the remainder in a large glass jar, covered, in the refrigerator. Treat yourself to a cup a day whenever you feel under the weather or just depleted of energy.

The spent herbs can also be folded into a small poultice and placed over any swelling or rash for 10 minutes of relief and healing.

YIELD: ONE 8-OUNCE POT OF TEA

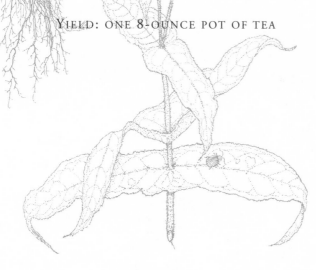

Fire Cider

1/2 cup finely chopped fresh onion

1/4 cup grated fresh horseradish root

1/4 cup grated fresh ginger root

1/8 cup finely chopped fresh garlic

cayenne pepper to taste

honey to taste

apple cider vinegar to cover all ingredients by 2 inches in a large glass jar

Stimulate the immune system and aid digestion with this classic creation, especially inspired by Barrie Sachs and Dr. Rolf Martin, and other herbalists who have personalized this. A warming, decongesting tonic, fire cider can be enjoyed daily to aid digestion, clear the sinuses, and warm the system.

Assemble all ingredients in a large glass jar and blend together well. Cap jar tightly. Let liquid rest for two weeks, shaking the jar every day.

Strain off the liquid and sweeten with honey, if needed. Save the solid ingredients. Take 1 teaspoon of the liquid every hour or as needed to treat head colds, sore throats, and sinus problems.

Serve the chopped, pickled ingredients to season vegetables or rice, especially if you enjoy spicy foods. This tasty condiment is great for sinus congestion and sore throats.

YIELD: ABOUT 8 OUNCES

Medicine Wheel Lightning

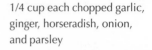

For chili lovers, here is a great general tonic that also makes fine vinegar for salad dressing and for pepping up your favorite vegetables and pasta dishes. If you feel a cold coming on, stir a teaspoonful of this tonic into 4 ounces of warm water and drink it right down!

Pack chopped vegetables and herbs into a 1-quart jar and fill to the top with vinegar. Put the lid on tight and shake this daily for the next two weeks. After two weeks, strain through a fine coffee filter, pressing out all liquid. Bottle the liquid.

Spread the filtered ingredients on a warm skillet and roast slightly; then add this to a big salad or pasta dish as a topping.

YIELD: ABOUT 1½ CUPS

If you make this with cayenne or paprika peppers you can also use 1 teaspoon of the liquid in a glass of water (stirred well) to cure a headache. This is a most refreshing tonic! My friends Jay Unger and Molly Mason developed their own special "fiery" formula as a "fiddle sauce" based on Jay's passion for habanero chilis and international fame as a fiddler/composer. It is so deliciously hot that compatriots wait in line to get a bottle.

1/4 cup each chopped garlic, ginger, horseradish, onion, and parsley

1/4 cup each chopped angelica stems and bergamot leaves

1/8 cup chopped or powdered chili or cayenne peppers

apple cider vinegar to cover all ingredients

Carrot-Horseradish-Strawberry Relish

3 cups grated fresh carrots

1 cup grated fresh horseradish root

2 cups chopped fresh strawberries

1/4 cup apple cider vinegar

2 tablespoons raw honey

 Open sinus passages and stimulate circulation with this delicious combination of roots and fruits. Barrie Sachs, herbalist and owner/founder of Happy Rainbows Tea & Apothecary Shop in Sherman, Connecticut, inspired this recipe. The ingredients are high in vitamin C and minerals.

Place all ingredients in a medium glass bowl and stir well until completely blended. Serve with carrot and celery sticks and toast. This is also an excellent accompaniment to soups and rice dishes.

YIELD: ABOUT 6 CUPS

This is a valuable winter remedy for sore throats, colds, and congestion. Eating several tablespoons of this relish should promote perspiration and loosen phlegm and congestion.

Steamed Purslane and Wild Onions

1 large handful purslane stems and leaves

1 small handful green wild onion tops

Water or vegetable broth

This may help to lower cholesterol and tone the kidneys. Both of these wild vegetables are delicious, therapeutic, and usually prolific by midsummer.

Wash leaves thoroughly and chop coarsely into a medium saucepan. Add about an inch of clear water or vegetable broth to this, cover, and steam over medium heat for 10 minutes. Remove from the heat and allow to cool for 10 minutes. Pour this into a serving bowl and dress lightly with cider vinegar.

YIELD: 1–2 PORTIONS

Berry Herbal Smoothie

This is as delicious to drink as it is good to daub on your nose and face to tone your skin! Fresh fruits and herbs from the medicine wheel garden make this drink alive with optimum nutrition, but frozen strawberries, raspberries, blueberries, and cranberries are also excellent, and right from the freezer they act as tiny ice cubes.

Place all ingredients in a blender container. Cover and blend on high for 10 seconds. Pour into a glass and enjoy.

Daub some of the smoothie from the blender container on your face and smooth it into your skin, especially if you have a cold sore or any trouble spots. Wash this off after about 10 minutes. This is especially cool and soothing, both to wear and to drink, on hot days.

YIELD: ABOUT 1 GLASS

You might want to save the banana peels to place in your medicine wheel garden, where they will add extra potassium to the soil.

1 peeled banana

1 cup soy milk

3 tablespoons plain yogurt to taste

1 tablespoon uncooked oatmeal, or 2 tablespoons cooked oatmeal

6 fresh bee balm leaves, or 3 dried

6 fresh or frozen unsweetened strawberries

1 small fresh lemon wedge

pinch dried ground ginger root

Bayberry-Chili Seasoning

10 dried bayberry leaves

10 dried ripe chili peppers

5 dried bee balm leaves

1-inch slice dried ginger root

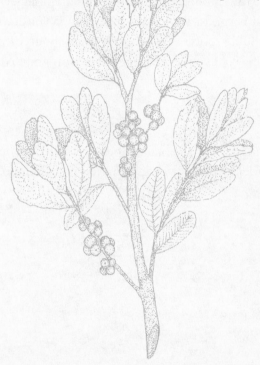

Here is a simple seasoning you can make directly from the summer harvests from the medicine wheel garden, bringing the essence of your work elegantly to your table. You may develop several variations on this recipe if you like it well enough.

Place ingredients one at a time in a clean coffee grinder and grind fine. Then place them all together in a small glass seasoning bottle. Shake to blend well. Adjust this mixture to suit your taste. Use a pinch at a time to season salads, pasta, and poultry dishes.

CHAPTER TWELVE

Cosmeceuticals

Health and Beauty Aids from the
Medicine Wheel Garden

RING YOUR MEDICINE WHEEL garden inside and into your everyday life with soothing remedies from your creative kitchen. Try making balms, creams, and salves to provide nourishing rejuvenation for your skin and chapped lips. Tinctures, ointments, and herbal steams help to further your personal healing treatments internally and externally. These herbal formulas also make great gifts.

You, whose day it is, make it beautiful. Get out your rainbow colors, so it will be beautiful.
—Nootka song to bring fair weather

Remember that you'll get the best results if you wear a smile, feel happy, and express gratitude as you are working. The more love you put into your creations, the more effective they'll be. I begin by smudging the kitchen and work areas, my utensils and myself with fragrant sage and white cedar. This helps me to feel very centered.

It is important to lay out all your ingredients and tools in advance of beginning each preparation. Sterilize your equipment and jars. This will help to ensure maximum benefits from your work.

Bayberry-Bergamot Facial and Head Steam

1 medium handful bayberry leaves, or 1/2 cup dried

1 medium handful bergamot leaves, or 1/2 cup dried

A few bayberry twigs (optional)

Water

Big towel

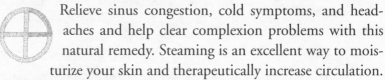

Relieve sinus congestion, cold symptoms, and headaches and help clear complexion problems with this natural remedy. Steaming is an excellent way to moisturize your skin and therapeutically increase circulation. The steam also carries the volatile oils from the herbs directly to your face and respiratory system.

Keep things easy and safe by preparing your space before you begin. Place a folded towel on the table where you will set the steaming pot. Put a hot plate on top of this. Place a large Turkish towel beside this, to arrange over your head and drape down around you and the steaming pot.

If using fresh leaves, wash them. Place leaves in a 1-gallon pot half filled with fresh water. Put this on high heat and bring it to a boil for about 1 minute. Turn off the heat.

While the water is actively steaming, transfer the pot from the stove to the hot plate on the table. Sit down with this in front of you. Lean over the pot carefully and position your face about 2 feet above the rim of the steaming pot, or where it feels most comfortable for you. Place the big towel over your head and the steaming pot, making a tent. Close your eyes and relax, breathing deeply. Enjoy this fragrant steam as long as you like. You can refresh the pot after it cools down by simply placing it back on the stove and reheating it to boiling. Three consecutive 10-minute sessions feels right to many people.

Afterward, using a slotted spoon, carefully lift out the botanicals and place them in a small towel. Fold this up and dampen it with the herbal decoction to use as a warm compress on any area of your body that seems to need attention, especially the back of the neck. Leave this on for 20 to 30 minutes, until it cools. Discard the well-used botanicals on your compost pile, with gratitude for their healing energies.

Arnica-Plantain-Bergamot Foot Bath and Compress

Relieve bruises, sore muscles, aching feet, and tired hands and feet with these therapeutic herbs. My dear friend Dale Carson the Abenaki artist, inspired this easy-to-make pain-relief formula.

Look around your property for narrow- or broad-leaf plantain (it often appears as a weed in the grass or near the patio and walks).

1 handful arnica leaves, or 1/2 cup dried

1 handful bee balm leaves, or 1/2 cup dried

1 handful narrow- or broad-leaf plantain, or 1/2 cup dried

Place the leaves in a 4-quart saucepan, cover with 2 quarts of fresh water, and bring to a rolling boil over medium-high heat. Reduce heat and simmer for 10 minutes, covered. Remove from the heat and allow to cool slightly.

Prepare a basin half full of tepid water for the footbath. Place this on a towel on the floor in front of your favorite chair. Or you might place this outside near your medicine wheel garden in a place where you can sit comfortably, with your bare feet soaking in the herbal water, for 15 minutes.

Also prepare a soft towel in which you can place these spent herbs. The towel will be soaked in the tea decoction, so don't choose a fancy towel; the liquid will stain it.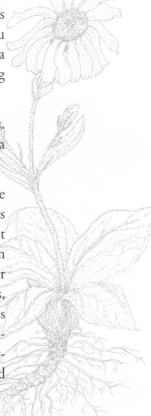

Now strain the herbal decoction into the footbath and place the spent leaves in the towel. Fold the towel flat, enclosing the herbs like an envelope, and briefly wet it in the herbal water. Wring out the towel. Sit down comfortably and ease your feet into the warm footbath; settle back and relax. Place the wet compress on your forehead and temples for soothing relief of anxieties, headaches, or tension. If you have a swollen knee, aching joints, or problems elsewhere on your body, place the compress gently over the trouble spot. Hold it lightly in place for 10 to 15 minutes. As the footbath and compress slowly cool off, visualize your pains and problems fading away with this action.

This is a valuable restorative all year round. You may choose various herbs to suit your needs, like jewelweed, heal-all, and sage with a tablespoonful of sea salt for poison ivy; or bayberry, bee balm, and chili pepper to enhance circulation. Always add a few leaves of broadleaf plantain for greater therapeutic effects. Try a cool footbath and compress in the heat of summer to cool the body down fast and relieve heat distress.

Jewelweed Complexion Cubes

1 healthy fresh jewelweed plant, cut off just above the roots

20 ounces water

 Soothe skin irritations and treat poison ivy and other skin rashes with this easy trick. Harvest jewelweed in late summer, when the plant is at its climax.

Bend or break the jewelweed so that it fits into a clean blender jar. Cover the herbs with the water. Cover and blend for 10 seconds or until thoroughly macerated. It should look like frothy green soup.

Pour the liquid into clean ice cube trays and freeze it overnight. The next day turn out the jewelweed herbal ice cubes into several clear zip-lock freezer bags. Label and date each bag. Refreeze them immediately. The frozen herbs retain their potency, so make enough to carry you through winter and the following spring.

These herbal ice cubes are excellent for many uses. One jewelweed ice cube rubbed over irritated, swollen skin or poison ivy patches will provide great relief. A cube added to a hot footbath will help to relax tired feet and treat foot fungus (athlete's foot or toenail fungus). Or use a cube as a brief facial massage, to close the skin pores after steaming has opened them. You will probably think of additional ways to use these icy treasures.

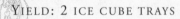
Yield: 2 ice cube trays

This same process also works well with bee balm, coneflower, and heal-all. Making your own herbal ice cubes allows you extended seasons of use. You might melt several of these herbal cubes during the winter to add to salves and lotions.

Strawberry Skin Cream

Enhance your skin's natural glow and feed the epidermal layers with this essential cosmeceutical. While you enjoy eating some of the fresh strawberries from your medicine wheel garden, gather a few more to use in this soothing recipe.

Measure all but the last two ingredients into the top of a double boiler. Heat at a low simmer for three hours. Stir frequently to blend ingredients.

Strain out the strawberries and pour the hot mixture into a clean bowl. Add the oil of wintergreen and tincture of benzoin, and whip the mixture continuously with a wire whisk or fork until it cools.

Spoon the whipped cream into sterilized glass jars, label, and refrigerate. Use within three months.

YIELD: ABOUT 14 OUNCES

Emulsifying wax and glycerin are easily ordered from most herbal catalogs if you cannot find them at a local health food store or pharmacy.

5 ounces emulsifying wax (see note)

2 1/2 ounces fresh strawberries, chopped

2 1/2 ounces glycerin (see note)

2 1/2 ounces water

2 ounces sweet almond oil or coconut oil

9 drops essential oil of wintergreen or bergamot

6 drops tincture of benzoin

Quick Strawberry Facial

3 tablespoons plain yogurt

4 strawberries (fresh or frozen without sugar)

1 thin slice lemon

Luxuriate for about 20 minutes with this restorative time-out. Strawberries contain a light glycolic acid, which helps exfoliate and rejuvenate your skin. Try this with chilled ingredients, especially in the heat of summer, to cleanse skin and close pores.

Place all ingredients in a blender or food processor. Blend for a few seconds into a smooth pulp. Smear these whipped ingredients all over your face and neck and hands. Now stretch out and relax for 10 minutes. Clear your mind. Think of your medicine wheel garden, and replenishing your body, mind, spirit, and emotions. Make this a special meditation.

Splash your face, neck, and hands with clear, cool water to rinse off the strawberry mixture. Pat almost dry with a clean cloth (the moisture retained is essential to rehydrate your skin). Finish by applying some of the Strawberry Skin Cream.

YIELD: 1 FACIAL

This facial can be varied by adding a 1-inch slice of fresh cucumber or avocado to the yogurt in place of the strawberries. Or you may substitute a ¼ cup of blueberries, elderberries, or chopped bee balm leaves and blossoms. Several drops of vitamin E oil are also good to add. You can use dried powdered bayberry, bee balm, heal-all, or yarrow leaves. Several plantain leaves will strengthen the healing potential.

Dragonfly Hand and Facial Rejuvenating Oil

Nourish your skin with these tantalizing oils in a delicate formula inspired by herbalist Vanessa Nesvig of Bar Harbor, Maine.

Place all ingredients in a Pyrex measuring cup and stand this in an inch of water in a saucepan. Warm this over medium heat, stirring to blend thoroughly. Simmer for 5 minutes, stirring frequently.

Carefully pour into three 2-ounce amber bottles; allow to cool for several minutes. Cap tightly, label, and date.

Shake well before using. Several drops on the back of the hands, rubbed together and across the forehead, are very nourishing.

YIELD: ABOUT 6 OUNCES

3 tablespoons sweet almond oil

3 tablespoons fresh aloe vera gel

3 tablespoons cold-pressed castor oil

3 tablespoons sunflower seed oil

1 tablespoon jojoba oil

1 teaspoon powdered ginger root

9 drops vitamin E oil

6 drops essential oil of cedar wood (or your favorite)

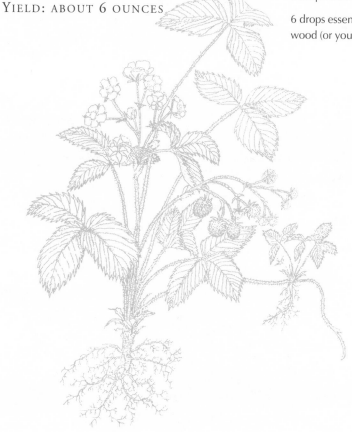

Algonquian Lip Gloss (Lip Balm)

3 tablespoons grated beeswax

2 tablespoons sweet almond oil

2 tablespoons fresh aloe vera gel

2 tablespoons honey

8 drops vitamin E oil

6 drops lanolin oil

5 drops essential oil of wintergreen

Protect chapped lips and rough skin with this simple formula. The next time you make clam chowder or clams on the half shell, save the twelve best medium-small clamshells and wash them thoroughly to use as receptacles for this easy creation.

Place the clamshells on a layer of paper towels on a flat pan. Place the beeswax in a Pyrex measuring cup in the microwave and heat on high for 15-second intervals until melted. Add the remaining ingredients in the order listed, blending them well with a butter knife. Heat again in the microwave for 20 seconds. Stir well and promptly pour the hot mixture into 12 medium-small clamshells. Allow the shells to rest, untouched, to cool completely.

YIELD: 1 DOZEN

Quahog clam shell filled with Algonquian lip gloss

Each one can be tied up in a square of clear plastic wrap, fastened with red ribbon or raffia. These make wonderful gifts.

Angelica-Strawberry Facial Mist

Use this mist/spritzer directly from the refrigerator for cooling rejuvenating pleasure on hot summer days.

1/2 cup fresh strawberries, stemmed and coarsely chopped

1/2 cup chopped angelica stems

2 cups fresh water

1 teaspoon fresh lemon juice

Place the chopped strawberries and angelica in a saucepan with the water. Bring just to a boil over medium heat. Reduce heat and simmer, stirring, for 10 minutes. Remove from the heat and cool slightly. Strain off the herbs and add the lemon juice, stirring well.

Pour this liquid into five small 2-ounce glass bottles, cap tightly, label, and refrigerate.

YIELD: 10 OUNCES

An easy variation of this recipe can make an herbal tick and insect repellent. Substitute bayberry bark, leaves, and stems for the strawberries; substitute fresh ginger root for the angelica. Add a sprig of chopped sage, and a few drops of essential oil of wintergreen at the end for extra cooling insurance.

Bee Balm–Heal-all–Strawberry Bathtub Tea

1 generous handful bee balm
and heal-all leaves

10 ripe strawberries

4 quarts water

 Soak away your muscle aches and stress with this medicine wheel garden "gift of healing." Betty Loiacono, spa director at the Norwich Inn and Spa in Norwich, Connecticut, inspired this herbal therapy.

Tie herbs and strawberries together into a small cloth pouch. Place this and the water into a large saucepan and bring to a boil. Reduce the heat and simmer for 5 minutes, while you run a nice bathtub full of water for yourself. Light a small candle and put on soft music. Pour the pan of hot tea water, with or without the tea pouch, into the prepared tub. Test the water for comfort, then slip into the water and enjoy a therapeutic, relaxing soak.

YIELD: 1 BATH

Sage-Cornmeal Facial Scrub

1/2 cup dried sage leaves

1/2 cup natural oatmeal (not instant)

1 cup fine cornmeal

 This soothing, cooling mixture can be used all over your body, but it is especially kind to the face. The sage makes this mildly antiseptic—thus it's good to daub on bug bites and other skin irritations, with caution.

Coarsely grind the sage and oatmeal, separately, using a clean coffee grinder or food processor. Mix together with the cornmeal in a medium glass jar with a tight lid. Shake to blend thoroughly. When ready to use, take a 4-inch square of cheesecloth or muslin. Place 1 tablespoon of the mixture in the center and tie it securely with ribbon. Wet the bag and your face. Using a gently circular motion, carefully scrub your face with this face dauber. Rinse your face with cool water and pat dry.

YIELD: 2 CUPS

Medicine Wheel Herbal Skin Scrub

Here is another way of bringing your garden into your shower. My good friends Joanna and Amanda Seitz inspired this nourishing skin scrub.

Mix all ingredients in a large glass jar. Shake out a small handful of this herbal skin scrub and massage your body with it during your next shower. Keep the remaining ingredients in a sealed glass jar.

YIELD: 3 CUPS

For a coarser rub add more rock salt; for a smoother rub add more Epsom salts. Enjoy substituting various herbs to suit your personal pleasure. Try incorporating ¼ cup dried ground bayberry leaves, or yarrow leaves and blossoms, or skullcap leaves, or sweetgrass.

1 cup Epsom salts

1/2 cup rock salt or sea salt

1/2 cup dried heal-all leaves and blossoms, coarsely chopped

1/2 cup dried bee balm leaves and blossoms, coarsely chopped

1/4 cup dried orange zest, coarsely chopped

1/2 cup baking soda (optional)

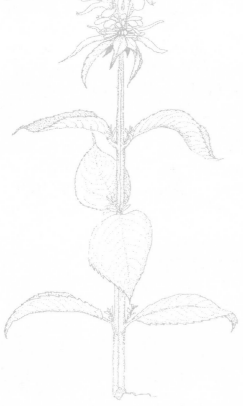

Goldenseal-Cayenne-Echinacea Cold-Care Capsules

1 ounce powdered goldenseal root

1 ounce powdered echinacea root

1 ounce powdered slippery elm bark or marshmallow root

1/2 ounce powdered bayberry bark

1/4 ounce powdered cayenne pepper

1/4 ounce powdered myrrh

100 vegicaps (see note)

Swallow one of these healing capsules whenever your body is feeling under siege, as though a cold or sore throat is coming on. This folkloric formula works wonders to strengthen your immune system. Try digging the goldenseal and echinacea from your garden, drying them, and powdering them for this recipe. Or you can purchase the loose powders at your local health food store and assemble these easy capsules at home.

Suggested dosage: 1 or 2 capsules each hour if you feel you are coming down with a cold or sore throat. Do not take more than 10 capsules a day, or use more than 3 days in a row. Continued regular use may overstimulate your immune system.

Mix the powders all together in a medium-sized glass bowl. Be careful not to make too much dust, and don't breathe it in; it could be irritating. One at a time, take vegicaps apart. Holding one half in the fingers of each hand, slide them together, scooping up the powdered mixture to fill each one. Press caps together again. Place the filled capsules in clean glass jars or zip-lock bags. Continue until you have filled all capsules and used up the powdered mixture.

YIELD: ABOUT 100 CAPSULES

Vegicaps are available from Trinity Herb, P.O. Box 1001, Graton, CA 95444. These are made of kosher gum from all-vegetable sources. Most herb suppliers can provide both capsules and tea bags for your home uses.

Arnica Lotion

Arnica blossoms can be picked fresh to make this soothing skin lotion to treat sprains and muscle pains. This is also valuable to reduce bruising, speed healing, and improve the local blood supply. *Do not use on broken skin.*

10 fresh arnica blossoms

2 cups boiling water

For compresses: Place the fresh arnica blossoms in a glass bowl and pour the boiling water over them. Cover and infuse for 10 minutes. Strain out the spent blossoms and place them in a damp cloth or towel and fold this into a compress to place on any bruised or aching place on the body. Cool compresses are good for soothing inflammations; hot compresses can help reduce bruising and swelling from some sports injuries. Soak and reapply both hot and cold compresses frequently for maximum benefit.

For skin lotion: Cool the strained arnica infusion (lotion) and pour all but ½ cup into a small basin to soak tired feet or hands. Use the remaining lotion to wash the body to stimulate surface blood circulation and soothe any inflammations.

YIELD: 2 CUPS

You can make a simple lotion by adding ½ teaspoon arnica tincture to 2 cups water in a bowl and stirring well. Make this stronger or weaker by adding more or less of the arnica tincture, depending upon your needs.

Follow this same procedure for making a simple arnica massage oil. Add ½ teaspoon (eye dropper full) arnica tincture to 1 cup almond oil. Pour this into a bottle and cap tightly. Shake this well before each use. You might blend in several drops of other essential oils for fragrance, such as wintergreen, bayberry, bergamot, sweetgrass, or lavender.

Witch Hazel Lotion

10 large witch hazel leaves,
fresh or dried

2 cups boiling water

Witch hazel is one of the most useful Native American astringent herbs to treat eczema, inflamed skin, and problem veins. Commercial witch hazel lotion is distilled from the winter wood and is preserved in a 13 percent alcohol solution. You can make your own lotion from the infused leaves or decocted twigs and bark, either fresh or dried.

Follow the same procedures for preparations and use as in the previous recipe for arnica lotion. The witch hazel lotion can be an effective eyewash (in this nonalcohol version) to clear inflammation of the eyes. It is also valuable to treat damaged facial veins, varicose veins, and hemorrhoids. The astringent properties help it to tighten distended veins, helping to restore their normal structure.

The lotion can be refrigerated or frozen for later use to make witch hazel creams, ointments, and salves.

Yield: 2 cups

A variation uses 20 six-inch-long witch hazel twigs and 3 cups of boiling water. Place the twigs in a medium pan and cover with boiling water. Simmer this over medium heat for 15 minutes, stirring occasionally, to make a decoction. Remove from the heat, cover, and allow to rest and cool for 20 minutes. Strain off the botanicals and use the strong liquid lotion to bathe the skin, especially over patches of eczema, to help prevent infection. This lotion has also proved helpful in treating the skin over underlying cysts and tumors. Make a small poultice to apply over irritated areas. Refresh this every 10 minutes for a 30-minute period twice or three times each day until the problem has cleared.

Yucca Root Medicine Wheel Shampoo

1 cup coarsely chopped yucca root, fresh or dried

2 cups warm water

Yucca is also called soapweed because its large, fleshy roots are easily pounded into a fine lather, which was used to treat dandruff and baldness as well as bring healthy shine to hair. Many Pueblo Indians wash their hair in yucca root suds before kachina ceremonies for purification and to honor the earth spirits.

Place the yucca root and water in a food processor and blend on high for 15 seconds, or until you get a good lather. Pour this into a large sterile jar; cap tightly, label, and date. Shake well before each use. Use about ¼ to ½ cup of this, depending upon the length and thickness of your hair, to shampoo, massaging it well into your scalp and working it through your hair. Allow this to remain on your hair for 3 to 5 minutes, then rinse out thoroughly. Comb and dry your hair naturally. See if you notice a healthier shine and softer feeling in your hair after repeated use.

YIELD: 2 CUPS

This is also the opportunity to add additional fragrant herbs from your medicine wheel garden to your shampoo. Make a strong tea of 10 bayberry or bee balm leaves, sweetgrass, heal-all, sage, or yarrow leaves and blossoms. Strain this and make this the 2 cups of liquid used to create the shampoo.

Bayberry-Yarrow Deodorant Powder or Talc

10 dried yarrow leaves, chopped very fine

10 dried bayberry leaves, chopped very fine

1 cup cornstarch

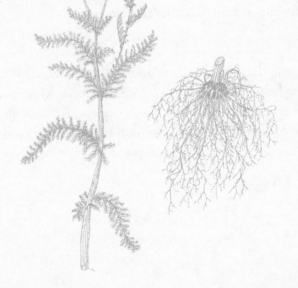

Bayberry leaves and bark are commonly used to keep bacterial infections in check, and to increase circulation. Yarrow is a mild antiseptic and anti-inflammatory. Both herbs have many virtues and each brings in mineral-rich nutrients from the garden. Do not use during pregnancy.

Measure these ingredients into a sterile jar; cap securely and shake well to blend. Label and date this fine body talc and keep it in the bathroom to use as a choice dusting powder or carry it with you in your gym bag.

YIELD: 1 CUP

You may want to make herbal variations of this simple recipe using dried calendula, coreopsis, marigold, sage, elderberry, or evening primrose blossoms.

Bee Balm–Bayberry–Sage–Yarrow Tooth Powder

Because bayberry leaves and sage leaves help to check bacterial infections, and infusions help to strengthen gums and check sore throats, these are natural additions to tooth powders, gargles, and throat sprays. This is a wonderfully cleansing and refreshing mixture of goodness from the medicine wheel. Make this tooth powder in small amounts and use it right up. Use it daily and alternate use with your conventional toothpaste.

Measure all ingredients into a small glass or ceramic (not metal) dish that you can cover tightly. Blend together well.

Sprinkle a pinch of this powder on your toothbrush and brush normally. If you have sensitive teeth and gums, place a small daub of aloe gel on your toothbrush first and then add the tooth powder.

To use this as a mouthwash and gargle, stir a teaspoon of the mixture into a cup of warm water. This is very effective during the cold and flu season in winter.

YIELD: ABOUT 2½ TABLESPOONS

1 tablespoon baking soda

1 tablespoon sea salt or kosher salt

1/2 teaspoon dried powdered bee balm leaves

1/2 teaspoon dried powdered bayberry leaves

1/2 teaspoon dried powdered sage leaves

1/2 teaspoon dried powdered yarrow leaves

Bee Balm–Yarrow Breath Freshener

You can make a quick, easy digestive aid and breath freshener by simply picking and slowly chewing a leaf or two of bee balm and yarrow. You can infuse a tea of several additional leaves of each to use as a gargle, mouth rinse, or throat spray.

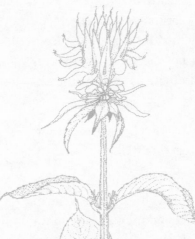

CHAPTER THIRTEEN

Aromatherapy
Bath Salts, Soaps, and Herbal Baths

On damp days I can really smell the sweetgrass. It perfumes our whole house as it waits for Sara to braid it and be woven into baskets. It is Mother Earth's hair. Folks say it keeps its perfume for over 100 years.
—Irene Richmond, Snipe Clan, Akwesasne Mohawk basketmaker, Hogansburg, New York, 1983

IN MANY WAYS WE have been experiencing aromatherapy every step of the way through this book. Herbal aromas and fragrances from combined herbal formulas fill our senses with pleasure and relax (or stimulate) our minds in the garden and in the home. Let's go more deeply into this ancient science that has become a modern multibillion-dollar business.

Fragrances tantalize many of our sensory feelings and thoughts. Certain aromas can trigger emotional memories of special childhood events, like the fragrance of strawberries or the smell of hot popcorn, or cool wintergreen. Perhaps these aromas remind you of certain parties or trips to the movies or memorable meals. Fragrances have the power to stimulate memories and change moods. Balsam fir, white pine, and hemlock exude the clean, irresistible aromas of cool forests and winter holidays.

The highly aromatic qualities of sweet flag and wintergreen may trigger thoughts of soothing medicines and cooling lotions.

American Indian Sacred Fragrances

The aromatic smoke rising from a tobacco, sage, or sweetgrass smudge evokes memories of special ceremonies and feels soothing. These are fragrances associated with Native American prayers and meditations as well as sweat lodge rites. Just the fragrance of tobacco alone (burning or not) conjures respect among traditional people, who associate it with prayer and making special offerings to the spirits. Tobacco is one of the most highly valued ceremonial herbs. It is used for praying and making offerings, and it is given to show respect. Periodically we offer a pinch of tobacco to a drum and other ceremonial objects.

The fragrances of bayberry, sweetgrass, and sweet fern can create the woodsy recollections of camping trips and summer hikes through coastal regions.

The therapeutic benefits of aromas are many; they can relax, soothe, energize the senses, and alter one's moods in positive ways. Aromatherapy is actually an ancient practice—many peoples have realized the benefits of using natural aromas to stimulate the senses. Think about the fragrances that trigger certain of your memories—the aromas of soul foods and fresh coffee brewing. What fragrances stimulate you to do your best work?

Total relaxation should bless the end results of all your work. Imagine stretching out in a steaming hot herbal tub bath. You are restored by your own homemade bath salts, and your hand-crafted herbal soaps cleanse your skin. Herbal candles guide your meditations to gratitude for all that the earth and your medicine wheel garden have provided. Sweet earth energies surround you and permeate your thoughts. What could be better?

Herbal Medicine Wheel Candle

a half-full bucket of fine damp sand

a round bowl or flowerpot to use as a mold, or a large French jelly glass

a medium wick, cut to the length of the depth of your hole plus 1 inch

paraffin wax

wax thermometer

wax dye (optional)

large spoon or stirrer

wicking needle

bayberry or strawberry essential oil, or candle perfume essence

 Flickering candlelight is perfect for relaxation and meditation. Imagine that you can surround yourself with handmade herbal candles that bring in yet another essence from the medicine wheel garden. Here is a medicine wheel sand candle you can make in many variations.

Tamp the damp sand down firmly with your fist. Push the bowl or candle mold down firmly into the center of the damp sand, and press the sand all around this. Carefully remove the candle mold, and measure the depth of the hole so that you can cut the wick to the proper length, plus an additional inch.

Unless you purchased primed wicks, prepare your wick. It is easy—simply heat a small amount of paraffin in the top of a double boiler and soak your wick(s) in this for about 5 minutes. Remove the coated (primed) wick(s), straighten them out, and leave them to dry on a flat plate.

Heat the paraffin wax in the top of a double boiler and add a dye color, if you desire, mixing thoroughly. Heat to about 127° F. Remove from the heat and stir in the fragrance to suit your tastes.

Pour the hot wax gently into the center of the sand, letting it trickle over the back of a metal spoon. You want the sand to hold its shape as much as possible. The wax will seep into the sand in 5 minutes, so heat the wax again and top up the candle. A well will form in the middle of the wax within 2 hours. Top this up with a bit more hot wax.

Push the wicking needle down through the center of the well. Withdraw the needle and use it to push the primed wick down through the center hole. Lay the needle across the top of the wax candle and rest the top of the wick against it to keep it centered and straight. Leave this to cool for another 3 to 4 hours or overnight. Lift the finished candle out of the sand and smooth the outer surface. Trim the wick, if necessary, so that it is not more than 1 inch above the top of the candle. Check the candle base

Origins of Essential Oils and Aromatherapy

The Arab physician Abu Ali Ibn Sina, known as Avicenna (980–1037), is credited with the discovery of the method of extracting essential oils by distillation. By the medieval period, essential oils were used as remedies for many problems. Modern research underscores their antiseptic and antibacterial properties. They are used in baths, compresses, inhalations, lotions, massage oils, and ointments.

and make sure it will sit securely on a candle plate or in a small dish of fine sand.

You may be inspired to make other natural and colored variations of this sand-cast candle. Try pressing tiny bits of medicine wheel herbs and blossoms around the outside of the warm wax. Or make simple round candles to sink into clean clay flowerpots partially filled with bearberry and bayberry leaves. The clay pots can also be embellished with acrylic paints and American Indian pictographic symbols. Enjoy exploring these artistic realms.

You can also purchase beeswax sheets in various sizes that are designed to be rolled into fine candle tapers around a central wick. These are the quickest and easiest of all to make—and no cooking is involved. These candles can be embellished with either a few drops of bayberry or strawberry essential oils, or your favorite candle fragrance, then worked into an arrangement of medicine wheel flowers.

Strawberry Herbal Bath Oil

1/2 cup olive oil

1/2 cup sweet almond oil

1/2 cup corn oil

1/2 teaspoon strawberry essential oil

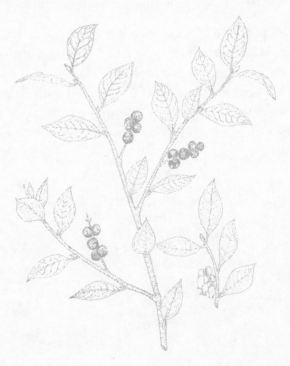

Busy gardeners need to relax and soak in a hot herbal bath after long days of garden work. What could be better than to enjoy some of the fruits of our labors in the bath? This simple basic recipe invites many variations based upon your own special preferences. *Bath oils can make the tub slippery, so be sure to use a secure rubber bath mat, and get in and out of the tub carefully.*

Pour all ingredients into a sterile bottle and cap tightly. Shake well to blend, and shake well before each use. Add 1 tablespoon to hot bathwater in the tub, or 1 teaspoon to a hot footbath in a foot basin.

If you enjoy a spicy or citrus smell, you might also add lemon verbena leaves, fennel seeds, or allspice berries, or perhaps several long, thin strips of fresh lime, lemon, and orange rind to the bottle of bath oil.

Blueberry–Ginger–Heal-all Bath Salts

Relieve sunburn, treat skin rashes and blemishes, and soothe the entire body with this natural formula, inspired by my daughter Kim Kavasch, who is an herbalist and naturopath in Albuquerque, New Mexico, and Maya Cointreau, herbalist and computer wizard, of Roxbury, Connecticut.

Bath salts offer a number of healing benefits. Sodium salts, which include table salt, borax, and baking soda, react with the minerals in hard water, making it feel soft and silky. This increases the effectiveness of soap. Sea salt adds trace minerals to your water and may give your bath a "spa" atmosphere. Epsom salts (magnesium sulfate) work well to soothe sore muscles and ease away stiffness. It is best to keep your specific needs in mind and formulate accordingly.

Place fresh ingredients together in a small pot with 2 cups of water. Bring to a boil over medium heat and simmer for 10 minutes.

Add remaining ingredients to 1 tablespoon of this herbal decoction.

Place all ingredients in a medium mixing bowl and blend well with a whisk. Pour the mixture into a large glass jar and cover. Next time you need to refresh body and spirit, add a handful of these salts to your hot bath.

Geranium relieves stress and anxiety, lifts depression, and promotes balance. Cedar stimulates spirituality, healing, and encourages deep relaxation. Blueberry and heal-all are cleansing astringents that help to heal chapped skin. Ginger stimulates the blood flow and tones the skin.

5 blueberry leaves

5 heal-all leaves

1-inch piece of fresh ginger root, chopped

3/4 cup baking soda

3/4 cup table salt

1/2 cup sea salt

35 drops essential oil of geranium

25 drops essential oil of cedarwood

1/4 teaspoon green food coloring

1/4 teaspoon blue food coloring

Medicine Wheel
Bayberry–Heal-all Soap

8 ounces warm water

4 tablespoons pure lye (such as Red Devil brand; found in the drain-opener section of the supermarket or hardware store)

1 pound lard (found in the baking or meat sections of many supermarkets)

20 drops essential oil of bayberry

1 tablespoon dried powdered bayberry leaves

1 tablespoon dried powdered heal-all leaves and blossoms

1 teaspoon ground cloves

2 glass or ceramic mixing bowls, one small and one medium (see note)

a Pyrex measuring cup

a large bowl half filled with ice

a wooden spoon

a plastic or wooden tablespoon

an 8-inch-square glass dish or mold

vinegar

Soothed skin and shining hair are benefits from this creation, inspired by Cheri Senieur, art therapist, of Middletown, Idaho, and Maya Cointreau of Roxbury, Connecticut.

Making soap is a time-consuming activity that requires advance preparation and a bit of caution. This is especially true when handling lye, which is traditional to the art of soap making. This recipe yields about 8 generous bars of soap with a spicy, woodsy scent and a smooth, silky texture.

Note: (1) Never use aluminum when making soap: not bowls, spoons, or foil. Lye dissolves aluminum. (2) If at any time lye comes into contact with your skin, flush the area with vinegar, and then wash well. Lye will feel slippery on your skin.

Measure 8 ounces of warm water into the smaller bowl. Carefully add 4 tablespoons lye. *Always add lye to water, never the other way around!* The water and lye react together to create quite a bit of heat. Stir the solution and let it sit to cool. Do not inhale the fumes. Work with good ventilation.

Heat the lard in a medium bowl until it liquefies. You can microwave it in the bowl for about 40 seconds.

Allow the two bowls and their contents to cool to room temperature. This may take half an hour or more. When they have both cooled sufficiently, slowly add the lye to the lard, stirring constantly.

Place the container in the ice bath and continue to stir until the soap "traces." Tracing occurs when you can dribble soap from the spoon and it leaves its mark on the soap in the bowl. At this point the soap will have a consistency like sour cream.

Add the remaining ingredients to this mixture, blending well, and pour the soap into the mold. Cover the mold with a cloth and store in a dry place for 24 hours.

Uncover the mold. After another 48 hours, unmold the soap. Cut it into individual bars and let them cure for 4 weeks in plastic bags. After this, enjoy and use your homemade soap!

Arnica, Bee Balm, Heal-All, and Strawberry Bath Balm and Tub Teas

Take a large clean bandana or 12-inch square of muslin out to the medicine wheel garden along with sharp cutters. Spread it out in a basket. Select and cut 6 good arnica blooms and place them in the spread fabric. Cut 6 nice bee balm and heal-all bloom stalks. Cut 10 healthy strawberry leaves. Add several blades of sweet flag and sweetgrass, and a large angelica leaf. Squeeze these all together firmly and tie them up in the fabric square. Bring this inside.

Place this herbal bath balm bouquet in a large pot of fresh water and bring it to a boil over medium-high heat. Lower the heat and simmer, uncovered, for 10 minutes, until a nice aromatic tea has developed. While you are doing this, run a nice hot bath for yourself. Light a few scented candles in the bathroom and put on soft music, or simply tune in to the sounds of nature. When this is all set, carefully pour the herbal bath tea—cloth, herbs, and all—into the bathtub. Test the water for comfort and stir the herbal tea in well. Then carefully ease yourself into this aromatic tub tea and relax. Use the herbal bath balm (cloth bag/bundle) to gently rub your skin, squeezing out the herbal essence on sore places and tired muscles.

Use this basic recipe to vary the tub teas and bath balms seasonally from your medicine wheel garden. If you are suffering with poison ivy or other skin rashes, you will want to use jewelweed and the astringent blueberry and bayberry leaves in a hot tub bath and poultice.

Note: Do not use arnica if you have any open cuts or sores on your skin.

Medicine Wheel Garden Foot Bath

This recipe is a variation of the previous one. Gather and prepare this healthy, fragrant foot soak from your medicine wheel garden. Take a clean bandana or 12-inch square of cotton cloth out to the garden. Clip a small handful of angelica, sage, jewelweed, and strawberry leaves. Tie these up securely within the bandana, making a little herbal sack. Bring this in and place it in a medium pan full of water. Simmer this over medium-low heat for 15 to 20 minutes.

Cool slightly and add this to a clean foot bath partially filled with water, herb-filled bandana and all. Blend thoroughly and test for temperature. Then sit and relax with your bare feet soaking in this fragrant, antiseptic herbal bath. This is a great time for healing meditation or to read your favorite book.

Enjoy your own variations on this formula using arnica flowers and elderberry flowers in early summer, or heal-all and sweetgrass in late summer, or wintergreen and sweet flag in winter. One of the finest herbs to relieve foot fatigue is broadleaf plantain, which is why I always plant it in the medicine wheel garden.

Medicine Wheel Garden
Dream Pillow

You may choose to make large and small versions of this aromatic pillow. You can place the small one on the back of your easy chair and slide the larger one into your pillowcase or on top of the pillow. You can harvest or purchase some of the additional sleep herbs beyond what you have grown in your medicine wheel garden. All herbs should be carefully selected, checked over, and well dried.

Select a pleasing calico or muslin fabric, double it, and cut through both layers to create two identical 6-inch squares and two 11-inch by 5-inch rectangles. Use pinking shears to keep the fabric from unraveling. Place the wrong sides together and carefully stitch around three of the sides. Now turn the pillows inside out so the seams are on the inside, and top-stitch around the three sides about ¼ inch from the edge. Next, carefully stuff them with a choice mixture of the listed herbs, which are also thought to enhance dreams.

Blend these all together well in a large bowl or plastic bag. Stuff the two pillows moderately full, then tuck in the edges of the fabric and whipstitch the last end closed. Make sure this is securely finished so none of the herbs leak out.

You will enjoy these pillows for many months, even years. I have one that has been through the washing machine and dryer and still has fine aromatic qualities.

1 cup dried bee balm leaves and blooms

1 cup dried angelica leaves

1/2 cup dried heal-all leaves and blooms

1/2 cup dried sweetgrass blades

1/2 cup dried mugwort leaves

1/2 cup dried catnip leaves and blooms

1/2 cup dried peppermint leaves

1/2 cup lavender flowers

1/2 cup flaxseeds

Medicine Wheel Garden Eye Mask

 This is a variation of the dream pillow and is made the same way. Select a soft piece of calico, silk, or flannel and double it. Using pinking shears, cut out two rectangles about 8 inches long by about 4 inches wide. Stitch three sides of this eye mask together with the wrong sides together, leaving the last short end open. Turn it right side out and top-stitch around the three stitched sides about a quarter of an inch from the outer edge.

Carefully fill this medium-full with the mixed herbs of your choice. You may want to increase the flaxseed, as it is cooling and soothing for the eyes and can help relieve puffiness and redness; if so, add an additional ½ cup flaxseed to this mixture before you stitch the final edge. Then tuck in the outer edges and whipstitch it closed.

As you use and enjoy this eye mask, you may decide to make more of them. These make wonderful gifts!

Complexion and Hair Spritzers

These treats from the medicine wheel garden can be made two ways: with fresh or dried herbs, or with purchased essential oils. My daughter Kim inspires these refreshing creations.

Method 1. Snip a handful each of fresh angelica, bayberry, and bee balm leaves, or you may use 1/2 handful each of the dried leaves. Place the leaves in a medium pot and cover with 1 quart of water. Simmer over medium-low heat, stirring frequently, for 20 minutes, uncovered. Cool and strain through a coffee filter or other fine filter. Bottle the resulting strong tea in 2-ounce spray bottles. You might also add a teaspoon of apple cider vinegar or lemon juice to give this a slightly acid pH, which is best for skin and hair. Label and date each bottle. Store in the refrigerator for maximum keeping qualities and ultimate refreshment during the heat of summer.

To use, simply point the spray nozzle at your face, holding the bottle about 12 inches away, close your eyes, and spritz your face and hair with this aromatic medicine wheel herbal spray. I keep one small bottle by my computer for an instant refresher.

Method 2. Easier yet, fill a 2-ounce spray bottle almost full with spring water. Add 8 drops, more or less, of your favorite essential oil—try sandalwood, rose, patchouli, lavender, or bergamot. Place cap securely on bottle and shake well. Then, with your eyes closed, mist your face and hair, holding the bottle about 12 inches from your face.

Once you decide on your favorite herbal blends, you can make your own aromatic formulas. One of my favorite invigorating spritzers is 6 drops each of essential oils of rose, vetiver, balsam, bergamot, sandalwood, and patchouli in an 8-ounce bottle of spring water. This makes an intensely fragrant spray mist that is quite revitalizing.

several large leaves of angelica

a small handful each of pennyroyal and cardinal flower leaves and flowers

a cup each of bayberry leaves and boneset leaves and flowers

as many bearberry leaves as the plants shed

a cupful of bee balm leaves and blossoms

a handful of heal-all leaves and blossoms

a handful of sage leaves and blossoms

a large handful of sumac leaves and berries, and joe-pye weed leaves and blossoms

a generous handful of sweet flag and sweetgrass blades

a generous handful of tobacco leaves and blossoms and yarrow leaves and blossoms

Kinnikinnick is an old Cree Indian word meaning "botanical mixture." Kinnikinnick was often used for smoking and smudging. It is basically like potpourri. Traditionally these mixtures have a great fragrance and are often carried in a special pouch. We have the benefit of making our own seasonal kinnikinnicks from selected botanicals harvested from our medicine wheel garden. Harvest fairly equal amounts of the leaves and blossoms.

Pick the fresh ingredients from your medicine wheel garden and dry them separately. It is important to dry each ingredient separately. Each herb requires a different drying time, and mixing them too soon may invite mold or mildew. You may take an entire season to collect and dry all these ingredients. You will certainly enjoy savoring the unique fragrance of each different plant that develops as water is lost and the constituents become more concentrated.

When the herbs are dry, crumble or cut the material into a fine mixture. Place the herbs in a large bowl or bag and mix everything well together. You may want to put this in a series of smaller bags for storage or gift giving.

Some Great Lakes Indian kinnikinnicks were made from over thirty different botanicals. Each blend has different therapeutic and spiritual properties. You may find that you prefer to use your own medicine wheel garden kinnikinnick rather than sage and other commercial blends for smudging and for rituals. Use this basic recipe as your springboard to create your own kinnikinnick formula. Try adding rosemary, lavender, oregano, marjoram, willow bark, and sumac bark.

When you are ready to use this fragrant blend of medicine wheel herbs, place a small handful in a fireproof glass or clay dish or a large seashell. Ignite this, and as it catches fire, blow out the flames so that it will just smoke. This is the smudge, this fragrant smoke, that each person gently sweeps over himself or herself to help wash away impurities, sadness, anxieties, or anything unwanted. Use your cupped hand or a feather to draw the smoke around and over you, or to sweep it into the corners of a room. This is the process we use also to "secure the circle or room" before a special gathering: One person walks around the perimeter of the room directing the smoke throughout the space, up and down and into corners. Smudging is a special prayer of gratitude for whatever you wish to undertake. It can also be a simple blessing of a space, or of a place and time. We usually begin our circle gatherings with a brief time of smudging, centering, and quiet. This helps to focus our minds and hearts on what we have come together to accomplish.

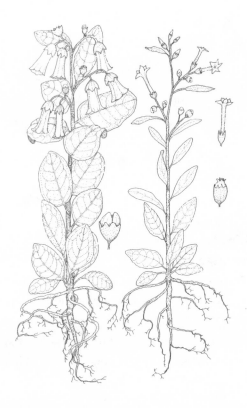

CHAPTER FOURTEEN

Ceremonial and Ritual Items

Smudge Sticks, Prayer Feathers, and Spirit Shields

I don't know why these traditions mean so much to me, more than my own life. I don't know what childhood incident, if any, programmed me in this direction, but if I am not doing these things, making these things, speaking of these things, I feel as if I don't exist.

—Claude Medford Jr., Choctaw-Apache artist, basketweaver, historian, Louisiana, 1982

MY FRIEND CLAUDE MEDFORD Jr. was a gifted basketweaver, and he taught me many things about native traditions and respect for the environment. He always enjoyed collecting herbs and weaving botanicals into lasting works of art. Many of his herbal infusing baskets are in private collections and in the collection of the Smithsonian Institution. One of his older "Texas Star" Choctaw food baskets appears on the cover of my previous book, *American Indian Healing Arts*.

I think of Claude and the many native elders I have studied and worked with each time I gather healing herbs or gather a group of friends together in a healing circle. Their spirits continue to guide my work with respect.

Our ceremonies are blessed with spiritual intent and sweetened with chants, prayers, and songs. Raising our voices together is bonding and reaffirming. Here I share several universal little refrains and offerings for your benefit. Use them with a happy heart.

Our group joins hands in a circle to sing. The general pattern is right hand palm down, left hand palm up, or thumbs left. This way the energies are equally shared and move around our circle freely. Our simple dances, directed by Pamela Redmer (our song keeper), move clockwise and then counterclockwise in step with the easy tempo of the chant. Then we drop hands, spin individually, and rejoin hands in conclusion.

We generally close each drumming circle and shamanic drumming circle with this old Arapaho song fragment from a Ghost Dance song:

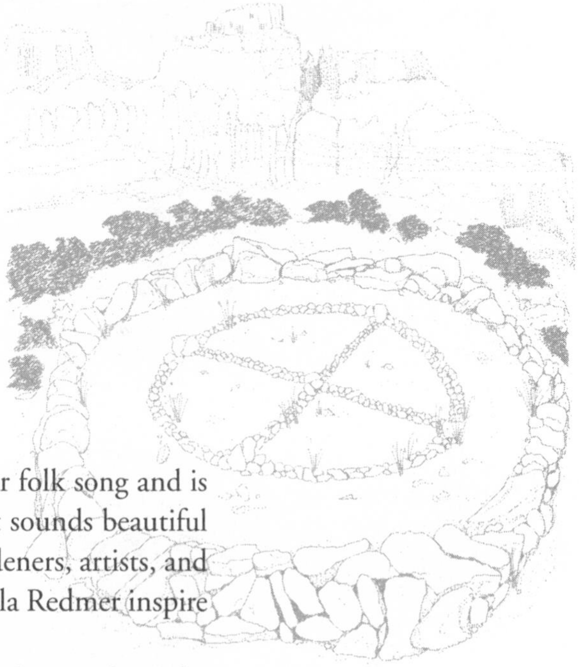

Long Wing Feathers
I circle around, I circle around
The boundaries of the earth,
I circle around, I circle around
The boundaries of the earth;
Wearing my long wing feathers as I fly,
Wearing my long wing feathers as I fly,
I circle around, I circle around
The boundaries of the earth.

This marvelous chant has become a popular folk song and is even listed in the *Sloop Clearwater Songbook*. It sounds beautiful with many voices singing in unison. Gifted gardeners, artists, and shamanic practitioners Missy Stevens and Pamela Redmer inspire this work.

Our ceremonies are also enriched by the ritual items that I describe in this chapter. For me, the making is often as valuable as the using. Perhaps as you collect and create the following items you too will find old memories or glimpse a new vision, or hum a song while you focus on the tasks ahead.

SWEETGRASS–SWEET FLAG BRAID

Fragrant natural perfume from these two botanicals makes this a fine ceremonial item for a personal altar. Or place a fresh braid in your car as a token of good luck.

Go to the medicine wheel garden in late summer and carefully cut a small handful of sweetgrass and slightly less sweet flag. Cut them with clean scissors just above ground level, for maximum length. Spread the long green blades to dry for a day in a cool, shady area on a blanket or paper. Do not dry in the sun. You do not want them brittle, just wilted.

Gather the blades all together and tie them securely at the base with a twisted piece of sweetgrass, leather, or string. Secure this to a table leg or chair back so that you can pull gently against it as you braid. Distributing the blades into three groups, braid them together snugly and make one long braid. Tie the end, or make a slipknot to hold it.

These braids smell heavenly and keep their fragrance for more than a hundred years. They smell especially wonderful on damp days, as the moisture seems to activate the aromatic substances in them. You may also dampen the braid slightly with water to bring up the fine perfume.

This braid can be burned or smudged for ceremonial use, or kept for an altar and house blessing. Place the sweetgrass–sweet flag braid in a place of honor.

We gather in a circle of thirty to sixty friends for some rituals and smudge every individual in the circle from head to toe, front and back. Usually one person will smudge everyone, but sometimes the braid is passed around the circle and each person smudges his neighbor.

When I smudge people I generally say a quiet blessing to each person as I finish; I place the smoking braid gently above their eyes, saying, "May your eyes see better than they have ever seen before." And then I gently place the smoking braid on their chest (below their throat), saying, "May you hear the wisdom of the ancients in your heart." There are many words of wisdom you can call upon while smudging. Enjoy finding your own.

Smudging with a Sweetgrass Braid

Sweetgrass imparts a beautiful vanillalike, earthy fragrance that is both soothing and stimulating at the same time. Native Americans have always delighted in the aromas of sweetgrass as well as its strength and holiness. This is a tenacious perennial grass that symbolizes (and is) the hair of Mother Earth.

Many of us carry braids and coils of sweetgrass and weave the blades into various ceremonial items. Sweetgrass braids are also used to smudge and pray with. Ignite one end, and when the flame has caught, immediately blow it out so that it will slowly smoke instead of burn. Carefully move the smoking braid all around you, front and back, especially around your hands, head, and heart.

You may use only an inch or two of the braid in a particular ritual. Simply stub out the remaining fire and save the braid for another occasion.

SAGE-SWEETGRASS SMUDGE STICK

Aromatic fresh herbs are bundled together here to provide smudge sticks for rituals. These can be made all during summer and early autumn.

Plan to cut your botanicals for this after the sun has dried the morning dew off the plants, about midmorning. While sage and sweetgrass are traditional, you might also use sweet flag, goldenrod, bee balm, sumac leaves, or yarrow. Spread the botanical cuttings out on paper or a towel in the shade to dry for a few hours or a day before creating the smudge stick bundles. They don't need to be thoroughly dry, just wilted.

For each smudge stick, select a generous handful of one or more of the herbs. Clasp them together securely and fold them back on each other one or two times, until you have folded and broken all the stems to a six- or eight-inch length in a nice fat handful. Place the herb bundle diagonally across the corner of a single piece of newspaper. Begin to roll the herbs up in the paper, using it like a cigar wrapper, fitting it snugly around the herbs and tucking in both ends. Secure the roll with a rubber band.

Allow this to dry overnight. The next day unroll it, tuck in any loose pieces, roll it up again more tightly, and replace the rubber band. Place the roll in a shady, airy spot to dry completely, for perhaps a week or two. Unwrap and recycle the paper. Tie the well-shaped smudge stick with cotton thread or embroidery thread.

Your medicine wheel smudge sticks can be saved in a basket for use during ceremonial and social occasions. They also make wonderful, fragrant gifts to special friends. These smudge sticks are also excellent insect repellents, so make enough for outdoor use with family and friends.

HERBAL PRAYER TIES

Celebrations are enhanced with your prayers when you make these simple offerings. Prayer ties are a great way of weaving herbs from the medicine wheel garden into all your ceremonies. All you need for this is small squares (or circles) of red cloth, red string or thread, and some loose tobacco or other dried herbs. Sometimes I start with a three-foot-long cord and make a dozen prayer ties or more to tie onto it at intervals.

A Prayer While Smudging

Creator, Great Mystery,
Source of all knowing and comfort,
Cleanse this space of all negativity.
Open our pathways to peace and understanding.
Love and light fills each of us and our sacred space.
Our work here shall be beautiful and meaningful.
Banish all energies that would mean us harm.
Our eternal gratitude.

Cut or tear pieces of red cloth about two inches square. Lay out your squares near each other. Take a pinch of tobacco or herbs and hold it to your heart while you make a brief prayer. Then put this in the center of a red square and tie it up into a little bundle with a small piece of red thread. It is just this simple, yet it is also profound.

I make a string of many prayer ties when I am working on problems. The long string loops around each little prayer bundle, tying it on with a slipknot. It helps me stop and work out special details, one by one, letting go of anxieties. I also make a string of prayer ties when I have much to celebrate. I make prayer ties for each member of my family and tie them all together with lots of love.

Native people make prayer ties before going into the sweat lodge, the Sun Dance, or an important ceremonial gathering. This is a patient, meditative way of communicating with the spirits in prayer. Every tribe has its own unique way of fashioning prayer ties.

Each season we make small prayer ties for our drums in the drumming circle. This renews our energies and expresses gratitude for progress. The prayer ties are special blessings for the spirit of the drum.

HERBAL FEATHERED PRAYER STICKS

The Indians of the Southwest make prayer sticks to invoke supernatural aid and to convey their prayers to the deities and the Creator. The Navajo refer to prayer sticks as *ke-tan,* or "place where it is feathered." Each stick serves as an offering and as protection for the one who carries it, and it is a symbolic prayer in itself. We choose special beads, feathers, gemstones, and colors of string, yarn, or cloth to symbolize aspects of our prayers—so the prayer stick becomes a living symbol of the prayer. They are lovely additions to your winter garden or to your indoor garden and altar.

Good friends at Zuni Pueblo, in Zuni, New Mexico, inspired these creations. These should be created in a prayerful, thoughtful

Wishi Ta Duewe Ya

This old canoeing song comes down to us through centuries of rhythmic use. It is a good working song, one that I often sing in the garden. We frequently sing this in our circle.

> *Wishi ta duewe ya, duewe*
> *ya, duewe ya,*
> *Wishi ta duewe ya, duewe*
> *ya day.*
> *Ya ta te nea ya, hey ya hey*
> *ya,*
> *Ya ta te nea ya, hey ya hey.*

Repeat over and over, liltingly.

manner. You actually visualize a prayer in each step of the activity. This way, when your prayer stick is completed, it is filled with prayers. Focus on renewal and gratitude.

Begin by collecting and saving cast-off bird feathers and special small sticks or branches that you clip in your garden or find in your travels. Clean each item well and smudge it with sage. Keep them in an attractive grouping or display them standing in glass jars or pottery bowls until you are ready to begin using them. It is important to honor their spirits. Save and dry the stoutest plant stems from your medicine wheel garden, especially yarrow, blue flag pods, sumac, and tobacco. Trim them to about twelve to eighteen inches in length.

You will need:

one or several small sticks, six to eighteen inches long
several feathers for each stick
fine red string or thread to tie them onto the stick
a tiny bundle of sweetgrass, sage, or cedar for each stick
   (other herbs are optional)
a small bead or piece of turquoise, or other precious
   object
a small capful of white glue (optional)
red or colored ribbon, perhaps a foot or two, or leather
   scraps to cut into leather ties

When you are prepared to begin, assemble the items you will need. Smudge everything, including yourself, with sage, and offer a prayer of gratitude. Think and work in a meditative, prayerful attitude.

Select a small stick. Hold it and decide which end will be the top, where you will fasten the feathers to it.

Brush a small amount of white glue around the top half inch of the stick. Use your fingers or a small brush, or another stick. Place the quills of one or two feathers in this glue at the top of the stick. Take a short length, twelve inches, of red thread and bind these feathers snugly in place. You might tie a small piece of leather around this, too.

Ancient peoples knew the importance of ceremony. Throughout the year they would celebrate different parts of the earth through this vehicle. They would have seasonal ceremonies, deer dances, strawberry festivals, corn festivals, bear dances, full moon ceremonies, and thanksgiving celebrations. These were not arbitrary events; rather they were well-planned ways of keeping the balance of the sacred circle.

—Sun Bear, 1991, of
Chippewa descent

Make a tiny smudge stick or bundle of the special herbs you have chosen, and tie this with another short length of red thread to the stick just below the feathers. Add beads if you like.

When you are finished, use the smudge again to express your gratitude, and draw each prayer stick through the smudge to bless it and secure your work.

PRAYER FEATHERS

You can also make prayer feathers using this same plan. If you find long wing feathers of crow, raven, sea gull, Canada goose, pheasant, or wild turkey, clean and smudge them. Cut or tear foot-long strips of red cloth, about one-half inch wide. Dab a small amount of white glue on the base of the quill, wrap it with the folded strip of red cloth, and tie it securely. You may want to attach a small herbal prayer bundle to this also at the base of the quill. I usually keep my prayer feather standing in a large hollow bone so that I can admire it and pick it up readily to use.

I make a new prayer feather every time the wild turkeys bless me with another molted feather. I save these and use them for smudging ceremonies, to draw the smoke around and to wipe the anxieties away from myself and other individuals whom I smudge.

Prayer feathers are beautiful blessings. They honor the spirit of the bird who created each feather. They have a spirit of their own, which they contribute when they become a ceremonial instrument. Prayer feathers make beautiful gifts. I have one friend, Vanessa, who walks with her daughter along a lakeshore that Canada geese frequent, and they pick up the molted feathers. She cleans them in soapy water, dries them, and restores them to make prayer feathers for our circle of friends.

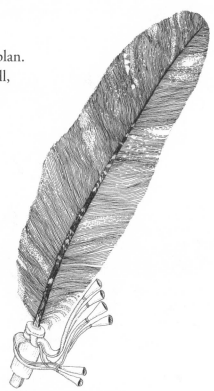

Put your ear to the ground and listen and you will know the ceremonies are all around us. We just have to be patient and listen.

—Mohegan elder, Connecticut

The summer and winter solstices and the spring and autumnal equinoxes are important quarterly points to mark in each year's calendar, regardless of where you live. These age-old reckoning points are also fine times to create long new prayer ties to hang out in the medicine wheel garden amidst the other ribbons and prayer ties. This can clearly become the most festive garden!

To take one example, winter solstice crowns the year's achievements, signaling a time of slumber in most northern regions. Cold weather begins in earnest, and the sun is at its farthest distance from the northern regions. Many Indian tribes held elaborate ceremonies at this time to "call the sun back" from its journey and ask the Creator for good health and enough food for the winter months of thin sun and deep cold. Beautiful gifts were made

Solstices and Equinoxes

Earliest tribal calendars counted the moons between one winter solstice and the next. Plains Indians painted mnemonic symbols of important events that occurred during each moon period on elaborate buffalo robes; some of the finest of these robes are called "Winter Counts." Similarly, tribes around the Great Lakes and in the desert Southwest carved symbols in fine wooden calendar sticks.

The two solstices mark the periods when the earth is at its farthest points from the sun in its journey. The summer solstice occurs about June 22, when the sun is in its zenith at the tropic of Cancer. The winter solstice happens about December 22, when the sun is over the tropic of Capricorn. Yet long before this was scientifically understood, earlier peoples often found the winter solstice a fearful time of diminishing daylight and increasing cold. By contrast, the summer solstice crowned the planting season with increasing daylight and warmth.

The two equinoxes mark the periods when there is relatively equal day and night. The autumnal equinox occurs about September 22 and the vernal equinox occurs about March 22. These positions are measured from the celestial equator. We mark these points as the time when days begin growing longer with more daylight in spring, and shorter days with longer nights begin after the fall equinox.

The two equinoxes and two solstices mark the quarter points of each year, and these were important ceremonial times among earlier tribal peoples. Native ceremonies usually began several days before the key event and lasted four to nine days or more. These were among the few times when everyone would come together to celebrate with their finest foods and best songs and dances.

and placed outside on earth altars to reassure Father Sun that all those who lived on Mother Earth remembered the importance and marriage of these two "life sustainers."

Making a winter solstice flag is a good opportunity to host a solstice lunch or dinner, gathering a few special friends together to reflect on the period just ending and the new one just beginning. During these festivities, I welcome each guest to write a prayer or thought for the next season on three-foot-long, one-inch-wide strips of white cotton sheeting (yours can be much larger or smaller, depending upon your own taste). Everyone writes, using waterproof ink in various colors, their own unique prayer, and then we all take the strips out and fasten them to the peace pole, cardinal poles, or a suitable tree branch. Then we make a circle joining hands and bless our efforts into successful being. We enjoy watching the prayer flags, like "wind horses," flutter in snow and rain, wind and sleet—knowing that our prayers are traveling a cosmic path to fulfillment.

I select a yellow banner for spring, a green banner for summer, and a purple banner for fall, and often repeat the festivities, hosting friends and family for a meal of favorite foods and spiritual reflections. We always incorporate a drumming circle and end with a group prayer. Perhaps you will embellish these times with your own intriguing rituals of celebration in the medicine wheel garden. The various plants and animals living here certainly seem to thrive on celebrations!

We Are the Stars That Sing

This old Passamaquoddy spirit song from the late 1800s is another rhythmic "earth song" that sounds beautiful when sung together in a circle of friends.

We are the stars that sing
We sing with our light.
We are the birds of fire
We fly over the heaven
Our light is a star.

We sing on the road of the spirits
The road of the Great Spirit.
Among us are three hunters
Who follow the bear.
There never was a time
When they were not hunting.
We look upon the mountains.
This is a song of the mountains.

SPIRIT STICK

My friend Richard Reilly in Brookfield, Connecticut, creates the most beautiful spirit sticks, which he gifts to his friends. Each one is made in a prayerful manner while thinking about the person for whom it is destined. I was greatly honored to receive mine.

Select an unusual stick that you find among nature's discards. Once you begin looking, you will notice the amazing variety of

Talking Stick

A talking stick is an elaborate, feather-embellished staff often wrapped with soft leather and tied with an arrowhead and special beads. These take time, patience, and more materials to make, and are often sold in museum shops and galleries. A talking stick signifies respect. This item is often taken to board meetings, because the one who holds it carries the attention of the group. As the talking stick is passed from one person to the next around the group, the significance is carried also. It is a reminder that one person at a time should talk and be listened to with respect.

downed wood. I gravitate to "spalted wood"—wood that has some decay beginning in it, which has created unusual patterns just beneath the bark. I have an old sugar maple that continually drops amazing twigs and branches, and the inner wood looks almost like calico or a jaguar's spotted coat. Spalted apple wood is also beautiful.

Look for sticks at least one to one and a half feet long and perhaps an inch thick. Peel the bark off carefully and clean the stick. Saw off the ends and sand them smooth. Marking off about one inch below the top of the stick, lightly draw with pencil a circle around the top. Duplicate this six more times until you have seven circles about one inch apart descending the stick. You may carve these in a little bit, perhaps a quarter of an inch or less, or use a wood-burning tool to incise a small groove around the pencil line. These will eventually hold the seven primary colors. Two inches below this you may incise double lines, patterns, your initials, or any special designs that appeal to you. You may want to darken this work with black ink or paint, or any color of your choice.

Select yarn or string and matching color beads for each of the cardinal directions: traditionally, yellow for east, red for west, blue for south, white for north, green for zenith, and black for nadir. You, or the person you are giving this to, selects the last color along with matching beads and fastens it on last. Fasten one end of a ten-inch length of each color around the grooved slot you made for it. Slip two beads of matching color onto the free end, and finish with a knot to hold them in place. When you are finished these cords will hang down like beaded fringe and gently strike against the stick.

The spirit stick is somewhat like a talking stick except for feathers. It is an item of honor and spiritual potency. You may want to stand it beside your altar, or lay it nearby. Hold it when you are talking, praying, chanting, and telling stories.

HEALING SPIRIT SHIELD

My friend Mitzi Rawls, a Choctaw artist who lives in Melbourne Beach, Florida, makes beautiful spirit shields and often leads classes in shield making at the Institute for American Indian Studies. The American Indian spirit shield or power shield was often conceived first in a dream or series of dreams, in which the dreamer would see exactly how it is supposed to look. The design and ideas would reflect this vision as the dreamer gathered the materials to make the shield. The power shield embraces the symbols and items that each person visualizes as his personal power or energy. One's favorite nature symbols and animal guides would be represented here.

Harvest a sturdy length of willow or grape vine—perhaps three feet long—and carefully ease it into a circle about one foot in diameter, bending it back upon itself and weaving its ends in and out together like a wreath. I often make a dozen of so of these at a time and stack them in the studio to dry for a week.

Healing spirit shield made with sweetgrass, sage, tobacco, antler, deer toes, and feathers on leather

Cut a circle of canvas, cotton, or leather slightly larger than your hoop. Whipstitch this on around your hoop using heavy thread or artificial sinew. (See Appendix 2 for suppliers where you can order leather, beads, fetishes, and artificial sinew.) Use long running stitches that show on the back but not on the front. Make sure the shield cover fits the hoop snugly. The circle may be stretched over the edges of the hoop, or it can fit within and be laced with an open stitch, whichever suits your fancy and your materials.

You may want to paint your shield (acrylics work well), or leave it natural and fix selected items to it. Perhaps you have a vision of thunder and lightning purifying you, targeting your illness or a disorder; perhaps you want to depict some aspect of your medicine wheel garden. Or you may simply want to sew on a particular feather, small medicine bag, or group of small shells.

I have laced a small deer antler to one edge of my shield and suspended a dozen deer toes beneath this as a dance rattle. I fastened a nice long sweetgrass braid at the other edge with a cluster of sage tied onto it. I have fastened a tiny turtle fetish to the center bottom, and tied several tiny herbal prayer ties onto the back. Two large wild turkey feathers are suspended from the bottom of the shield, which signify fertility, endurance, and abundance.

Your healing spirit shield is a beautiful item to hang on the wall in your studio or meditation room. It is also a fine focus for meditation.

MEDICINE WHEEL HOOP

The medicine wheel hoop is considered sacred by Plains Indians, who fashion small ones out of quilled leather (used as personal adornments) and also create larger ones on a bent willow hoop. The latter is the one we can most easily create—much like the beginning hoop for a dream catcher. You might like to suspend the medicine wheel hoop above your altar, where it can hang free and turn in the breeze. Like a multidimensional mandala, it may become a meditation point and a focus for prayer. My friend Wendell Deer with Horns, Lakota pipe carrier from Cheyenne River Reservation in Eagle Butte, South Dakota, created a fine one for me many years ago. It is a symbol of protection and prayer.

A traditional Plains Indian medicine wheel hoop was decorated with eagle and hawk feathers, symbols of highest bravery and honor as well as keen sight. But to protect these endangered birds, today it is illegal for anyone other than American Indians to possess these feathers. I recommend substituting other feathers you have collected. Or you can draw a feather or cut out a picture of one, glue it on art board, and trim this. Some American Indian artists are painting and crafting amazing replicas of sacred feathers for just such use.

It can take a while to collect all the items and draw (or paint) the sacred feathers to suspend from the hoop. Yet this is what makes this project such a thoughtful one.

You will need:

A medicine wheel hoop made with feathers from the snowy owl, turkey, crow, and hawk

a fresh green three-foot-long willow rod, bark peeled off
a ball of twine or artificial sinew
four long narrow strips (about twelve inches) of sinew or twine
four small squares of red wool or cotton cloth
two fourteen-inch leather thongs or pieces of cord
    select herbs in tiny bundles from the garden
four distinctive feathers: turkey, Canada goose, or whatever you prefer (these can be long wing or tail feathers)
small cuttings of sage, sweetgrass, and bearberry from your garden
assorted beads, bones, and small special items (optional)

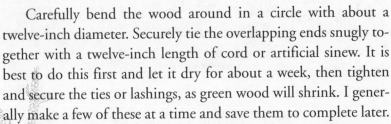

Carefully bend the wood around in a circle with about a twelve-inch diameter. Securely tie the overlapping ends snugly together with a twelve-inch length of cord or artificial sinew. It is best to do this first and let it dry for about a week, then tighten and secure the ties or lashings, as green wood will shrink. I generally make a few of these at a time and save them to complete later.

Tie one end of the leather cord at the overlap joining and secure it. Then stretch it straight across the middle of the circle hoop and tie it securely at the other end. Repeat this with the other strip of leather, so that it intersects with the first cord at a 90-degree angle in the middle of the circle. Loop it once around the other cord, making the center of the medicine wheel, before tying it to the opposite rim. Your hoop will then be divided into quarters, just like your medicine wheel garden.

Create four red herbal prayer ties and fasten one to each of the four cardinal directions where the leather ties are attached to the hoop. Next tie the four long red streamers onto the bottom rim of the medicine wheel. These can be adorned with beads, if you wish, and the four feathers can be tied to the ends of these red ties. Or the four feathers can be embellished with a small bundle of herbs and tied on close to the rim of the medicine wheel across the bottom. Create a loop on top of the hoop to use to suspend it.

Place selected herbs from your medicine wheel garden in a small leather medicine bag or six-inch square of red wool or cotton and tie them securely at the top of your medicine wheel hoop. If you have additional feathers, you may tie them together and fasten them to the center of the hoop. Finally light a smudge of sage and cedar, or kinnikinnick, and smudge the whole creation thoroughly. Repeat the smudge whenever you wish to renew your hoop's power.

MEDICINE WHEEL HEALING MANDALA

A mandala is composed of circles and other geometric figures representing cosmic forces in world order. (The word *mandala* is

The Ghost Dance Religion

The Ghost Dance religion was born of visions and hope in 1888 when a Paiute Indian from Nevada received a mystical vision during a solar eclipse. Wovoka, son of the mystical leader Tavibo, claimed that the earth would soon perish and be reborn again in a pure state, free from suffering, along with the Indians' resurrected ancestors. Much of this movement was based upon peace and understanding. The gospel proclaimed that the Indians must cleanse themselves, shun the destroyer alcohol, and renounce violence. It was vital to gather to dance and pray and celebrate the earth. This new religion spread quickly among the conquered and despondent western tribes.

Among the Plains Indians there were a number of mystics who sought to take the Ghost Dance religion and personalize it for their own people. Kicking Bear and Short Bull were two Miniconjou Teton Sioux leaders who espoused confrontation and elimination of the white settlers who continually harassed their people. The U.S. government became concerned about this religious fervor tinged with activism and banned the Ghost Dance on Sioux reservations in November 1890. Panic laced with passions and misunderstandings followed, leading to the brutal, unnecessary violence at Wounded Knee, South Dakota, on December 29, 1890, where more than 150 Indian men, women, and children were murdered in their harsh winter camp by the Seventh U.S. Cavalry. This effectively ended the Indian wars, yet "Remember Wounded Knee" became an enduring rallying cry and birthed a new century of passionate activism. Many of the old Ghost Dance songs and symbolism, especially the mystical circles, continue to inspire countless individuals well beyond the lens of memory.

Sanskrit for "circle.") Mandalas appear in sacred art all over the world, and especially in Navajo and Tibetan sand paintings. A mandala can be painted, drawn, fashioned in collage, and even developed in three dimensions.

Creating your own mandala can be a valuable aid to meditation and prayer. I use a mandala to bring more of my medicine wheel garden into my artwork and personal reflections. Every three months, I make a new mandala around the times of each equinox and solstice. I place on it or fasten to it designs and drawings of the most essential things I wish to accomplish during this period of time. It is a personal tool for positive growth.

I cut a one-foot-diameter circle of art board and lay it down in my work area like a tray. I design it as if it will be a mirror for my life these next three months. Sometimes I place a favorite picture

Making a mandala is a discipline for pulling all those scattered aspects of your life together, for finding a center and ordering yourself to it.
—Joseph Campbell, *The Power of Myth*

in the center of this circle and fasten it down. Then I surround this with beautiful beads and feathers or a favorite necklace. I draw, paint, or fashion in clay miniature examples of the things I want to have in my life. Placing these items all around the center of my mandala is a thoughtful process. I finish by making a tiny medicine bag out of leather and putting a tiny crystal inside along with tiny selections of sacred herbs from my medicine wheel garden. This is placed near the heart of the mandala. A braid of sweetgrass and sweet flag surrounds the outside of my mandala.

This is a fine project to incorporate into personal puberty rites for young people in the family, or for someone who is going through difficulties. It also makes a wonderful group project for a circle of close friends and family. The mandala becomes an energized symbol of hope, encircling our heartfelt needs and desires. We know that we can attain what we can visualize!

You might even wish to buy cement and plastic forms to design your own garden stepping-stones and make each one a special mandala for healing and enlightenment. The possibilities are endless—bounded only by your time, energy, and imagination.

MEDICINE WHEEL HEALING MANTRA

My friend Sandra Cointreau taught me to use healing mantras as a form of meditation. The ritual words and phrases of the mantra sound out the forces representing universal energy, and can help us bring forth a positive new reality. I have a classic mantra, which I repeat several times daily and even write out and tape to my bathroom mirror. At times of special need, I create a positive, loving mantra to address the situation and repeat it morning, noon, and night.

Keep your mantra fairly short and straight to the point. It helps if you can phrase it poetically or as an easy prose piece. Remember to smile while saying it. This is an everyday mantra:

Among the Navajo Indians, healing ceremonies are conducted through sand paintings, which are mostly mandalas on the ground. The person who is to be treated moves into the mandala as a way of moving into a mythological context that he will be identifying with—he identifies himself with the symbolized power. This idea of sand-painting and for meditation purposes appears also in Tibet. Tibetan monks draw cosmic images to represent the forces of the spiritual powers that operate in our lives.

—Joseph Campbell, author of
The Power of Myth

I am a beautiful, loving person. I love my life.
I am surrounded and protected with healing energy.
My body, mind, and spirit grow healthier and stronger every day.
My balance within nature and family is healthy and gratifying.
My work grows steadily more wonderful and appreciated.
I have everything I need in life without harming anyone.
Thank you, dear God—Great Mystery!

Here is a mantra to help banish anxieties, depression, and turmoil from your life:

I am a beautiful, loving person. I love my life.
I send love and gratitude to everyone around me, especially my
  family.
All anxiety, turmoil, and unhappiness is banished from us.
We reflect the beauty and understanding in each other.
I breathe in peace and harmony and give this to everyone
  around me.
My gratitude and love to you, dear God—Great Mystery!

The following mantra may help you to manifest the money you need in your life. Often we must change our attitudes about things in order to manifest what we want.

I am a beautiful, loving person. I love my life.
I allow money to flow into my life in sweet abundance.
Money is an important means of exchange in my life.
Money allows me to balance and accomplish what is best in my
  life.
Abundance is mine—with harm to no one.
Thank you, dear God—Great Mystery!

We all know the power of positive thinking, which enables us to manifest our highest good. I often repeat my mantra while standing or sitting in my medicine wheel garden. Here it becomes a prayer. Then I usually sing the Navajo Beauty Way, which seems like a perfect mantra for living one's life.

MEDICINE WHEEL WISDOM CARDS

Create your own set of wisdom cards by developing positive mantras to address each of the various concerns in your life. You will need a stack of twenty-eight blank cards. These might be three-by-five-inch file cards, or fine card stock from your favorite craft store. You can also cut them from larger sheets of art board.

Carefully hand-letter a short mantra on each blank card. These mantras might represent a positive mental gift and affirmation for each day of the lunar month, from one full moon to the next. You may even want to illustrate them yourself or with artwork cut from another source. Get creative and fashion a different animal, bird, and plant for each mantra; coordinate them with your medicine wheel garden. You might even take them to a place where you can have them laminated. If you are inspired by these mantras and suggestions, see what magic you can create!

You have probably seen such cards, yet how much more powerful it is to create your own. You can determine the shape, size, colors, and uses of your set of cards. I use my cards daily. I draw one card each morning to greet the new day. Sometimes I will draw a spread of three or four cards in order to gain perspective on a problem or project that I need help with. Occasionally I will lay the cards out like a medicine wheel hoop around one central card in order to gain an overview of where I am at that time in my life.

MEDICINE WHEEL HERBAL HEALING PRAYER BEADS

A simple fragrant craft dough can be used to shape beautiful prayer beads embellished with blossoms and herbs from the medicine wheel garden. You might even roll it out into a large circle and inlay it with selected stones and flower petals from the medicine wheel garden, creating a small medicine wheel mandala or altar. My talented friend Lydia Granitto inspires this work; it is born from ideas she has shared with our Healing Circle.

Place in a medium saucepan and mix together well:

1 cup flour
1 cup water or strong herbal tea (bee balm, heal-all,
    strawberry leaf, or sage)
½ cup table salt
1 tablespoon corn or sunflower seed oil
2 teaspoons cream of tartar

Cook over medium heat *just until it begins to bubble*. Remove from the heat and blend in one or more of the optional ingredients below:

6 drops essential oil of bergamot or wintergreen
4 tablespoons fresh or dried flower petals or chili pods,
    chopped fine, or dried powdered citrus rind

Place the dough on a clean platter or tray and knead for five minutes until smooth and plastic. This should yield about 8 ounces of warm, silken dough.

Working quickly, pinch off small bits of dough and roll them into little balls for beads. Each bead may be given a special prayer or mantra. Use a wooden toothpick to make central holes. Place the beads on a clean paper towel over a tray and dry overnight or for several days, depending upon the humidity in the air. You may also dry the beads in a warm (not hot) oven overnight.

When the beads are thoroughly dry you may paint or spray-varnish them, or leave them natural. (The salt content absorbs moisture, so it is best to protect them by varnishing or painting them.) String these beads on fine cord or ribbon, according to your wish. You may want to wear them or place them on your altar.

Store the remaining dough/clay in an airtight container. It should last for months. You may knead in food coloring and different essential oils at any time. Your dough can be used to shape little *milagros* or holiday ornaments, or may be embellished into Little People sculptures for gifts and for your medicine wheel altar.

Tree of Life

Once again the tree of life
Grows on the land,
Once again its roots
Stretch to the four directions.
Once again the sacred
Hoop is dancing.
Once again we're safe
Within her warm embrace

Growing along with your medicine wheel garden can be exciting. Tending it by hand and making small offerings of prayers and stones to the prayer cairns will build amazing energy over time. You have created your own sacred space, and it blesses you and all who come to visit you. Within this circle there is continual give-and-take and growth. Your medicine wheel garden is a living space filled with therapeutic benefits, and surprises will always await you within there.

I bring back a small round rock from every place that I visit, and I set these somewhere within my medicine wheel. This adds more universal energies to my sacred space. I host a Fire Ceremony once a year, usually at the summer or winter solstice, and burn the old ribbons and prayer flags; then I immediately replace them with new ribbons and prayer flags.

Your garden has become a crucible of healing that can nurture you and others for many years. It is also a spiritual center, an altar, an energy center, and a meeting space around which to celebrate life. As you look after the various plants and energies in your medicine wheel garden, you continue to enhance sacred space and your own spirituality. I hope that your garden will always reflect joy, growth, and healing for you.

Appendix 1

Native Plant Suppliers

You can find many of the right plants for your medicine wheel garden locally. Your area garden centers and nurseries will enjoy helping with your plant and soil requirements. There are also a number of nurseries that can supply your needs by mail. Their catalogs are especially fascinating to page through for more details. Some resources listed here specialize in native plants and organic medicinal herbs.

Many suppliers across the country and in Canada can provide native plants, seeds, mulch, and other garden needs. Here are just a select few.

Burgess Seed & Plant Company   1-309-663-9551
905 Four Seasons Road
Bloomington, IL 61701

Henry Field's Seed & Nursery Co.   1-605-665-9391
415 North Burnett   www.henryfields.com
Shenandoah, IA 51602

Gurney's Seed & Nursery Co.   1-605-665-1930
110 Capital Street   www.gurneys.com
Yankton, SD 57079

Johnny's Selected Seeds
1 Foss Hill Road
RR 1, Box 2580
Albion, ME 04910-9731

1-207-437-4301
Fax: 1-800-437-4290

Miller Nurseries
5060 West Lake Road
Canandaigua, NY 14424-8904

1-800-836-9630

Penn Herb Company
10601 Decatur Road, Suite 2
Philadelphia, PA 19154-3293

1-800-523-9971
Fax: 1-215-632-7945

Pinetree Garden Seeds
Box 300
New Gloucester, ME 04260

1-207-926-3400
www.superseeds.com

Prairie Moon Nursery
Route 3, Box 163
Winona, MN 55987-4515

1-507-452-1362
Fax: 1-507-452-5238
pmarsy@luminet.net

Richter's Herb Specialists
357 Highway 47
Goodwood, Ontario
LOC 1A0 Canada

1-905-640-6677
Fax: 1-905-640-6641
orderdesk@richters.com
www.richters.com

Seymour's Selected Seeds
P.O. Box 1346
Sussex, VA 23884-0346

1-803-663-3084
Fax: 1-888-739-6687

Shepherd's Garden Seeds
30 Irene Street
Torrington, CT 06790-6658

1-860-482-3638
www.shepherdseeds.com

Spring Hill Nurseries
110 West Elm Street
Tipp City, OH 45371

1-800-582-8527
Fax: 1-800-991-2852

Territorial Seed Company
P.O. Box 157
Cottage Grove, OR 97424-00611

1-541-942-9547
FAX: 1-888-657-3131
www.territorial-seed.com

BIOLOGICAL SUPPLIERS FOR GARDENERS' NEEDS

These suppliers offer a broad variety of garden supplies, including biological products, natural insect controls, and live insects that contribute to a rich and healthy garden.

ARBICO
P.O. Box 8910
Tucson, AZ 85738-1247

1-800-827-BUGS
www.arbico.com

Gardens Alive!
5100 Schenley Place
Lawrenceburg, IN 47025

1-812-537-8650
Fax: 1-812-537-5108

Appendix 2

American Indian Craft Suppliers

These good folks provide remarkable catalogs and supplies for your creative needs. Great varieties of beads, feathers, leather supplies, and other items are available here for your special sacred and ceremonial items.

Crazy Crow Trading Post
P.O. Box 847
Pottsboro, TX 75076
1-800-786-6210

Grey Owl Indian Craft Sales Corp.
P.O. Box 1185
Neptune, NJ 07754-1185
1-800-487-2376
greyowlinc@aol.com
www.greyowlcrafts.com

Wandering Bull
247 South Main Street
Attleboro, MA 02703
1-800-430-2855

The World Peace Prayer Society

Founded in 1955 in Japan but now based in the United States, the World Peace Prayer Society is dedicated to bringing the message of the simple prayer "May peace prevail on earth" to all people. They also provide a list of peace pole suppliers from around the world on their website.

800 Third Ave., 37th floor
New York, NY 10022   www.worldpeace.org

The Peace Pole Makers of the U.S.

Recommended by the World Peace Prayer Society, the Peace Pole Makers of the U.S. manufacture durable wooden peace poles featuring the message "May peace prevail on earth" in several different languages.

3534 Lanham Rd.
Maple City, MI 49664, 1-616-334-4567   www.peacepoles.com

Cultured Stone Products

Suppliers of over 120 different colors and textures of stone, Cultured Stone Products is a good resource for stone for large-scale medicine wheel gardens.

Owens Corning Corporation
Napa, CA 94590, 1-800-255-1727   www.culturedstone.com

Sacred Circles Institute

Gives instructions on "walking the sacred wheel," a year's journey of initiation in sacred practices, incorporating American Indian tribal wisdom and Earth-based wisdom into teachings from around the world.

P.O. Box 733
Mukilteo, WA 98275, 1-425-353-8815   www.sacredcircles.org

Appendix 3

Some Sacred Sites

Many Native American sacred sites are located in remote wilderness areas and on private property. Some sites are now controlled within the national parks and their Canadian counterparts. The majority of these sites do not have formal addresses. Keep in mind that many sites are considered sacred and are closed to the visiting public when Native American rituals are taking place. Check in advance for special regulations regarding visits. Here are some of the more prominent sites you might want to visit. I have also included as many Indian-owned sites and museums as possible because these are remarkably worth visiting.

Check with your own regional and state museums and historians to learn about special prehistoric and sacred sites near you. Most states and Canadian provinces also have welcome centers along major highways where you may stop to get additional ideas, maps, and brochures on special locations.

Canada

ALBERTA   1-800-661-8888

Homelands of the Inuit (Eskimo), Blackfeet, Shoshone, and Cree Indians are here.

Writing-on-Stone Provincial Park   1-403-647-2364
Highway 500, follow signs, on the Milk River
Milk River, AB
Massive stone outcroppings bear the largest concentration of pictographs and petroglyphs by nomadic Shoshone and Blackfeet Indians.

BRITISH COLUMBIA

Homelands of many Northwest Coast tribes.

Haida Kwagiulth Museum and Culture Centre   1-604-285-3733
3 km south of Quathiaski Cove, BC
Indian-operated center presenting cultural heritage and tours of nearby rock art sites.

ONTARIO

Territories of many northern tribes, especially the Iroquois, Huron, Ojibwa, Cree, and their ancestors.

Royal Ontario Museum   1-416-586-5551
100 Queen's Park Crescent W.
Toronto, ON
Massive totem poles, remarkable exhibits, and details about several pictograph sites. Canada's largest museum.

United States

ALABAMA   1-800- ALABAMA

The Heart of Dixie State is the home of the yellowhammer woodpecker, the southern pine, and the homelands of the Creek, Cherokee, Choctaw, and Chickasaw Indians.

Desoto Caverns Park   1-800-933-2283
Desoto Caverns Parkway, near Childersburg in the northern region.
Enormous twelve-story caverns once used by Native Americans.

Indian Mound and Museum   1-256-760-6427
1028 S. Court Street
Florence, AL 35630
Large Mississippian mound, forty-three feet high; Native American artifacts from the Paleolithic to historic periods.

Moundville Archaeological Park   1-205-371-2234
1 Mound Parkway
Moundville, AL 35474
Twenty-six large prehistoric platform mounds in a 320-acre park, including temple mounds near Black Warrior River.

Oakville Indian Park and Museum   1-256-905-2494
1219 County Road 187
Danville, AL 35619
Largest Woodland ceremonial Indian mound in the region, plus Cherokee council house museum.

Russell Cave National Monument   1-256-495-2672
3729 County Road 98
Bridgeport, AL 35740
Archaeological cave shelter preserves record of more than nine thousand years of Indian occupation.

Shell Mound Park   1-334-861-2882
2 N. Iberville Street
Dauphin Island, AL 36528
Prehistoric Indian mounds.

Woodland Ceremonial Mound and Copena Burial Mound
                                      1-256-905-2494
1219 County Road 187
Danville, AL 35619
Woodland Indians ceremonial mounds covering 1.8 acres, and twenty-seven feet high.

ALASKA   1-888-805-6234

The Last Frontier State is the homelands of the Aleut, Athapaskan, Haida, Inuit (Eskimo), Tlingit, and Tshimsian People.

Denali National Wildlife Preserve
Denali Mountain and Denali Lake

Alaska's great wildlife heritage and countless sacred sites are protected here.

ARIZONA 1-888-520-3434

The Grand Canyon State is homeland of the Apache, Navajo, Tohono O'Odham (Papago), Pima, Mohave, Hualapai, Chemehuevi, and Hopi Indians.

Canyon de Chelly 1-602-674-5436
P.O. Box 588, on the Navajo Indian Reservation
Chinle, AZ 86503
Red sandstone walls rising a thousand feet above the valley floor hold Canyon de Chelly, twenty-six miles long, joining Canyon del Muerto, twenty-five miles long. Sites span several periods of Native American culture and include White House, Antelope House, Standing Cow, and Mummy Cave.

Casa Grande Ruins National Monument 1-602-723-3172
1 mile north of State Road 87
Coolidge, AZ
Impressive site: group of six-hundred-year-old remains from the Hohokam culture.

Casa Malpais 1-602-333-5375
1 mile west of Springerville, AZ, off U.S. 60
Elaborate Mogollon village complex of 1,250 years ago.

Montezuma Castle National Monument 1-602-567-3322
50 miles south of Flagstaff on I-17, then 2.5 miles east, near Camp Verde, AZ
Remarkable Sinaguan prehistoric ruin of five-story, twenty-room dwelling of A.D. 1125.

Petrified Forest National Park and Painted Desert
1-602-524-6228
73 miles from Gallup, NM, in northeastern AZ on I-40
Anasazi culture including Puerco Ruins, a 150-room site six hundred years old; Agate House ruin and Newspaper Rock petroglyphs.

Pueblo Grande Museum 1-602-495-0900
Phoenix, AZ
Large Hohokam mound site plus two ball courts.

Tonto National Monument　　　　　1-602-467-2241
4 miles west on U.S. 60 from Globe, AZ, then 28 miles northwest on State Road 88
Two remarkable Salado Province cliff dwellings, A.D. 1300, two-
story pueblos built in large caves.

Tusayan Ruin and Museum　　　　　1-602-638-2305
22 miles east of Grand Canyon Village
Grand Canyon National Park, AZ
Small pueblo site, late-twelfth-century occupation.

Tuzigoot National Monument　　　　　1-602-634-5564
2 miles east of Clarkdale
Clarkdale, AZ
Ruins of a hilltop Sinagua pueblo occupied about A.D. 1100

Walnut Canyon National Monument　　　1-602-526-3367
7 miles east on I-40 from Flagstaff, AZ, then 3 miles southeast
Series of masonry cliff dwellings built into overhangs along the
canyon rim.

Wupatki National Monument　　　　　1-602-556-7040
32 miles north on U.S. 89 from Flagstaff, AZ
Amphitheater, ball court, and three-story structure with hundred
rooms near Sunset Crater.

ARKANSAS　　　1-800-628-8725

The Land of Opportunity is the homeland of unique prehistoric
Mound Builders cultures, ancestors of our historic Indian cultures of
the rivers and plains.

Hampson State Museum　　　　　1-501-655-8622
U.S. 61
Wilson, AR
Artifacts from the late Mississippian Nodena site, a fifteen-acre
palisaded village.

Toltec Mounds State Park　　　　　1-501-961-9442
U.S. 165
Scott, AR
Prehistoric earthworks built as early as A.D. 400; complex site in
the lower Mississippi Valley.

CALIFORNIA   1-800-462-2543

The Golden State holds a great concentration of Native American sites. About twenty Indian missions, plus many special sites.

Anderson Marsh State Historic Park   1-707-279-2267
Off SR 53, between Lower Lake and Clearlake
Kelseyville, CA
Ancient archaeological sites and petroglyphs plus Pomo Indian dance house used for spring ceremonials.

Chumash Painted Cave State Historic Park   1-805-968-3294
Painted Cave Road, in Santa Ynez Mountains near Santa Barbara, CA
Amazing ancient multicolored cave paintings and carvings, numerous pictographs.

Providence Mountains State Park   no phone
Off U.S. 95 near Blythe, CA
Giant desert figures, 100 to 150 feet long, called *intaglios,* represent stylized hunters and game animals. Many think they relate to a form of shamanic hunting practice.

Rock Maze   1-619-326-4591
Off I-40, Fort Mojave Reservation, near Needles, CA
Indian-operated site; field furrowed in a mazelike fashion over about two acres. Sacred symbolism.

COLORADO   1-877-735-6336

The Centennial State is graced with the lark bunting and the Rocky Mountain columbine, and is the homeland of various Northern Plains People, especially the Ute.

Anasazi Heritage Center   1-303-882-4811
State Road 184
Dolores, CO
Site of an extensive archaeological project.

Lowry Ruins   1-303-247-4082
9 miles west of Pleasant View
Cortez, CO
Largest great kivas known in the area; eleventh-century Anasazi ruins.

Mesa Verde National Park　　　　　1-303-529-4465
U.S. 160
Mesa Verde, CO
Several Anasazi villages and more than forty cliff dwellings.

CONNECTICUT　　1-800-282-6863

The Constitution State is graced with mountain laurel, white oaks, and robins, and is the homeland of the Mohegan, Paugussett, Pequot, and Schaghticoke Indians and their ancestors.

The Appalachian Trail system cuts through the state and one edge of the Schaghticoke Indian Reservation in Kent, CT.

Institute for American Indian Studies　　　1-860-868-0518
38 Curtis Road, just off State Road 199
Washington, CT 06793
www.birdstone.org
Documents more than ten thousand years of the area's Native American prehistory, plus replica of Eastern Woodland Indian village, garden, and trails. Medicine wheel garden with healing plants, peace pole, and prayer cairns.

Mashantucket Pequot Tribal Museum and Research Center
1-800-411-9671
Mashantucket Pequot Tribes Nation
Ledyard, CT 06339
www.mashantucket.com

FLORIDA　　1-888-202-4581

The Sunshine State is the homeland of the Seminole and Miccosuki Indians, plus earlier Native Americans. Among numerous special sites are:

Crystal River State Archaeological Site　　　1-904-795-3817
North Museum Point, off U.S. 19
Crystal River, FL
Diverse mound site just inland from the Gulf.

Indian Temple Mound Museum　　　1-904-243-6512
Route 139
Ft. Walton Beach, FL

Site of temple mound illustrating ten thousand years of Indian occupation on the northwest Florida coast.

Lake Jackson Mounds State Site   1-904-562-0042
2 miles north on I-10, at southern tip of Lake Jackson
Tallahassee, FL
Major mound and village site with seven mounds, a plaza, and village middens.

GEORGIA   1-800-VISIT-GA

The Empire State of the South is graced with the Cherokee rose, brown thrasher, and live oaks, and is the home of early Algonquian people.

Etowah Indian Mound State Historic Park   1-404-387-3737
State Road 61/113, 6 miles south of I-75
Cartersville, GA
Major Mississippian ceremonial center.

Kolomoki Mounds Historic Park   1-912-723-5296
Off U.S. 27, 6 miles north of Blakely, GA
Large mound complex: seven mounds on 1,293 acres, plus a museum charting Indian cultures in this region from 5000 B.C.

Ocmulgee National Monument   1-912-752-8257
I-16 exit 4, U.S. 80 east
Macon, GA
Spectacular center showing 10,000 years of Native American cultures, ceremonial centers, mounds, and museum.

Rock Eagle Stone Effigy Mound   no phone
Eatonton, GA
Enormous stone effigy of an eagle dating back about five thousand years.

IDAHO   1-800-847-4843

The Gem State is home to the Shoshone, Bannock, Paiute, Kootenai, and Coeur d'Alene.

Nez Perce National Historical Park Museum   1-208-843-2261
7 miles from Lewiston, ID
www.nps.gov/nepe/
Only national park dedicated to a Native American tribe, preserving their culture and history.

Shoshone Falls   1-208-733-3974
In south-central Idaho
www.twinfallschamber.com
Higher than Niagara Falls and a place of prehistoric significance.

Snake River Birds of Prey Natural Area   1-208-362-3716
www.peregrinefund.org
Half a million acres surrounding the Snake River; many sacred
areas now embraced within this sanctuary.

ILLINOIS   1-800-226-6632

The Prairie State is graced with native violets, cardinals, and white
oak, and is the homeland of the Illini and Kickapoo Indians and
their earliest mound-building ancestors.

Cahokia Mounds State Historic Site   1-618-346-5160
Collinsville Road, 6 miles east off 1-55/70
East St. Louis, IL
Site of the largest city in prehistoric North America, established
about A.D. 700. Monks Mound and Woodhenge celestial obser-
vatory. Late Mississippian complex.

Dickson Mounds Museum   1-309-547-3721
State Road 97, 60 miles northwest of Springfield
Springfield, IL
Site of a large Mississippian community of villages, camps, and
work stations starting in A.D. 1100, abandoned by A.D. 1350.

INDIANA   1-800-800-9939

The Hoosier State is home of the cardinal and the tulip poplar,
and the homeland of the Wyandotte and their ancestors.

Angel Mounds State Historic Site   1-812-853-3956
8215 Pollock Avenue
Evansville, IN
Best-preserved Mississippian site in North America, dating from
about A.D. 900, including temple.

Wyandotte Cave   1-812-738-2782
State Road 62
Leavenworth, IN
Prehistoric quarry and sacred site; source of Wyandotte chert.

IOWA   1-800-345-4692

The Hawkeye State, graced by the eastern goldfinch and wild rose, is homeland of the Mesquakie, Sac, and Fox Indians and their ancient ancestors.

Effigy Mounds National Monument   1-319-873-2356
State Road 76, 3 miles north of Marquette
Marquette, IA
Spectacular site of two hundred mounds, including twenty-six animal effigies and the "marching bears." Covers the past 2,500 years of Effigy Mound Culture work.

LOUISIANA   1-800-33-GUMBO

The Pelican State is Cajun country and homeland of the Choctaw, Chickasaw, Houma, Tunica-Biloxi, Caddo, and Natchez, and their ancestors.

Marksville State Historic Site   1-888-253-8954
837 Martin Luther King Drive
Marksville, LA 71351
Earthen mounds dating from A.D. 400. Evidence of two thousand years of Native American culture.

Poverty Point State Area   1-318-926-5492
6859 State Road 577, about 6 miles out of Epps, LA 71266
A four-hundred-acre site of Archaic-period earthworks.

MINNESOTA   1-800-657-3700

The Gopher State is home of the lady's slipper orchid and the common loon. It was settled over ten thousand years ago by ancestors of today's Ojibwa (Chippewa) and other Great Lakes Indians.

Grand Mound Interpretive Center   1-218-285-3332
State Road 11, 17 miles west of International Falls, MN
Largest burial mound in the Upper Midwest, almost two thousand years old.

Indian Mounds Park   1-612-296-6157
East of the business district, overlooking the Mississippi River, in St. Paul, MN
Several remarkable ancient mounds.

Pipestone National Monument   1-507-825-5464
At the north edge of Pipestone, MN
Native Americans mined much of these three hundred acres for centuries for the fine red catlinite (pipestone); mining still continues. This is a very sacred site.

MISSISSIPPI   1-800-WARMEST

The Magnolia State was settled over ten thousand years ago by ancestors of the Choctaw, Chickasaw, Creek, and Natchez Indians, who created the trails, or traces, that have become our main highways.

Emerald Mound   1-800-305-7417 or 1-601-680-4025
Natchez Trace Parkway
Built around A.D.1400 by ancestors of the Natchez Indians; second largest ceremonial mound in the United States, covering nearly eight acres.

Grand Village of the Natchez Indians   1-601-446-6502
400 Jefferson Davis Boulevard
Natchez, MS
National Historic Landmark, ceremonial mound center from A.D.1200 until A.D.1730.

Nanih Waiya Historic Site   1-800-467-2757
Coy community, Philadelphia, MS   1-601-773-7988
Ancient sacred mounds, legendary birthplace of the Choctaw Indians.

Natchez Trace Parkway   1-800-305-7417 or 1-601-680-4025
RR1, NT 1143
Tupelo, MS 38801
Headquarters and museum/visitors center. This scenic byway, part of the national park system, began over eight thousand years ago as an Indian and buffalo trail. It stretches from Natchez, MS, to Nashville, TN, with many historical markers to stop at along the route and incredible natural beauty to enjoy. This cuts through the state diagonally from the northeast to the southwest. Check out the First Mississippians Tour, which zigzags to sites across the state from the northeast corner to the Gulf.

Winterville Mounds Museum State Park   1-601-378-5559
2415 Highway 1 North Drive
Greenville, MS
One of the largest Indian mound groups in the Mississippi Valley. Numerous artifacts are on exhibit.

NEVADA   1-800-638-2328

The Silver State is graced with mountain bluebirds, sagebrush, and single-leaf piñon, and is the homeland of the Paiute and Ute Indians and their ancestors.

Valley of Fire State Park   1-702-397-2088
State Road 169, 14 miles Southwest of Overton, NV
Red sandstone walls show numerous examples of prehistoric rock art.

NEW MEXICO   1-800-733-6396

The Land of Enchantment is graced with roadrunners, yuccas, and piñons, and is the homeland of nineteen Pueblo Indian groups, along with the Apache and Navajo.

Acoma Pueblo Sky City   1-505-252-1139
State Road 23, about 3 miles northeast of Acoma
Sky City, NM
Enchanted Mesa towers 430 feet above the surrounding plains; one of the oldest inhabited cities in North America.

Aztec Ruins National Monument   1-505-334-6174
Off U.S. 550, about 1 mile north of Aztec, NM 87410
Twelfth-century ancestral Pueblo ruins, including the Great Kiva.

Bandolier National Monument   1-505-672-3861
State Road 4, well beyond Pojoaque Pueblo
Santa Fe, NM
Remarkable monument; a number of pueblo and cliff dwellings, particularly a circular community village.

Chaco Culture National Historical Park   1-505-786-7014
Via NM 371, 40 miles north of Crownpoint, NM
World Heritage Site, twelfth-century Ancestral Pueblo; thirteen major ruins; forty-five campsites; prehistoric economic and ceremonial center.

El Morro National Monument   1-505-783-4226
State Road 602, 43 miles southwest of Grants, NM, via SR 53
The two-hundred-foot-high Inscription Rock holds many
petroglyphs; two Anasazi villages once thrived atop this
mesa.

Gila Cliff Dwelling National Monument   1-505-536-9461
Via NM 15, 44 miles north of Silver City, NM
Remarkable Mogollon ruins, A.D. 1275, and thirteenth-century
cliff-dwelling ruins.

Nuestra Señora de Guadalupe de Zuni   1-505-782-5581
Zuni Pueblo, NM, 40 miles southwest of Gallup.
Impressive paintings of Zuni kachina dancers adorn the walls of
this chapel, painted by Alex Seowtewa and his sons.

Petroglyph National Monument   1-505-899-0205
Off Unser, 3 miles north of I-40, near Albuquerque, NM
Large collection of prehistoric rock art images on West Mesa vol-
canic escarpment, plus nature trails.

Puye Cliff Dwellings   1-505-753-7326
State Road 30, 11 miles west of Espanola, NM
Extensive Anasazi occupation of this Pajarito Plateau complex in
the twelfth century.

Salmon Ruins and Heritage Park   1-505-632-2013
Via U.S. 64, about 2 miles west of Bloomfield, NM
Eleventh-century Ancestral Pueblo ruins and museum.

Three Rivers Petroglyph National Site   1-505-585-9597
Via U.S. 4, 17 miles north of Tularosa, NM
Stunning petroglyphs and nature trails.

NORTH CAROLINA   1-800-VISIT-NC

The Tar Heel State is graced with cardinals and dogwoods, and is
the homeland of the Cherokee, Creek, and Catawba Indians and
their early ancestors.

Town Creek Indian Mound State Park   1-910-439-6802
State Road 31, 5 miles southeast of Mount Gilead, NC
Important center during the sixteenth century.

OHIO 1-877-787-7473 or 1-800-BUCKEYE

The Buckeye State has abundant beauty and ancient sites. These are the homelands of the Shawnee, Mohican, and Delaware people and their ancestors, the Hopewell Culture.

Adena State Memorial 1-800-413-4118
Hopewell Culture National Historical Park
P.O. Box 353
Chillicothe, OH 45601
One of the most amazing prehistoric mound sites and huge complex.

Flint Ridge State Memorial Museum 1-614-787-2476
State Road 688, 3 miles north of U.S. 40, near Brownsville, OH
Site of the famous Ohio pipestone quarry, important in native traditions since Hopewell times.

Fort Ancient 1-513-932-4421
State Road 350, 7 miles off Middleboro Road, near Lebanon, OH
A Hopewell settlement site, about one hundred acres, atop the bluff overlooking the Little Miami River.

Hopewell Culture National Historic Park 1-614-774-1125
Chillicothe, OH
Remarkable thirteen-acre complex with twenty-three interpreted mounds. One of the most important Hopewell sites.

Miamisburg Mound State Memorial 1-614-297-2300
State Road 725
Miamisburg, OH
Huge Adena Mound, sixty-eight feet high.

Mound Cemetery no phone
Fifth Street
Marietta, OH
A thirty-foot-high aboriginal mound, once part of an extensive earthworks complex.

Newark Earthworks 1-614-344-1920
State Road 79
Newark, OH
The Mound Builders State Memorial includes one very large earthwork and numerous smaller mounds.

Seip Mound State Memorial   1-614-297-2301
U.S. 50, 3 miles east of Bainbridge, OH
Great Hopewell mound and related exhibit.

Serpent Mound   1-513-587-2796
State Road 73, 4 miles northwest of Locust Grove, OH
Spectacular, enigmatic ancient mounded earthworks site; prehistoric origins remain a mystery.

OKLAHOMA   1-800-654-8240

Indian Country, the Sooner State, is home to the scissor-tailed flycatcher, redbud, and mistletoe, and more than sixty different American Indian tribes.

Spiro Mounds Archaeological Park   1-918-596-2700
State Road 9
Spiro, OK
Includes mounds complexes linked to the Southern cult in Mississippian times.

SOUTH DAKOTA   1-800-732-5682

Mt. Rushmore State is graced with Black Hills spruce and pasque flowers, and is the homeland of the Sioux Nation and their ancestors.

Bear Butte State Park   1-605-347-3176
Sturgis, SD
One of the most sacred places for the Sioux and many other Plains Indians.

TENNESSEE   1-800-462-8366

The Volunteer State is graced with iris, tulip poplars, and mockingbirds, and is the homeland of the Cherokee and Chickasaw Indians, and their ancestors.

Chucalissa Indian Museum   1-901-785-3160
Mitchell Road, next to Fuller State Park, Memphis, TN
Interesting mounds site, more than a thousand years old.

Old Stone Fort State Archaeological Area   1-615-723-5073
U.S. 41
Manchester, TN

A two-thousand-year-old ceremonial site; mounds and walls were combined with cliffs and rivers to form an enclosure around more than a mile of natural terrain. A mystical site for Indian people.

Pinson Mounds State Archaeological Area   1-901-988-5614
460 Ozier Road, off U.S. 45
Pinson, TN
One of the largest Hopewell mound groups in North America.

Shiloh National Military Park   1-901-689-5275
10 miles southwest of Savannah, TN
More than thirty Mississippian mounds built between A.D. 1100 and A.D. 1300.

TEXAS   1-800-452-9292

The Lone Star State is home to the mockingbird, pecan, and blue-bonnet, and is the homeland of many southern tribes, including the Seminole, Cherokee, Caddo, Comanche, Cheyenne, Kiowa, Arapaho, Alabama, and Coushatta.

Caddoan Mounds State Historic Site   1-409-858-3218
State Highway 21, 6 miles southwest of Alto, TX
Two mounds and a thousand-year-old village.

Hueco Tanks State Historic Park   1-915-857-1135
38 miles east of El Paso, TX
These *huecos* (rock basins) have collected water since Paleoindian times; thousands of rock art elements remain.

Seminole Canyon State Historical Park   1-915-292-4464
U.S. 90, 40 miles northwest of Comstock, TX
Spectacular limestone rock shelters with amazing pictograph murals from prehistoric times.

UTAH   1-800-200-1160

The Beehive State is graced with blue spruce trees and sego lilies, and is the homeland of the Ute, Navajo, and early Anasazi people.

Capitol Reef National Park   1-801-425-3791
On State Road 24, 5 miles east of Torrey, UT
Canyon walls are alive with pre-contact rock art.

Fremont Indian State Park   1-801-527-4631
At the junction of I-70 and State Road 89
Richfield, UT
Exhibits of the Fremont culture from nearby Five Fingers Hill.

Hovenweep National Monument   1-303-529-4461
Straddling the Utah/Colorado boundary, near Pleasant View, UT
The Ute word *hovenweep* means "deserted valley." Visit the remains of multiroom pueblos, small cliff dwellings, and towers.

Newspaper Rock State Park   1-801-587-2141
At Indian Creek Canyon, in Canyonland National Park, Monticello, UT
A massive cliff mural of ancient rock art.

WEST VIRGINIA   1-800-225-5982

The Mountain State is graced with sugar maples, cardinals, and big rhododendrons, and is the homeland of eastern Algonquian tribes and their early ancestors.

Grave Creek Mound   1-304-843-1410
801 Jefferson Street
Moundsville, WV
This mammoth mound is a seventy-foot-tall Adena structure; adjacent to it is the Delf Norona Museum.

WISCONSIN   1-888-577-5052

The Badger State is graced with sugar maples, robins, and wood violets, and is the homeland of the Oneida, Ojibwa, Stockbridge-Munsee, Lac du Flambeau Chippewa, Winnebago, Hochunk, and other native peoples and their ancestors.

Lizard Mound County Park   1-414-335-4445
County Road A
West Bend, WI
Numerous animal effigy mounds.

Sheboygan Mound Park   no phone
Off Panther Avenue
Sheboygan, WI
Thirty-three mounds effigy shaped like panthers and deer constructed over a thousand years ago.

WYOMING   1-800-225-5996

The Cowboy State, where the Great Plains meet the Rockies, is a state of immense beauty, with meadowlarks, cottonwoods, and Indian paintbrush. These are the homelands of the Crow, Cheyenne, Blackfeet, and Shoshone people and their ancestors.

Bighorn National Forest   1-307-672-0751
Off U.S. 14A, beyond Burgess Junction, near Sheridan, WY
The Big Horn Medicine Wheel is located near the western rim, above the headwaters of the Tongue River; the medicine wheel is a mountaintop shrine of stone, seventy feet in diameter.

Devil's Tower National Monument   1-307-467-5283
28 miles northwest of Sundance, off WY 24
Devil's Tower, WY 82714
America's first national monument; giant rock columns rising 1,280 feet above the valley at the western edge of the Black Hills.

Selected Bibliography

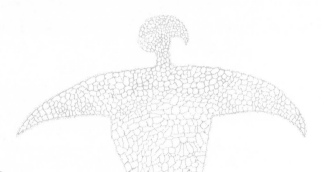

HEALING

Alford, Lori Arviso, and Elizabeth Cohen Van Pelt. *The Scalpel and the Silver Bear: The First Navajo Woman Surgeon Combines Western Medicine and Traditional Healing.* New York: Bantam, 1999.

Chevallier, Andrew. *The Encyclopedia of Medicinal Plants: A Practical Reference Guide.* London: Dorling Kindersley Ltd., 1996.

Corlett, William Thomas. *The Medicine-Man of the American Indian and His Cultural Background.* Springfield, IL: Charles C. Thomas, 1935.

Kavasch, E. Barrie, and Karen Baar. *American Indian Healing Arts: Herbs, Rituals, and Remedies for Every Season of Life.* New York: Bantam, 1999.

Lyon, William S. *Encyclopedia of Native American Healing.* New York: W. W. Norton & Co., 1996.

Mehl-Madrona, Lewis. *Coyote Medicine.* New York: Scribner, 1997.

Newcomb, Franc Johnson. *Hosteen Klah: Navaho Medicine Man and Sand Painter.* Norman: University of Oklahoma Press, 1964, 1980.

Thomas, Richard, with Peter Albright. *The Complete Book of Natural Pain Relief: Safe and Effective Self-Help for Everyday Aches and Pains.* Buffalo, NY: Firefly Books, 1998.

Van Straten, Michael. *The Family Book of Home Remedies: A Practical Guide.* London: The Ivy Press, Ltd., 1998.

HERBS AND HERBALISM/HERBOLOGY/ETHNOBOTANY

Dunmire, William W., and Gail D. Tierney. *Wild Plants of the Pueblo Province.* Santa Fe: Museum of New Mexico Press, 1995.

Elliott, Doug. Wild Roots: *A Forager's Guide to the Edible and Medicinal Roots, Tubers, Corms, and Rhizomes of North America.* Rochester, VT: Healing Arts Press, 1995.

Gilmore, Melvin R. *Uses of Plants by the Indians of the Missouri River Region.* Lincoln: University of Nebraska Press, 1991.

Green, James. *The Male Herbal: Health Care for Men and Boys.* Freedom, CA: The Crossing Press, 1991, 1997.

Hobbs, Christopher. *Handmade Medicines: Simple Recipes for Herbal Health.* Loveland, CO: Interweave Press, 1998.

Kavasch, E. Barrie. *Native Harvests: American Indian Wild Foods and Recipes.* Revised ed. Washington, CT: Institute for American Indian Studies/Birdstone Books, 1998.

———. *American Indian Earthsense: Herbaria of Ethnobotany and Ethnomycology.* Washington, CT: Institute for American Indian Studies/Birdstone Books, 1996.

———. *Earthwise: American Indian Traditional Uses of Trees.* Washington, CT: Institute for American Indian Studies/Birdstone Books, 2000.

Kindscher, Kelly. *Medicinal Plants of the Prairie: An Ethnobotanical Guide.* Lawrence, KS: University of Kansas Press, 1992.

Moore, Michael. *Medicinal Plants of the Mountain West.* Santa Fe: Museum of New Mexico Press, 1979.

———. *Medicinal Plants of the Desert and Canyon West.* Santa Fe: Museum of New Mexico Press, 1989.

Soule, Deb. *The Roots of Healing: A Woman's Book of Herbs.* New York: A Citadel Press Book/Carol Publishing Co., 1995.

Tilgner, Sharol. *Herbal Medicine: From the Heart of the Earth.* Creswell, OR: Wise Acres Publishing, 1999.

GARDENING

Art, Henry W. *The Wildflower Gardener's Guide.* Pownal, VT: Garden Way/Storey Communications, 1987.

Druse, Ken. *The Shade Garden.* New York: Clarkson Potter, 1992.

Ellis, Barbara W., and Fern M. Bradley. *The Organic Gardener's Handbook of Natural Insect and Disease Control.* Emmaus, PA: Rodale Press, 1996.

Glattstein, Judy. *Waterscaping: Plants and Ideas for Natural and Created Water Gardens.* Pownal, VT: Storey Communications, 1994.

Jay, Roni. *Gardens of the Spirit: Create Your Own Sacred Spaces.* New York: Sterling Publishing Company, Inc./A Godsfield Book, 1999.

Mollison, Bill, and Remy Mia Slay. *Introduction to Permaculture.* Rev. ed. CA: Ten Speed Press, 1997.

Ondra, Nancy J., and Barbara Ellis, eds. *Soil Composting: The Complete Guide to Building Healthy, Fertile Soil.* Boston: Houghton Mifflin Company, 1998.

Smith, J. Robert, with Beatrice S. Smith. *The Prairie Garden: 70 Native Plants You Can Grow in Town or Country.* Madison: University of Wisconsin Press, 1980.

Stevens, David, and Ursula Buchan. *The Conran Octopus Garden Book.* London: Colour Library Direct/Conran Octopus Limited, 1999.

Streep, Peg. *Spiritual Gardening: Creating Sacred Space Outdoors.* Alexandria, VA: Time-Life Books, 1999.

Winger, David, ed. *Xeriscape Color Guide: 100 Water-Wise Plants for Gardens and Landscapes.* Golden, CO: Denver Water/Fulcrum Publishing, 1998.

NATIVE AMERICAN SPIRITUALITY AND SHAMANISM

Awiakta, Marilou. *Selu: Seeking the Corn-Mother's Wisdom.* Golden, CO: Fulcrum Publishing, 1993.

Bahti, Mark. *Spirit in the Stone: A Handbook of Southwest Indian Animal Carvings.* Tucson, AZ: Treasure Chest Books, 1999.

Black Elk, as told to John G. Neihardt. *Black Elk Speaks: Being the Life Story of a Holy Man of the Oglala Sioux.* Lincoln: University of Nebraska Press, 1932, 1979.

Blackman, Margaret B. *During My Time: Florence Edenshaw Davidson: A Haida Woman.* Seattle: University of Washington Press, 1982, 1990.

Connor, Sheila. *New England Natives: A Celebration of People and Trees.* Cambridge, MA: Harvard University Press, 1994.

Devereux, Paul. *Shamanism and the Mystery Lines: Ley Lines, Spirit Paths, Shape-shifting and Out-of-Body Travel.* St. Paul, MN: Llewellyn Publications, 1993.

Duncan, Barbara R., coll. and ed. *Living Stories of the Cherokee.* Chapel Hill: University of North Carolina Press, 1998.

Fawcett, Melissa Jayne. *Medicine Trail: The Life and Lessons of Gladys Tantaquidgeon.* Tucson: University of Arizona Press, 2000.

Grey Wolf, Amy Baggott, and Morningstar. *Earth Signs: How to Connect with the Natural Spirits of the Earth.* London: The Ivy Press, Ltd., 1998.

Mander, Jerry. *In the Absence of the Sacred: The Failure of Technology and the Survival of the Indian Nations.* San Francisco, CA: Sierra Club Books, 1992.

Meadows, Kenneth. *Earth Medicine: Revealing Hidden Teachings of the Native American Medicine Wheel.* Rockport, MA: Element, 1996.

———. *Shamanic Experience: A Practical Guide to Contemporary Shamanism.* Rockport, MA: Element, 1991.

———. *The Medicine Way: A Shamanic Path to Self-Mastery.* Rockport, MA: Element, 1990.

Miller, Jay. *Mourning Dove: A Salishan Autobiography.* Lincoln: University of Nebraska Press, 1990.

Milne, Courtney. *Sacred Places: A Journey into the Medicine Wheel.* New York: Stewart, Tabori & Chang, 1994.

Perkins, John. *Shape Shifting: Shamanic Techniques for Global and Personal Transformation.* Rochester, VT: Destiny Books, 1997.

Red Shirt, Delphine. *Bead on an Anthill: A Lakota Childhood.* Lincoln: University of Nebraska Press, 1998.

Rockefeller, Steven C., and John C. Elder, eds. *Spirit and Nature: Why the Environment Is a Religious Issue.* Boston: Beacon Press, 1992.

Spatz, Ronald, exec. ed. *Alaska Native Writers, Storytellers and Orators: The Expanded Edition.* Anchorage: University of Alaska, 1999.

Storm, Hyemeyohsts. *Seven Arrows: The Story of the Shield and the Medicine Wheel.* Cherokee, NC: Cherokee Publications, 1974.

Streep, Peg. *Altars Made Easy: A Complete Guide to Creating Your Own Sacred Space.* San Francisco: Harper San Francisco, 1997.

Summer Rain, Mary. *Dreamwalker: The Path of Sacred Power.* West Chester, PA: The Donning Co., 1988.

Sun Bear, Wabun Wind, and Crysalis Mulligan. *Dancing with the Wheel: The Medicine Wheel Workbook.* New York: A Fireside Book, 1991.

Villoldo, Alberto. *Dancing the Four Winds: Secrets of the Inca Medicine Wheel.* Rochester, VT: Destiny Books, 1990, 1995.

Wallis, Velma. *Two Old Women: An Alaska Legend of Betrayal, Courage and Survival.* Fairbanks, AK: Epicenter Press, 1993.

Wa'Na'Nee'Che (Dennis Renault) and Timothy Freke. *Principles of Native American Spirituality.* San Francisco, CA: HarperCollins/Thorsons, 1996.

Wilson, Gilbert L. *Buffalo Bird Woman's Garden.* St. Paul: Minnesota Historical Society Press, 1917, 1987.

REFERENCE

Artress, Lauren. *Walking a Sacred Path: Rediscovering the Labyrinth as a Spiritual Tool.* New York: Riverhead Books, 1995.

Bataille, Gretchen, and Kathleen M. Sands. *American Indian Women: Telling Their Lives.* Lincoln: University of Nebraska Press, 1984.

Brown, Simon. *Practical Feng Shui.* London: Ward Lock, 1997.

Brumley, John H. *Medicine Wheels on the Northern Plains: A Summary and Appraisal.* Medicine Hat, Alberta: Alberta Culture and Multiculturalism, Historical Resources Division, 1988.

Cajete, Gregory, ed. *A People's Ecology: Explorations in Sustainable Living.* Santa Fe: Clear Light Publishers, 1999.

Campbell, Maria. *Halfbreed.* Toronto: McClelland and Stewart, 1973.

Clottes, Jean, and David Lewis-Williams. *The Shamans of Prehistory: Trance and Magic in the Painted Caves.* New York: Harry N. Abrams, Inc., 1998.

Coe, Ralph T. *Sacred Circles: Two Thousand Years of North American Indian Art.* London: Arts Council of Great Britain, 1976.

Crosby, Harry W. *The Cave Paintings of Baja California: Discovering the Great Murals of an Unknown People.* San Diego, CA: Sunbelt Publications, 1997.

Eddy, John A. "Astronomical Alignment of the Big Horn Medicine Wheel," *Science* 184, 4141 (1974): 1035–43.

———. "Medicine Wheels and Plains Indian Astronomy." In A. F. Aveni, ed., *Native American Astronomy,* pp. 147–69. Austin: University of Texas Press, 1977.

Fagan, Brian. *The Science of Sacred Sites: From Black Land to Fifth Sun.* Reading, MA: Addison-Wesley/Helix Books, 1998.

Feest, Christian F. *Native Arts of North America.* New York: Oxford University Press, 1980.

Giddings, Allie Hungerford. *A History of Sherman: Records and Recollections.* Sherman, CT: The Sherman Historical Society, 1973–77.

Grinnell, George B. "The Medicine Wheel," *American Anthropologist* 24, 3 (1922): 299–310.

Highwater, Jamake. *Arts of the Indian Americas: North, Central, South: Leaves from the Sacred Tree.* New York: Harper & Row Publishers, 1983.

Martineau, LaVan. *The Rocks Begin to Speak.* Las Vegas, NV: KC Publications, 1972.

Mohen, Jean-Pierre. *Megaliths: Stones of Memory.* New York: Harry N. Abrams, Inc./Discoveries, 1999.

Perrone, Bobette, H. H. Stockel, and V. Krueger. *Medicine Women, Curanderas, and Women Doctors.* Norman: University of Oklahoma Press, 1989.

Rossbach, Sarah, and Lin Yun. *Living Color: Master Lin Yun's Guide to Feng Shui and the Art of Color.* New York: Kodansha America, Inc., 1994.

Thomas, David Hurst. *Exploring Ancient Native America: An Archaeological Guide.* New York: Routledge, 1999.

Wright, R. Gerald. *National Parks amd Protected Areas: Their Role in Environmental Protection.* Cambridge, MA: Blackwell Science, 1996.

Index

About the Author

E. Barrie Kavasch is an herbalist, ethnobotanist, mycologist, and food-historian of Cherokee, Creek, and Powhatan descent, with Scotch-Irish, English, and German heritage as well. She is the co-author of *American Indian Healing Arts* (1999, Bantam), and of two books on Native American foods, *Enduring Harvests* (1995, Globe Pequot) and *Native Harvests* (1979, Random House), which was hailed by *The New York Times* as "the most intelligent and brilliantly researched book on the foods of American Indians." She has studied with many acclaimed native healers—some of whom contributed to this book—and is a research associate of the Institute for American Indian Studies in Washington, Connecticut. Her work has been featured in *The New York Times, Martha Stewart Living,* and many other publications, and she has been a guest lecturer at the New York Botanical Garden, the American Museum of Natural History, and the Yale Peabody Museum.